FOR PITY'

Dedication

I dedicate this book to
Miss Audrey Brown,
a beautiful woman who has
enjoyed her life to the full,
with love and understanding,
and who now at well over 90 years
of age still plans for the future
and dreams her dreams,
and is once, twice, three times a lady.

Sadly, Audrey died just before the publication of this book, still dreaming at the age of 94.

Published by
Chipmunkapublishing
PO Box 6872
Brentwood
Essex CM13 1ZT
United Kingdom

http://www.chipmunkapublishing.co.uk

Compiled By Kalpesh Parmar

FOR PITY'S SAKE

In Westminster Abbey
When you look for me,
Don't try the nave
Try the WC.
William Carter is my name,
That's WC in the Hall of Fame
A gutter poet.....that's my game.

Dear John

Here is my first novel

Take care

William. Carter

FOR PITY'S SAKE

CONTENTS

FOR PITY'S SAKE

One More E-mail, One More Year

Introduction

Romance is almost dead. For most, it comes to life just once a year, on Valentine's Day, when the modern male of the species is bullied or forced into it. Love and marriage are said to go together, but in most cases, after three to five years sex and marriage don't seem remotely compatible!

In our hero Billy Clayton's eyes, the feminist concept of the emancipated modern woman has suppressed male romantic love as it is expressed in such works as King Arthur, Shakespeare's "Romeo and Juliet", and Bronte's "Wuthering Heights" (Heathcliff), and in classic films starring Rudolph Valentino, Errol Flynn, Clark Gable.

Influential novelist Fay Weldon recently stated that 21st-Century women have become too practical and independent to surrender to passion and love. They know that women who hold out for the fantasy of 'Mr Right' might now wait forever.

Even the woman who achieves marriage and children remains dissatisfied. Her husband leaves home promptly at seven-thirty each morning and returns at ten-thirty at night (if she's lucky). The "Pretty Woman" who stimulated him sexually and mentally, the sex kitten who drove him crazy with desire, is no more. Instead he is left with a good "mummy" who talks about baby-foods and nappy-rash, and who grows fat because she no longer has time to exercise because the children are a full time job. Of the forty-five percent of Western marriages which do not disintegrate in divorce, two-thirds exist in mutual stagnation. More and more couples today are willing to admit that they are in a "low sex" or "no sex" marriage. ("Low" is defined as making love once a month). Bored, he starts to be tempted by the ease of finding "working girls" on the internet, and the office secretary seems more alluring and worth the risk. Once he starts exploring, to his delight he finds that there are even online dating websites that encourage infidelity, such as "Excite UK" which has personal ads for married men and women seeking extra-marital affairs.

Is it surprising then that some girls look for rich mates who might be otherwise unsuitable but who can give them a pampered, stress-free life, enabling them to look after themselves while they pay other women to look after their homes and children? Or that some girls sacrifice the idea of a permanent union with a man in pursuit of an independent, fun-filled life? Those women can end up strong and alone; with many good memories but perhaps years of loneliness ahead of them (Western women have a life expectancy of about 82 years and outlive men in their age group by an average of six years.)

Deep in the recesses of the female psyche is a longing for a man who can be strong for her, a man who can support her in every way. She dreams of letting her hair down from the locked room in the tower so he will climb up and rescue her from her mediocre life. Our heroine Natasha was drawn to the near-perfect, rich, intelligent, chivalrous "Mr Smith" because he seemed to be a modern Mr Darcy (like the character in Jane Austen's "Sense and Sensibility"), the type of man she had been led to believe in her childhood actually exists.

The modern woman is pressurized by the air-brushed images she sees in magazines, in movies, and on television of perfect, sexy, size-zero models whom she can never hope to emulate in their £5,000 Versace dresses. She struggles to survive a week at a time, for months at a time, and for what stretches out to become lost years at a time, just keep a tiny pied-a-terre on the third floor of a Victorian block of flats in NW3, living on a measly £300 per week which she has to work 50 hours to earn. Her rent costs £120, her council tax and utilities another £40, not to mention food, travel expenses, toiletries… it never ends. She barely has enough left over to buy a pair of cotton knickers from Primark. She does what she can to look stylish and different each day, though she has little in her wardrobe.

She battles with bosses who don't appreciate her, and work colleagues who jostle for her position like predators ready to pounce the minute she makes a mistake. As time goes on she realizes that most of her friends and colleagues are of the fair-weather type, with hidden agendas. All is fair in love and war… and work, it seems. It takes a toll on her and she begins to suffer from nervous disorders, irritable bowel syndrome, ulcerative colitis, and allergies, and her longing for escape becomes overwhelming.

She tries to make new friendships after work at wine bars, clubs, and evening classes. It is difficult to meet new people this way; everyone seems either to have a pre-formed social group with impenetrable borders, to be suspicious of a pretty single woman, or to be socially inept.

Natasha

Sometimes Natasha made the journey to south London to visit her sister, who introduced her to her boyfriends' single friends and workmates. However, she found that most of them were completely unsuitable and it was no surprise that they were still single.

A girlfriend from her school days who came to England after she did had finally found a willing man, who was from the USA. After many disappointed loves she was desperate, so she married him, only to find out that his family was poverty stricken and she would have to work hard to support them as well as herself and her husband. Natasha's friend, even though she had the benefit of 20/20 hindsight, kept matching up our heroine to her husband's friends from America, in the hope that she might settle for one of them and, in the process, help her friend to feel less alone in her own hopeless situation.

While she welcomed any way to meet new men, the matchmaking created problems for Natasha because she did not want to upset her sister and friend, nor their partners, by rejecting the advances of the men they introduced her to. After these meetings, she returned home alone to the haven of her little rented room where she was comforted by her teddy bears, potted plants, and her cooking. To fall asleep, she escaped into chick-lit books with characters that she could identify with. They also gave her some hope for her own happy ending one day, despite the pitfalls of modern dating.

By this point, her ten-year love affair with Billy Clayton was nearly at an end. It was one of those rare relationships that combined a deep emotional love with an all-consuming physical passion for each other. The love they felt for each other would always live on, but the physical spark had naturally dimmed a little over the intervening years. They had had more than three thousand sexual encounters during their time together and had experimented with every position, location, and number of participants in their love-making. They had done it all together, and Natasha realized that she needed some new sexual excitement and thrills.

Nothing she tried in her real life to meet new men had worked, so she turned to the internet, a world where she could meet new people without having to put on makeup, dress up or spend money. Little did she know that she was opening herself up to a cyberworld that can be fraught with danger. Had Natasha paid more attention to the news around that time, she would have learnt some of the danger of using the internet to connect with people. Fiona Marshall (sister of Carphone Warehouse tycoon David Ross) and her lover, Richard Flippance, were reported to have been stabbed to death by Fiona's jealous husband Alex Marshall, who learnt about their liason after hacking into her email account.

So Natasha turned to a machine to find her knight on his stallion. Internet dating held out for her the promise of a new sexual excitement that would shake her to the core and rescue her from the long, lonely nights at home of watching dreary soaps which provided the questionable solace that some people's lives were even more dead-end than hers, baby programmes that only made her feel despondent and broody, and unrealistic romantic films which only stirred up her dreams of what might have been, what by rights should have been.

She was a girl seeking love as well as sex, but even in her excruciating sadness and loneliness she found everyday encounters with available, single men boring. She actively searched for the dangerous excitement of the married lover, the boss or a work colleague, her friends' boyfriends and husbands, and even the transient men who moved into and out of the rooms next to hers. Anything to get her juices flowing, anything that removed her from the mundane and offered forbidden fruits. In her tender years, after her parents divorced, she shared her mother's lover. The groping and touching in forbidden places, and the wild excitement at the thought of being discovered, had set a high threshold for Natasha's satisfaction.

Suddenly one day a letter appeared on the computer screen, one that would totally change her life. Had she not had a fight with her older, married lover Billy two months previously about an infidelity of hers that he had discovered, Natasha may not have taken up the offer when she received the first letter from the incredible, irresistible 'John Smith'. However, she was at a stage in her relationship with Billy and in her life as a whole when she had decided to take her chances on finding someone new amongst the millions of men who surf the internet each night looking for just her sort of girl.

As a means of alleviating her miserable, frustrating existence, she would become one of the masses of lonely women who responded to these possible knights in shining armour. If they encountered men who seemed clever, funny and good with words, they found it easy to develop an internet correspondence and sometimes be persuaded to have cybersex or webcam sex with them. But meeting these men in real life often resulted in finding that their Prince Charming was 5 feet tall, bald, fat, and flatulent, or permanently unemployed, or a married man looking for a one night stand in a cheap B&B.

With perhaps one in three or five or seven thousand internet exchanges, there might sometimes, just sometimes be a real-life "Mr Right" at the other end. A six foot five inch perfect specimen of a man; oozing testosterone, strength, and stamina from his magnificent body. He makes her laugh with his crazy sense of humour, he is "good on paper" with a coveted job in investment banking and a salary in excess of one million pounds a year, he drives a white Ferrari - the modern-day version of the white stallion, and he actually is looking for a steady girlfriend.

Hard to believe that such a man as this was in a lonely hotel room that night, surfing the internet and considering reaching out to a random, attractive young woman who caught his eye, to see what might develop. It was of course, on one of these lonely nights online that our hero 'John Smith' discovered 5 year old photos of the ravishing Natasha on an Italian working-girls site.

Billy

Of a different generation, background, and lifestyle, Billy Clayton might never have met Natasha amongst the eight million residents of teeming London. Billy was a fifty-something world-renowned photographer, poet and artist with a globe-trotting lifestyle and a string of glamourous ex-wives and lovers to match. Billy was never without a beautiful woman, and he sampled them from the world over. For example, he had been married to a gorgeous Miss World contestant, and had had a long-term committed relationship with an exotic Asian beauty featured in a James Bond film amongst other major roles. Despite all the enviable experiences and exciting relationships he had had throughout his life, however, it was not until he met the young Natasha Nemcova by chance one day in a West London hospital that he met the woman of his dreams.

Our old-school hero Billy was a man fighting to save romantic love from dying out entirely. A man who was enthralled with women – exploring them, pleasing them, teasing them, loving them, pleasuring them – he had passionate opinions about women and their pussys. Natasha was a woman who was complete, who was totally aware of her power and of her pussy and everything it meant to the man in her life. She had the most beautiful pussy he had ever found. He loved her with his whole being.

For Billy, breaking up was like dying, and he did not want to die yet. Many say that if you love something you should set it free and if it returns to you, it was yours all along and it if doesn't, it could never have been yours. Billy disagreed completely. He believed that a woman changes, challenges and tests the strength of a man's love-bond to see if he needs her, is as devoted to her, and is as willing to fight for her as he claims. Billy felt that women had much more respect for men when they fought for them and did everything they could to win them back if they were about to lose them, as in the days of old.

'Once you have found her, never let her go.
Once you have found her n – e – v – e – r let her go.'
--Roger and Hammerstein, 'South Pacific'

This gorgeous, beautiful, wonderful, titillating, fascinating and pleasure-giving true-life fantasy and reality that is between a woman's legs. Why concentrate on this particular part of a woman? The answer can be found in examining the lives of some famous women throughout history who have known and appreciated this part of themselves. All these powerful women had one thing in common: they realised that their pussy was their greatest asset, and learnt to use it to their advantage.

It has been hypothesized that forty to fifty thousand years ago women were unaware of their power over men, and unsurprisingly so. According to the anthropologist Leaky, women only came 'on heat' (as animals do), once in a 40-day cycle. However, the human female has become the most sexual animal on this planet. She is the only creature that is available for sex 24 hours a day, every day, 365 days a year. No more waiting to come "on heat", modern woman has evolved to become permanently ready for sex.

In our ancestors' society, women's lesser physical strength made it impossible for her to compete with men directly for meat. She needed a man to provide her with a portion of the group's kill. Every time she put her bottom up in the air men would have sex with her, would treat her more favourably, feed her, and invite her closer to the fire. This social change had a physiological and biological effect on the female body. Instead of coming "on heat" once every forty days, it was advantageous for her to remain receptive to sex throughout the whole of her cycle.

The so-called "woman's libber" may not have helped the progress of women, because the women who have appreciated their pussies and learnt to use them powerfully have always done better in life due to their femininity and receptiveness than women who have demanded to be equal. Those strident women often end up barren and living alone after several failed relationships or marriage breakdowns.

The modern pussy is an amazing pleasure machine designed to give infinite pleasure to both males and females during sex, and many intelligent woman have learnt how to get the best from this asset. These women become the most powerful in a society, and some have even earned a place in history on this basis. Cleopatra who helped bring about the fall of the Roman Empire, certainly bringing down Marc Anthony, Emma Hamilton, who was worshipped and adored by Lord Hamilton and Lord Nelson, and Nell Gwyn, the long-time mistress of Charles II are all examples of such women.

Helen of Troy had probably one of the most remarkable stories ever known. Ten thousand ships were launched to capture and return her to Menelaus, King of Sparta, and fifty thousand men lost their lives in the attempt. The moment Menelaus found Helen again, he drew his sword to behead her. Immediately Helen unclasped her dress which fell to her feet, and stood before him naked. The minute he saw this most exquisite creature disrobed, he spared her life and forgave her. She continued to live with him until the day he died.

This factor of female power is still eminent in the modern world. In the film "Scent of a Woman", Al Pacino is on an airplane with his young prodigy. As he is blind, he cannot see the flight attendant so asks his prodigy "What is she like"? The young man answers, "She's very beautiful, she smells beautiful, and has a wonderful figure, apart from her legs which are not all that good". Al Pacino replies, "Let me give you this lesson, never worry about her legs, never worry if they're piano shaped or pear shaped or too long or too short. It's what's in between them that's important."

It is the centre of a woman; it is used for urination and menstruation, she gives pleasure to herself and to her lovers through it, and she gives birth to the future human race through it. She adores it, pampers it, protects it, and dresses it with fine silks and satins.

Of course, it is but a part of the whole of a woman. It is her spirit, her heart, her intelligence, and her beauty, combined with her ability to appreciate and wield her pussy for pleasure and power that makes each woman unique.

It may be a magical element of a woman that makes men lust after her, but it may often be the case, that from true lust, grows true love.

FOR PITY'S SAKE

CHARACTERS

Natasha Monika Nemcova

She was a fresh, young girl from the Eastern Europe. Only 19 tender years of age, with not more than 200 words of English, she was working in London as an au pair for an old lady.

This was her second position after arriving in the country, and she found it when she was nearly at the point of desperation. She was down to her last British pound, so if it had not been for a randy Turkish boy who had taken her in for three weeks, Natasha would not have been able to find her current job.

She knew that all the boy wanted was sex, but she reasoned that at least she was not living on the streets. Natasha was worldly-wise, an instinctive animal, who knew that her only hope of survival would be the one asset which nobody could take away from her... So rather than get on the coach to head back to her homeland, she had given in to him.

In her mind, an early return home would make her a pathetic failure in the eyes of her relatives and peers. Anyway, according to her domineering, manipulating father, she already was a failure. His mean treatment of her had resulted in a low self-esteem. When she fled her home country, her three-year virginal relationship with her first real boyfriend also had died, and she wanted so badly to make a brand new life for herself in England. Her primitive jungle awareness had led her to run far from her homeland in Moravia in the hopes of finding her pot of gold, and a beautiful man to complete her life.

After the Turkish boy had finished with her, she was left lonely. She had little free time, working 12 hours a day for the old lady, and in snatched moments of time still writing letters to her first love back home.

Billy Clayton

An ageing lothario, Billy was the product of an aristocratic Irish mother, a champion boxer English father, with a French grandfather in the mix. Vastly experienced in the ways of sex and romance, he had slept with over a thousand women before the age of 25 and had lived with thirteen amazing women, including a Miss World contestant, a Bond girl, and a top-ranking Asian businesswoman (and along the way, he was married to four of them).

However, his skill and success with women did not make him flippant or shallow. He was an intelligent man with three degrees, including one from the prestigious and world-famous St Martin's School of Art. All of his relationships had been long & satisfying. Each of his four marriages had exceeded six years. Happily married when he met the beautiful Natasha, forming a new relationship had been the last thing on his mind.

John Smith

Smith was a brainy, sophisticated city trader, towered 6ft 5" in height, had a degree in psychology and sociology, and was a chartered accountant. His salary was in excess of three quarters of a million pounds, which afforded him with a luxury flat in Maida Vale and a full-time Spanish maid. He was a practising Roman Catholic. His father, an architect, was half-Polish and half-English. His mother was a window dresser of Irish heritage. He had one sibling, a sister.

He and his girlfriend Ruth had recently broken up after a five year relationship due to religious differences, but they remained good "fuck buddies". Two months after the split, on a business trip to Germany, he was scanning the internet for a hot working girl and came across pictures of the gorgeous Natasha on an Italian website. He immediately sent her an email.

Ruth Cohen

A stunning, Orthodox Jewish woman, Ruth was the owner/manager of a nail bar on Finchley Road which her father had set up for her. Their massive family home was in Hampstead Garden Suburb. She was the baby of the family, and had three older brothers.

Yuri Sakamoto

Yuri, Billy's wife, was a beautiful, smart, sympathetic Oriental lady who had a high-powered position with a major Japanese company. Having been married six years, they were the very best of friends who gave each other space and time.

Chris Ngengo

Chris was a 5ft 4in African man built like a brick house who was Natasha's lover for seven months in secret.

Jamie Rain

This 35 year old property developer, with a 2 million pound mansion in Buckinghamshire, managed to talk Natasha into six or seven "freebies".

Fran Smith

The sister of John Smith, she was a props lady in London's theatre district. She lived alone with six cats.

Simon Williams

A AS400 systems administrator and Linux system expert, Simon was a loner who had studied computers since the age of 15. Now at the age of 35, he was still unmarried and without a girlfriend. He lived by himself in a two bedroom luxury flat, directly opposite from Natasha's apartment building.

The Beginning

The beginning, the beginning, the beginning
Wherever there's a beginning
There must be a middle and an end
But we never think about the end
When we're at the beginning
And the beginning with a man and a woman
Is usually passion and sexual attraction
And the end
When the words have gone away
There's nothing left
Lovers come and go
She goes her way you go yours
Life is like that
A pretty flower
It nurtures
Blossoms, by the hour
But then it dies and fades away
After all the years
Tormented fears
You never want to say goodbye

FOR PITY'S SAKE

THE BEGINNING

Oh darling, beloved and best beloved
and reader of my words.

This is the story of a dream
for all older men. A dream that became reality.
A reality that became a fantasy.
A fantasy that turned into a love story.
A love story that turned into a friendship.
A friendship that became a soul mate.
A soul mate that became a memory.

When I close my eyes, I can take myself back to that night where fate took over.

It was almost as if it were yesterday. On the 9th October 1996, after a wonderfully, successful artistic and financial year, I dreamt up the idea of taking my two children and Yuri, my wife of 6 years, as well as 7 of my best friends, on a 10 day boat trip to Copenhagen and Gutenberg. I paid for the trip as a thank you gift, for all the help and friendship they had given me.

There was Stefan, his beautiful girlfriend Tsubasa, Tony and his exotic Somalian partner Soosoo, Jimbo, my carpenter, George, my agent, Michel, a sound and television mixer, Yuri and my son Ben and daughter Emma.

Stefan was an accomplished pianist, who could play anything by ear but usually used his fingers. Michel was a passionate sound mixer and music fanatic, and each night my close friends, family and I crowded onto the little dance floor on our boat to sway to the music. It was such a beautiful boat, and happened to be the same one upon which Polanski's "Bitter Moon" was filmed.

Little did I realise, how eventful and life changing this journey would become.

As we rolled and pitched our way to the pretty sea port of Kobenhavn, and the town centre Newhaven, the rough seas of the Skagerrak and the Kattegat started to throw the boat about, like a cork on a windy pond.

Many of the guests on board were very sick, but not our little group. We spent our time on cocktail fuelled mad dancing to the squealing of the Spice Girls, as this was, you know, what I really, really wanted. We were having a fantastically crazy time.

The events which were to change my life began to unravel and show themselves in the closing minutes of the boat trip. Harwich was in sight and "Mad Michel" suggested a mad race around the boat by all the males.

'Last one to reach the bar…' he screamed at the top of his voice, 'Buys the drinks!'

He shot off faster than the sea breeze, closely followed by Stefan & Tony.

They rushed across the deck, but an incident was inevitable and the silly bastard tripped and hit his head on a life boat in his hurry to the lead. When the boat finally arrived in Harwich, the ambulance was waiting on the quay, and he was swiftly taken away unconscious to it by stretcher.

He finally made his way back to a leading London hospital, chauffer driven in luxury, whilst the rest of us made our way home in our cars.

Some four days had passed and we all drew straws to take it in turns to visit him. My wife and I were the first.

When we arrived, he was sitting up in bed feeling very sorry for himself. How the great and the good had fallen. His head was heavily bandaged and he had had concussion since he arrived.

But the Devil helps his own. He was a big man, permanently randy and always on the look out for what he could pull, and how did we find him? In a mixed ward, with him being the only man in it.

On one side he had an old lady, on the other, a black nurse who had been admitted for some virus she had picked up on the ward. Across from his bed were three other women of various ages, between 40 and 70.

'What's this then?' I said to him jokingly, 'Sex on the national health?' He gave me a cheeky smile.

'I presume Michel, if you're not too sick, you can jump into other people's beds at night, when the ward supervision is at a minimum, with only a staff nurse and a sister to keep an eye on all of them?'

'Too right my boy!' he shouted out with glee.

It was then that I noticed her.

FOR PITY'S SAKE

While Yuri talked to Michel, I looked towards the bed by the window. And there she was. Sitting with a solitary teddy bear watching over her, was an angel, question marks, capital letters and stars flying all above and around her head. She was totally alone, despite it being peak visiting time.

My round, John Lennon glasses started to steam up. I was always the little boy who took in birds with broken wings as a child and she was the most beautiful, tragic, vulnerable creature I had set my eyes on.

She lay there like a broken doll on heaps of pillows, disorganized sheets with drip tubes and catheters everywhere. Her large brown eyes stared forlornly at her teddy on the window sill with the slight ghost of a Mona Lisa smile on her lips and a face whiter than Snow White.

'Who the hell is that!?' I said to Michel, 'She is beautiful! Devastating!' He looked up as me as if I were mad.

'She… She…' I kept repeating to myself.

'She is just some poor little Czech girl who speaks no English. She's just had some cancerous lumps cut out of her throat. One of them was so near her vocal chords, she nearly lost her voice.' He continued, trying to impress me with his knowledge of her condition.

'But anyway Billy, look closely and you'll see her face, arms and whatever you can see of her body, are all covered in big, white and weepy spots, or blackheads. She's obviously in a bit of a state and hardly has any visitors either. Apart from one Serbian boy who pops in for a chat once a week or so.' He paused and looked at me.

'Go and chat to her if you want mate... not that you'd get more than two words out of her.'

'But she's a goddess Michel!' I exclaimed. 'She's got a face to die for!'

'Crumbs, do you really think so Billy?' said Michel.

'I'm gonna talk to her Michel.'

Yuri just looked on with curiosity.

I might have hesitated, if I could have known the consequences of that one hello.

She was to become the famine and the feast, the light of my life, the pain in my loins, the Devil, an Angel, my reason to carry on living.

When I looked across at her from the other end of the room, somehow I just knew that she was someone I would be seeing again, and again and again...

'Hello.' I said. 'You are beautiful.' She smiled up at me with a mixed look of fear, anticipation and gratitude. There were tubes, which I presumed were for feeding, inserted in her nose, down her throat and in both her wrists. Another was in the ankle of her foot, protruding slightly from the sheets.

She looked so very vulnerable.

Her family were all back in the Czech Republic and it was painful for her to get any further information than that. Apparently she worked as an old lady's carer and au pair.

Outside the hospital, large scale building works were taking place and the racket coming from outside was intolerable, even through the double glazed windows.

I took her hand and when she squeezed mine back, it felt incredible. I sat on the empty bed next to her, still not letting go of her hand. The first touch is always the beginning of something special and this was to be no exception.

I glanced at my watch, it was exactly 8:30pm on the 20th October.

The case notes at the end of her bed told me that she was only 20 years old. I was fast approaching 55, though my passport lied about my age. Her dark brown eyes looked into me with hope and unknowing.

She was wearing an off-white paisley pyjama top, which just revealed her more than ample, young breasts.

I took the hand I was still holding to my mouth and kissed it, and told her I would visit in a couple of days.

Whether she understood or not was difficult to tell.

She was like a beautiful, friendless alley cat, caught by fate in a strange, foreign environment, with only her own jungle instincts to survive. No language or means of communication…totally alone.

Her eyes opened widely at me like a cat's eyes caught in the headlamps of a car on the road. I turned to go, looking back from the doorway and into the room one more time.

Four days later, I visited Michel again. Well, perhaps this was not quite true! I hardly gave him more than a nod of acknowledgment as I passed by his bedside clutching a large teddy bear and a bunch of flowers.

'Are they for me Billy boy?' he shouted from the bed.

'No Michel, you're far too ugly to deserve such nice things. These are for the Angel.'

Michel shouted, 'Would that be for the fallen angel Billy Clayton?'

'No Michel this is not Los Angeles, this is Paddington and the only bear is you!'

'Not true Billy, I got into bed with her last night and we had a cuddle while we watched television, until the staff nurse threw me out and back to me own bed.'

'You dirty bastard.' I said to him. I glanced up at the bed I was heading for and she was smiling at me. All the tubes and paraphernalia had gone, except for one in her wrist.

A large red raw scar ran across her swan-like neck, almost reaching from one ear to the other.

I placed the flowers and the teddy in her arms.

'For me?' she said. 'For me?' she repeated. Her dark brown eyes pierced mine. 'I Natasha.' She nodded her head from side to side. 'I... I Natasha Nemcova.' She used the strangest expression. 'Never in my life.' She said.

Her voice was soft and pretty, as she repeated it again .

'Never in my life, anyone be so kind...'

I already knew I was in love with her.

We spent a very long hour talking, but even with her limited vocabulary, I managed to decipher that she was from Moravia in the south of the Czech Republic, and that her family were very poor so none of them could come to see her or even afford to call.

One of the doctors was slightly worried about her, so I decided to phone her sister, who had surpringly good English, but expressed no desire to come to England. Natasha the angel had given me her sister's number so I could let her know how she was doing.

I realised then, after I'd put the receiver down, what the strange feelings I instinctively felt from the alley cat meant. There was obviously some conflict within the family which she would not want to speak of to a stranger such as myself.

Five days later, I returned again, clutching another teddy, but to my utmost horror, sadness and disappointment, the bed by the window was empty.

Nobody would tell me her address, or any information about her other than what I'd gathered from asking every doctor, nurse and cleaner in the hospital that she lived somewhere near Baker Street.

Michel, my so called friend, would tell me nothing. He was due to be discharged that day and I knew that he knew more than he was prepared to tell me.

Sherlock Holmes lived in Baker Street. I was about to become him, and was going to do everything in my power to find this girl.

THE SEARCH

Every day was madness. For the next six weeks, I chased every lead. I must have phoned every doctor, every nurse, and every hospital administrator, and anyone I could think of who might have had even the smallest clue as to where she lived, worked and slept.

All drew was a complete blank.

I took to walking the streets around the Baker Street area. I had given my card to the black nurse who was in the bed next to Michel but never heard from her. She had said she wanted some photos done sometime. I eventually resorted to phoning Michel again, but he was proving a right bastard. He was very peeved off indeed when he told me his story.

Apparently he had asked her out after he came out of hospital and got her number from her then. She had gone around to his house one early evening and he had somehow managed to get her into bed.

He inferred or tried to imply that he had in fact been revolted by her and claimed he had stripped her down to her knickers and then changed his mind. Her body was covered in weeping spots and old scabs and she was wearing large white cotton knickers that his grandmother probably would have worn.

She was quite reluctant to give in to him, but when he had put his hand inside her knickers, she became quite upset, so he ended up cooking her spaghetti bolognaise and throwing her out instead.

He also threw her phone number away after she had left, as he had already consigned her to the 3/10 category.

He insisted that this was the true story and that he had not fucked her, and that after she had gone through the door he had not even offered to take her home.

'Anyway,' he said triumphantly, 'I don't even know why you're bothering to try to find her. She's nothing special.' He then put the phone down on me.

It was December 6th, almost 6 weeks had passed, and it was 11 o'clock on a grey winter's morning. It felt eminently greyer in my heart. There was no sunshine for me. I'd lost her and the pain was unbearable.

Suddenly my phone rang.

My heart stopped, just for a second.

'Billy?'

A sweet voice whispered to me over the phone. I could hardly believe it. I was overcome with joy and I praised God like I had never done before. It was her, she had found me! Like I, she had been searching for me and had phoned the black nurse who had passed my number on.

I was ecstatic and my words were tumbling out. She began to laugh. She may not have understood me but could certainly feel my excitement and enthusiasm.

She told me that she would be at my place at 2.30pm at the latest and could stay till 5.30pm.

It was a Friday afternoon. The doorbell rang and my heart started to beat against my chest like a hammer. Even as she came up the spiral staircase, I could not control myself. I already had a hard on for her... one that was to last for 11 years.

She looks so incredibly pretty, I thought to myself. I made her tea and biscuits as she sat on my chesterfield inspecting the room with a natural curiosity and unmistakable intelligence.

She wore a simple knitted dress underneath a hand-knitted, short, thick, hooded woolen jacket, with a strong black and white pattern. She removed it and put it next to her neatly folded as she gazed at some photographs of my wife on the wall.

Of course she knew I was married, but yet did not seem to mind. As she chatted away in her limited vocabulary, mixing words upside down and inside out, I felt her irrepressible loneliness. I felt her need, her hunger to be held… and I felt the sex.

I asked her what kind of music she liked, and she told me she was quite keen on Phil Collins and Genesis, so I put on the track, 'I Can't Dance, I Can't Walk'.

She told me about her, her life, her dreams, her family and her background. It was a slow, and a little laborious but we managed to establish a little more than we has in the hospital.

I asked her if she wanted to see me again and she cried 'Yes!' with such enthusiasm, it blew me away.

'Okay then. Why don't you come around on Monday?' She was obviously disappointed and sadness welled up in her eyes. I was quick to realise the reason behind the tears.

'I can't see you on Saturday or Sunday Natasha. I have my

daughter and son coming for the weekend. I'm sorry... didn't I tell you about them?' She shook her head. 'My daughter's the same age as you. Well actually, thank god, 4 months younger than you.'

I looked at her sweet face and suddenly felt old. Fuck, I was old enough to be her father, and then some!

Her eyes glossed over just slightly. Not a tear but just a sadness. She said that she was pleased to have somebody.

The weekend was one of anticipation, I hardly enjoyed my children. I was fairly selfish and I hardly thought of them at all. Admittedly for the whole weekend, I could not get her out of my head, and a large part of me hoped that she felt the same way.

Monday the 9th December was to be a very memorable day indeed. In fact, when I look back on it, I t was the most memorable Monday ever. It was an aphrodisiac Monday a Viagra Monday, a hope for the future Monday

This was the first Monday I could ever imagine looking forward to. She phoned at 1.30, sweet bubbly and excited. Why did Macbeth keep coming into my head? Could it have been an instinctive warning against possible dangers. I had always had a hidden protection over me.

My name sake William like Shakespeare, bubble, bubble toil and trouble, fire burn and cauldron bubble. Liver of blaspheming Jew (am I really meant to be with you).

This was too special a day, not to save it forever.

So I got my movie camera out and placed it in the clothes cupboard in my bedroom with the door slightly open to reveal everything that may or may not happen if the bed was where history would be written that day what was meant to be. Would be.

In case I got real lucky, I wanted to keep that moment forever. Madness, madness. In my mind already I wanted this relationship to last. And I knew I was insanely willing to risk losing everything in my life that I held dear to me, for a young slip of a girl.

35 years younger than myself a lolita in cotton panties Vladimir Nabikov's reality, in my bedroom.

Natasha, Light of my life, fire and hunger in my loins, my heart , my hopes, having her.for as long as I could cling to her and damn the future..

She was Nat to her friends, a small flying insect. She was

Natasha to her mother, A first born Russian princess but to me, she was my dragon lady.
She was born on the 4th July 1976. A Cancerian born dragon, to match equally, my Capricorn dragon. We were two hot fire breathing dragons together, a perfect match in every way.

She walked in, put herself down on the chesterfield, and kissed me lightly on the cheek, her lips just straying, a little bit close to mine as she did the courtesy greeting.

I held her hand, pushed up the sleeves of her long woollen dress and stroked her bare arms. I put on Genesis again for her (probably the first time anyone's tried to seduce a woman to Phil Collins).

I played with her arms for almost an hour. They were slightly hairy but I tried not to notice.

Wow, 3.30 on the 9th December, a time to remember, a moment to savour till the day I die A no one day in numerology, a success day, a cocaine going around my brain day. She was hungry, hungry for me and my body. She had been a long time without regular sex, and was only 20 years old, and we were both new to each other, so the excitement was intense. When She came up the spiral staircase earlier and my arm had encircled her waist. Before she sat herself down, she clung to me for a moment like a marionette puppet ,as though we had got our strings entangled . She was lost and wanted me to do it all for her. Make it easy, make all the decisions, no guilt on her part. She let me orchestrate the whole seduction, so that in her mind she could think...."well , he did it to me."

I was happy to take on the task, to be her mentor, teacher, Svengali, her lover, master, Prof Higgins.

She washed her hands and face before she came...she did. Her eyes were dark brown pools locked into mine. A thought flashed through my brain " what are you to teach me proper then... can I come out of my garden into yours?"

The only two regrets in life is growing old and dying. I don't want to miss anything in life. The young say all the time that they are bored. There is no room ever in this life to be bored.
There is so much to do, so much to explore, so much to find in each other and the world .I took hold of her hand and led her to the bedroom. Her woollen dress hit the floor in 15 seconds flat.

FOR PITY'S SAKE

I went to the clothes cupboard and secretly turned on the movie camera. I wanted to record this moment for eternity, posterity. Something to play back over and over, even if I was reduced to a wheelchair.

I have always wanted to stop time, ever since I was a young boy in hospital. I spent 7 years in a tuberculosis ward.
I used to draw the doctors, nurses and the other kids

I spent my life stopping time, photography, film, paintings, moments preserved. I was fascinated by our ability to do that. The only true immortality.

I pulled off her thin white t-shirt over her head. That was under the dress she had white cotton knickers on , slightly too big, long white socks and a large black bra.

We were both kissing like mad, her tongue, like a dragon's serpent flicking in and out, Her mouth devouring mine. I prised her full breasts out of their captivity, pushed her bra up to her neck. I was lost in them sucking her nipples, licking her oreals. Suddenly she stopped me and pushed me away, and in her strong accent her finger pointing at the cupboard door which had swung wide open.

'No film! You are not filming us.' she screamed.

I turned the camera off apologetically. At least I had her down to her knickers on camera...

Satisfied that she was no longer being filmed she came back into my arms like a bat out of hell. I picked her up and threw her on the bed and followed her quickly with my pants around my ankles.
She turned her back on me quickly and I caressed her large breasts. Cupped them in my hands from behind. Then I played with her bottom, her thighs, she could feel my hard cock pressing against the crack of her arse. We must have spent 30 minutes this way, her with her back to me , playing .I slid my hands inside her cotton knickers and at last she turned to face me.

There was a waterfall on the bed, somewhere. She was squirting out her creamy juices like an Australian geyser
Her cotton knickers were so wet it would be impossible to wring them out.

I tried not to notice the hundreds of spots on her back, chest and tummy. Knowing that she had been really ill, I ignored them. And anyway, she was nice, and none of us are perfect. A silly thought I believed she had five spots for every year that I was older than her, so I think that was compensation enough for me and her. Life is give and take.

As her knickers came down, I had such a hard on, I could hardly contain myself. He was throbbing, the veins at bursting point, oscillating from side to side and up and down, like a conductor's baton. At last I gazed at her treasure box , but no I did not !? She was covered in a layer of thick black forest hair, some of it a full 20cm long! I was so shocked. I love to see a pussy, I love to suck a pussy, to get my whole head in there. I love it shaven, soft and smooth like a baby's bottom. I don't want to spend the next day picking black hairs from my teeth.

This was real black forest gateau. I couldn't even see her cleft. This had to go sometime, if this relationship were to continue seriously.

Her breathing was heavier and heavier as she started to moan. Her face was on fire, I started to get 3rd degree burns. She was a little gasoline station. The smell of her sex, her burning face and neck, she was a rich combustible mix of highly inflammable petroleum ready to explode.

My two fingers worked her pussy faster and faster, massaging her sweet tiny clitoris to insane madness.
Hitting her g-spot over and over again with the tips of my fingers.
And then it happens... she really came.

A loud drawn out whimpering scream, a cross between the cry of a seagull and an animal in pain. Her body was shuddering and she was screaming for a full 3 minutes, as my fingers carried on. She grabbed my hand to pull me away, as it was too much
She couldn't take it any longer, as the ecstasy had now become pain.

Her legs were wide apart now and her knees were slightly bent. Everything was wet her thighs, my hands, my arms, the sheets, everything.

We had shared a monsoon of pleasure, of tingling flesh, of skin touching skin, of me touching her, of her touching me. Her eyes wide , wide open, beautiful brown soft pools of desire.

It was 4.30, this was eternity for me ready to begin... I knew I'd been granted a glimpse of Heaven, Adam with the expectation to taste apple fresh in his mouth, this was an orchard it.

I knew with certainty.

Her beauty surpassed everything I had imagined in my wildest dreams. Her Pussy surpassed any expectation ever imaginable.

Pure Silk from Heaven with clotted cream inside.

The sensations I felt when first entering this paradise defies description sometimes words can so often be inadequate. It was Heaven and Hell all rolled into one gorgeous, beautiful succulent moment which responded willingly and eagerly as it opened to the touch of my fingers.

Nothing can ever replace in any dream I could ever have for the rest of my life, the moment my hard throbbing cock first slid all the way into the hot cauldron of fire heaven & hell of sensual delights of her adorable, lovable, eat for ever, vomit & eat it again Pussy.

Her amazing little Pussy was a sweet, petit void within a delicate flowering bud just blooming, only played with by three other men before me.

Almost virginal in it's delight & inexperience, crying out to be taught everything the older man could teach it on it's long road to sexual fulfilment.

Within three minutes of our first encounter my testicles were covered in her sweet honey dew, as was her thighs & the bed.

During one whole hour, her crazy excitement, mixed with my enthusiasm meant that the only thing that spoilt the magic of this, our first encounter, was the wiping of excess, sweet juices that flowed everywhere..

I fucked her on and on for a whole hour and a half. We were so crazy; we never even had time to think of putting on a condom. She was mad beneath me, insane beneath me, alternating continuously. Crying moaning, breathless, laughing, everything a man could dream about. A lifetime of memories, all into one afternoon.

Her pussy farting moaning and bubbling, like bottled Guinness that had been shaken. I fucked her on and on, never stopping.

Changing the angle and the depth of my penetration of her continually and then I filled her with my thick, creamy cum. I screamed and screamed in an orgasm of pleasure, I was sure that the whole world could hear me, as I ejaculated into her over and over again.

We both drowned in our juices. She was so happy, laughing with pleasure. Two dragons copulating, a rare sight to behold indeed…

I lifted her buttocks with my hands and fucked her hard again the second time. Nothing existed, the sun moon and stars fell through the window. A tear fell down her cheek, it hit the corner of her pretty mouth and continued on down her cheek then dripping onto her breasts. Then another, and another.

She held me more tightly kissing me with a passion that wasn't sexual anymore but a yearning for something else…Love, love, love.

We were drowning and I was her lifeboat and she the only one who could swim. Her navel was filled with water, we were both so wet. Her pussy was still contracting, fully dilated pouring out thick cream and giving little pussy farts.

Paradise found, ourselves lost, as we lay side by side, too hot to hold each other, too wet to touch. She glanced up at my large clock on the balcony opposite.

'Oh my god!... the time, the time!' she said.

We rushed out to my car throwing our clothes on without washing. We were the white rabbits, Alice in wonderland gone mad. We'd been in the garden, madder than the Hatter, the tea party was over. I drove my car like Schumacher to Baker St. 6pm rush hour and was there in less than 5 minutes. She pointed to a tiny window, high up in a large block of flats. "That's my bedroom. See you tomorrow.

'See you tomorrow,' she shouted as she jumped out of the car. She didn't ask or even know that I could. She assumed that I would. But love was on my forehead, neon lights flashing.

I turned the car around and headed for home. I glanced at the seat she had just occupied. There was a pool of liquid there. It must have seeped all the way through her knickers and her woolen dress.

This was sex and passion, love and commitment on two legs….this was a dragon lady.

THE BLACK FOREST
Tuesday 10th December

The most pleasurable thing you can ever do with a beautiful woman that you want to desire and love, is unwrap her slowly and sensuously until her naked body confronts you, which is my belief in the prelude to making love, even when I was only 19 years old.

That is why an older man, as a teacher for a younger woman, is the best experience she can have. Young men, as I was once, are crazy, frantic, and they hardly stop to un-wrap a girl sensuously. They want to get on the girl as soon as they can. An older man will take time to get her excited. Also an older man will have more experience of a woman's body and older men last longer. Where young men it's often over before it's begun. Or as one young girl described to me, when talking about a recent break-up with her young boyfriend, she said, when we did it, I had sneezes that lasted longer! Experience means technique. If the older man is intelligent and sensitive, he has learnt much of his years in pleasuring women. Also a little grey hair on a man's chest can be a real turn on for women.

Tuesday 10th December came, and she arrived; another unforgettable day, as I was soon to be 55, and she was just 20… She had her hair in a cute little pony tail, which bounced up and down as she walked, and swung permanently from side to side. She kissed me passionately as she arrived at the top of the spiralled staircase.

'Hi.' I said to her as we came out of the clinch.

'I need to use the bathroom.'

She said, 'okay' and walked straight up to the bedroom.

As she did so, in her excitement, the elastic came off the end of her ponytail, and her hair flicked out in a cascade of beauty. For me, she was an absolutely perfect creature, and I could not wait to join her on the bed.

After a quick scrub up in the bathroom, I took a shaving brush, soap, shaving cream and shaver. Naked, I ran up the stairs to join her. I was pleasantly surprised at her eagerness.

After our first encounter which had been very memorable, I found her lying on her back. Her dark, provocative hair framed her pretty face, and she intoxicated me with her dark, brown eyes, which would have pained me to have them blue.

She was only wearing a pair of tiny cotton knickers. Her eyes opened wide in surprise at me holding the shaving equipment. I said nothing at all to her. I walked straight to the edge of the bed, as she held out her hands for a cuddle. I ignored this completely. I had a job to do and I wanted to achieve it quickly. I wanted to do it before she could even think of refusing, so the element of surprise was most important. And also fun!

Her red nipples looked so good, inviting, teasing, screaming to me, 'Suck me please!' They were plump and ripe and full, like mad, rampant tomatoes, and when I touched them like her face, they were so fucking hot, I burnt my fingers on them.

Her whole body was translucent in the north facing studio light, and her pretty, small, pink tongue, darted in and out teased me into kissing her and trying to pull me on top of her. I pulled her knickers off in one smooth movement, and spread her legs wide. She lay there in wonderment, looking like a tiny little girl with her first big ice cream. I soaked her generously until her whole black bush of hairs were covered in thick creamy soap.

'What are you… do with me?' She said in her broken English. 'What are you do with me?'

I put a towel beneath her bottom, which in ten minutes was covered in thick black pubic hairs.

Then suddenly it was there before my eyes, the most beautiful little cleft, with a tiny little pearl of a clitoris glinting at me. Her pussy was already lying ready with excitement.

I left her lying and waiting on the bed as I got rid of the towel full of hairs and the shaving equipment. I was so eager, I simply threw it all in a black bin liner bag. By the time I had gotten into bed she was crazed with impatience and excitement.

I touched it and it was as soft and sweet as a baby's bottom. Thank God at last! I did not have to pick out her black hairs from my teeth the next morning. While I had shaved her, she trusted me so much that she said nothing.

Her legs were now tingling with excitement and her toes were curling and uncurling. The cream started to pour out of her, and it was nothing to do with the shaving soap I used. I was on the bed next to her now, and keen to give her an Oscar winning performance.

Her heart started to beat, and her breasts started to heave and pull. Her nipples were erect, and my hand felt the sweetness of God's creation, so beautifully formed.

My fingers started to play the Bohemian Rhapsody on her. For both of us, the ceiling, the room, everything, was filled with every colour of the rainbow.

My heart and hers were beating so fast and loud, we could hear them. She had her eyes closed, something she did not do quite so often in the future.

Oblivion!

Her breath came in gasps, her body was so hot, it glowed like hot lava pouring out of her. I was all too eager this time, and so was she, for me to suck and lick her to distraction. I placed her hands on my bottom as my cock went in and out of her rhythmically.

My cock bumped and nudged at her pussy, and slid in and out in long strokes. My balls slammed against her bottom cheeks with a loud noise, and her pussy grunted and groaned. As the rhythm built up, she held my head and kissed me deeply and swung her legs around my back. She felt now, she was being a bad, bad girl. The letters she sent home to her ex with love, meant nothing at this moment. She was lost with no map to get back. She was in a new dimension of love-making that she had never before experienced. Her bottom and her body moved in perfect rhythm with mine. We were making the most amazing music together.

This girl was born to fuck.

Who cared if her body had a few spots from hormonal problems? She was both sizzling and helpless, all at the same time. In total submissive surrender. At this moment I could have done anything with her. But she pulled me in harder and harder, tighter and slippery, she covered me in warm honey dew.

My balls were bouncing off her cheeks now like ping-pongs, and we were both groaning with excitement and exhaustion as it had already been a good two hours. I thought it was about time to go out and down on her beautiful pearl. Sucking it in and out of my lips like a vacuum cleaner, she exploded in seconds. Her knees knocking together, she would scream to the first of three orgasms she would have that day.

Her pussy was so swollen, as were her pretty lips, set in a face of an angel. She stood up and looked in the mirror.
'What will the old lady I work for say?' she said. Her mouth was swollen to twice its size. I had sucked and teased her and she stood looking in the mirror. I started to tease again, this time with my fingers.

First one finger, then two. She did not want to stand any more, so she wrapped her legs around me and we fell onto the bed. My fingers were now hitting her g-spot, and I went down to her again. I could not get enough of her. She is the best aphrodisiac in the world, Viagra on two legs, the dream of every older man.

I was kissing her frantically now. 'Please don't kiss me anymore!' she cried, 'The lady I work for… I could never explain this.'

Suddenly, I had gone from three fingers to a whole hand and she gasped with all her breath. I could not believe my eyes. It was the first time for both of us. My whole hand was pumping at her pussy, five inches up my wrist. I was literally holding her by her pussy.

She was now burning up, moaning and crying, and she orgasmed again. I licked her pussy with my tongue, trying to kiss it better after the almost painful torment she had endured from my whole hand. Unbelievably, she started to orgasm again.

Day almost turned into night as madness took over. Even though we were both weak and tired and had no energy left, I could not leave her alone. I pulled her on top of me and she bounced up and down, taking it deep inside her. She sucked me in, holding me even tighter and tighter.

Then for the first time she took me into her mouth, and I was so excited and crazy, I came down her throat over and over, as she swallowed it down like thick yoghurt.

My fingers played with her nipples. Everything was like before, wet, wet, wet… her legs, wide, wide apart. Tears were rolling down her cheeks now. She was so dependent on me. Her sadness and love were overwhelming.

This time it was awesome, massive, as I straddle her again. She moaned so loudly that I was afraid the people next door would hear. She had come again for the third time and we were both completely insane, lost in the magic of the moment.

Her head was almost touching the carpet, and her nails were digging into my shoulder. Unbelievably, I came again.

I have never ever, with any woman had four orgasms in one day. She lay shaking over and over like blamange. Her face, her body, every part of her was red hot. Her eyes were filled with tears.

'Never in my life have I had it so perfect.' She whispered.

She could not bring herself to use the word pussy or cunt, as she struggled to get the words out, so she used the correct medical term instead, which seemed incongruous after the love-making we had just shared together.

'My vagina is sore and on fire' she said. 'You make my head lost. You are not a boy, you are mature… intelligent. I love it with you! You are older, but have like young passion.'

I kissed her and told her her old lady would be waiting.

'But I don't want to go!' she said.

'You know I'm married.'

She nodded.

'I won't be trouble, I promise!.. I promise…'

I gave her some Vaseline from the bathroom to rub on her lips, and drove her home to Baker Street. She rubbed my back as I drove the car and held my hand as I held the wheel.

'I'm so sore.' She complained.

The thought floated through my mind. 'I'm not bleeding surprised!'

We arrived at Baker Street and I dropped her off. Her eyes looked at me filled with longing and want.

'Tomorrow?' She said, 'Promise. Please promise!'

'Okay, I will phone you tomorrow morning.'

As I drove away I saw her standing on the pavement, a vulnerable, beautiful, lonely little bird, who looked like she had lost her wings and her heart. She had fallen in love madly at last, but with an older married man. She was still a tiny speck in the mirror, still standing on the pavement looking after the car until she disappeared from sight.

Tears started to fall down my cheeks at the wheel, and my cock started to get hard just thinking about her. I glanced down at his direction, taking my eyes off the road for one second, and thought to myself, 'A right mess you've got me into! Where do we go from here?' But then I knew… I was in love with her.

TEN YEARS ON WE ARE WHERE WE ARE NOW

She was no longer a fresh young infatuated girl of 20. She had grown up fast in the last ten years and was now a mature, sophisticated, very sexy woman. Let's talk of it... No, let's not. An older man of 65 years – it had to go only one way. This thing had started to change. Love as it dies is like a pebble thrown into the water. Wings of pure soul grow wider and wider, till they reach the shore and break your heart.

The writing was on the wall, and I knew it. We had shared over three thousand sexual encounters together. We had talked over fourteen thousand times on the phone – sometimes four or five times a day. We had circumnavigated the world together. She had warm flesh for me, laughed for me, disappointed me, teased me, waited for me... And I her! We had been soul mates. Everything. She took the air from my lungs. How could I ever let her go?.. But after all we're going to loose everything in this world. In the end everything has to die and death is just a last exposure. The camera clicks for the last time – and all that is left are the images. All the egos are obliterated.

As you give the life up for the unknown you discover that love is a wish that hides in your heart and nobody has any idea about it. The hardest thing to control is your heart. If mercy has a human face let's all pity a human heart. But when you're asking all these questions to yourself be prepared to hear the truth. And I was facing it. Really facing it. Bang, wow! No more pain, no more jealousy, no more hurt... but no more her. Then I think I would rather had been punch-drunk and in love again.

Since her last two infidelities things are falling down here fast. I had lost control. How could I keep her for one more year? She wanted a baby, a home, a husband – the whole pack of it. But what could I do? Maybe if I'd managed to find a way of keeping her for one more year we could get a compromise?..

Her last boyfriend, her last love, her last secret had been 5'4 inches tall and black as the ace of spades. The other one had been 'a client' – he just wanted to have free sex from her without paying. And if she did come back to me again, if she did trust me again – could I trust her? The spring can be a new beginning. Maybe my heart would be singing. By the time the crocuses will have pushed up from the soil, love would find the way. Maybe all birth and rebirth has to come from hurt and pain. A time to laugh and cry, and hug, and sigh. Here she would be. And I as well.

For seven months she kept him in a secret, her little black lover. Of course she tries to dismiss it as nothing. It was only a stupid sex thing she tried to convince me. Just how seven months were. Just a long unfortunate accident. I can't fathom, but I'm sure that she shared the fun of seeing him like the excitement of tasting some forbidden fruits. He was an African with not much money. He maybe had rhythm and music in his soul, but he became happy only when she was on her back. My tears fall in pain. And she is washed away out to sea.

She always knew I was married but kept her love in a secret compartment. That was the problem, the deceit and the deceiving. She had magic but it turned out to be black. Could one more year be an impossible dream?

The last time we had sex was on the 9th of December. And then she flew home to her family. While she was away the whole story came out. When I picked her up at Stanstead on Boxing Day I wanted to kill her. How could I trust her again? The lips she turned to me were lips that lied over and over. It's now seven weeks since we've been to bed… Can a man cut out his heart? Yes, because I was having a one-sided love affair with myself. I was driving down a one way street, the wrong way. The traffic lights had turned red and I was bleeding to death. I needed the blood transfusion to catch more time. Another year maybe. But for what?..

January

From: john smith <appledogstime@yahoo.co.uk>
Date: 9 January 19:30:04 GMT
To: monika_nw3@yahoo.co.uk
Subject: you and possibly me

Dear Monika,

I work in the city and I have just returned from Germany. In Germany I saw a site with some beautiful pictures of you. I would love to spend some real good time with you. I live in ST JOHNS WOOD. I'm not sure where you would be, but this says nw3, so you must be close. I don't know what your charges would be for your time but to cut to the chase I have a budget of £600 an hour for a minimum of two hours. I am 29 years old, fit with dark hair, dark eyes and 5 ft 11 inches in height. If we get on I'd like to meet two times a month. I really hope you are still working, as you are wonderful.
John H Smith...call me john please x

From: monika_nw3@yahoo.co.uk>
Date: 10 January 09:49:16 GMT
To: john smith <appledogstime@yahoo.co.uk>
Subject: Re: you and possibly me

Dear John
Unfortunately I am not in the business anymore, though I thank you for your kind words. Could you please tell me which site it was that you saw my pictures on so I can have them taken down.
Hope you find what you are looking for.
Kind regards Monika xx

January

From: john smith <appledogstime@yahoo.co.uk>
Date: 10 January 14:12:22 GMT
To: monika_nw3@yahoo.co.uk >
Subject: Re: you and possibly me

Just got to my desk, I'm a city trader. Sorry to hear that this is the story, you look so nice and I would love to meet you some time. Me..I have just broken up from a four year relationship with a lady..and she is moving out on the first of feb..so no love. My life is empty so when I saw your pictures I fell in love..and I am sure you are just as nice in real life. Anyway lets keep in touch if you don't mind, it'll be nice to have such a charming pen friend..have you any sort of boy friend? You don't have to tell me?? I'm sorry about the website but I can't remember what it was called?? I was in my hotel room late at night, lonely and scanning the Internet. Hope we could co-respond. Thank you John x

From: john smith <appledogstime@yahoo.co.uk>
Date: 10 January 17:56:31 GMT
To: monika_nw3@yahoo.co.uk >
Subject: Re: you and possibly me

Forgot to say it's my birthday soon and it's going to be a BIG city party. I can try to get you an invite and you can bring a girlfriend along with you if you want? It's on the 19th of January. I was born in 1976. Think on it.
Thank you John

From: john smith <appledogstime@yahoo.co.uk>
Date: 17 January 10:55:38 GMT
To: monika_nw3@yahoo.co.uk >
Subject: Re: you and possibly me

Dear Monika,
I still think of you. Would love to have been your pen friend.
love john x

From: monika_nw3@yahoo.co.uk >
Date: 22 January 16:31:02 GMT
To: john smith <appledogstime@yahoo.co.uk>
Subject: Re: you and possibly me

Dear John,
I know you still think of me and believe me when I say that I don't need a pen friend right now. Hope your birthday party went well and I hope you find somebody soon.

Love M xx

From: john smith <appledogstime@yahoo.co.uk>
Date: 24 January 14:54:25 GMT
To: monika_nw3@yahoo.co.uk >
Subject: Re: you and possibly me

When you think, you're just so nice, I need you.

love John

From: john smith <appledogstime@yahoo.co.uk>
Date: 29 January 16:54:08 GMT
To: monika_nw3@yahoo.co.uk >
Subject: Re: you and possibly me
Come on don't be a party pooper, write to Johnny. Tell me nice things to make me more up beat. I work hard and play hard. A beautiful girl like you sending me the odd letter five times a year is all I need to get me through the long empty nights and the long days on the hard time stocks market. love john

January

From: john smith <appledogstime@yahoo.co.uk>
Date: 11 February 20:10:40 GMT
To: monika_nw3@yahoo.co.uk >
Subject: Re: you and possibly me
Dear Monika
Long time no hear from you, can we have a nice meeting for a drink on valentines say at ten fifteen at that nice little pub on England's lane...if it's near to you that is. It's just been refurbished.
love john x (one drink cant hurt)

From: monika_nw3@yahoo.co.uk >
Date: 12 February 10:49:58 GMT
To: john smith <appledogstime@yahoo.co.uk>
Subject: Re: you and possibly me
Hi John,
You are right one drink would not hurt if I didn't already have a program sorted. I am not sure what planet you are from but you can remind me. Valentines day date with a man I have not met or seen?... Hope you find somebody nice to have that drink with you, sorry it can't be me. All my love M xx

January

ROSES IN THE AIR

She may have been a woman of the night at one time to pay her way through school, but she was my friend in the day. However, I could not help her at that time out of her financial difficulties, as I had problems of my own, with legal bills running into thousands over a property I owned. Sometimes I wished I was blind or less sensitive rather than feel the hurt or the infatuations that she had also started. Sometimes it was even another woman. When she got infatuated, there was no stopping her for three weeks or so. But it was obvious to me she did not love me in the same way anymore. But she was in love with me enough still not to let me go. I hadn't been in her flat for months but I managed to persuade her to let me take her out on Valentine's Day.

We went to the sea, had fish and chips on the beach, and ended up in a little restaurant in Suffolk, before the long three hour drive back to London.

What a fool was I!

After all the pain and all the infidelities, I still could not get enough. She was like a drug. She was carrying a lot of guilt.
I finally met her black lover and when he met me, you couldn't see him for dust. He ran so quickly, he vanished never to return. Why is it that modern men do not fight for women anymore? Maybe because they do not love them so deeply anymore. Anyhow, he just wanted her for sex, and she had come to terms with it.

He was a never-was-er
Who never was and never would be
Yes, the only success he ever had in bed
Was in his head

We sat in the little restaurant scattered with red roses and valentine's couples, but there was an uneasy feeling. It was our first real date since the beginning of December. The barriers between us, felt like a ten foot high brick wall. But she tried to get things on a good footing, and to be honest with her life as it was now.

Then she dropped the bomb. It was Hiroshima and Nagasaki, all rolled into one. I was almost half expecting it, but it was still a shock to hear from her pretty lips.

'I'm writing to someone on the internet' she said. She searched my eyes deeply for a reaction. I only gave her pain, and even more pain. But could I keep her for one more year?

'Who?' I said.

'No one important,' she said, 'He found my old site of years ago and offered me £600 a night to go to bed with him,'

'Will you see him?' I asked, trying to be cool.

'I don't think so.' she said. Yes, she was still the same girl, more mature now, but always reluctant to tell the whole story.

'So will you keep writing to him?'

'I might.' She said, knowing my jealousy was inflamed. I looked at her and said, 'Well I don't care a shit if you do or not. 80% of all people on the internet are invented anyway. If you want to go and hurt yourself again, that's up to you... Will you talk to me about it? Will you be honest for a change?'

'I might.' she said, teasing me and driving me mad again. She knew she had power over me, and she could keep me dangling on a string. The silk of her underwear was less than a millimetre thick, but she knew that unless she wanted to, a centurion tank could not have gone through it. Trying to get the right magic formula to rip those silk panties to one side for a man... it is impossible for the female brain to understand the enormous helplessness and frustration the average man feels when caught in this sort of trap. They instinctively know the power that they hold. They have something that every man wants. The only time you can be sure of it is when you buy it, or when she is hopelessly in love with you. On the first, you just get the pussy, and on the second, you get all the strings, the commitment and the emotion.

Life on Earth is about getting to the other side of the Universe. In the end, all the poems, the books, the love songs, the pretty underwear bought to please her, the dresses, the candlelit dinners, are all to charm her, coax her, persuade her, to let you in. A million subterfuges so that she would give in and let you take her.

Every night, especially on Valentine's night, (who knows the figure? 20 million? 30 million?) beautiful women give in to a man, because on that one night of the year, every man tries to fulfil his destiny as she sees it. You have to woo her, seduce her, make her laugh, make her cry, and shower her with pretty things to persuade her that you love her.

January

She was strangely silent on the long drive home, and gave nothing away.

We had places to go
Things to do people to see
Our world falls apart I'm not with you
Go away, leave me alone
Where's my mind?
It's not at home
Love on the rocks
We are both alone

And so we were. We reached her home at 11:45. It had been a long day. She kissed me on the cheek, made it obvious that there was no invite. She smiled as she got to her gate, and turned her head and looked at me in the car, and said, looking impish, coquettish, and again teasing me to get her revenge on some hurt that she thinks justified it,

'Yes I will write to him.'

She left me to hang on her words.

Millions of men throughout the world were pulling knickers off at this moment, but not this one! The roses are all stripped and bare, and all the petals are left drifting in the air, and all I am left with are words.

February

From: john smith <appledogstime@yahoo.co.uk>
Date: 18 February 13:15:41 GMT
To: monika_nw3@yahoo.co.uk >
Subject: Re: you and possibly me

So sorry, I did not mean to upset you. All you had to say was you had a date and I would have understood. You seam very upset or hurt, I hope it's not me. Are you not happy at this time? Anyway, would you like lunch if you feel unsafe? or dinner where ever you want...please I just would like to meet you. Your face is so kind.

My regards john x

From: john smith <appledogstime@yahoo.co.uk>
Date: 22 February 15:30:11 GMT
To: monika_nw3@yahoo.co.uk >
Subject: Still think of you

...AND the beautiful girl I saw in the pictures and I hope for a meal or
drink with her...John

From: monika_nw3@yahoo.co.uk >
Date: 23 February 17:49:10 GMT
To: john smith <appledogstime@yahoo.co.uk>
Subject: Re: Still think of you

Think of me? No you think of the fantasy of me you have built in your head. Go out and try to chat up somebody real! You might even like them after a while. Stop wasting your time..(and mine). Though I find your E-mails endearing it is not going anywhere fast with us is it, do something mad and talk to a blonde girl in the bar you haven't been to before. If she doesn't respond, talk to the brunette. No luck there, it wasn't your lucky day. Don't give up. Stop messing and do something... Love Me

February

From: john smith <appledogstime@yahoo.co.uk>
Date: 23 February 19:26:04 GMT
To: monika_nw3@yahoo.co.uk >
Subject: Re: Still think of you

It just goes to show what ever you have in this world means nothing. Here I am a city trader, nice flat, nice car, told you I'm good looking, £250,000 a year and more but still the girl I have passed a dozen emails with is the one that I can't even get to go out for a drink with me!! How hard is that????? Can't you even let me get you a quick drink? Half hour tops and bring a friend if you wish.

John xxx

From: monika_nw3@yahoo.co.uk >
Date: 24 February 09:32:26 GMT
To: john smith <appledogstime@yahoo.co.uk>
Subject: Re: Still think of you
So what is the problem with such a nice guy like you? Who has a good job, nice car and flat? Where has it gone wrong for you? And don't tell me you don't have time to go out and meet people. Anyway can you imagine what a disappointment it might be with us meeting, two strangers in a public place trying to make a conversation they probably don't want to have? I have still not seen a photo of your face so how would I recognise you. Also I'm still very torn as my ex still loves me very much, and I him. If I can find a way to reach a compromise so that we may still have something…

February

From: john smith <appledogstime@yahoo.co.uk>
Date: 24 February 13:06:15 GMT
To: monika_nw3@yahoo.co.uk >
Subject: love and all that jazz
I don't have a problem?? I just felt what one hundred people a week feel..I fell in love at first sight with some one I saw. What's wrong with that? People do that every day. I have lots of offers but I can't get the girl in the picture out of my head. It's natural, it could happen on a tube, a bus, anywhere. With me I saw your picture and fell in love and wanted to get to know the girl...all quite normal. So when? I would just would love to meet you, as I know the girl in the picture is as nice in real life.. xxxx John X

From: john smith <appledogstime@yahoo.co.uk>
Date: 1 March 14:20:12 GMT
To: monika_nw3@yahoo.co.uk >
Subject: Re: Still think of you all the time

We don't have to meet public...how about a very private discreet restaurant at finchley rd or at st johns wood? As you wish. Also you know more of me then I know of you so I'm not a complete stranger for you. I could never be disappointed in you ever. You look and sound great from your emails. I think you're very smart and intelligent. Come on take a chance in life...meet me???

From: john smith <appledogstime@yahoo.co.uk>
Date: 5 March 18:07:52 GMT
To: monika_nw3@yahoo.co.uk >
Subject: How can I forget you?
You look wonderful, you sound wonderful and from the picture I have of you on my desk, which I downloaded, all those months ago I can say you're wonderful. So what more can I say, I'm in love and spring is on the way. How about a meet in a beautiful garden ...john

March

From: monika_nw3@yahoo.co.uk
Date: 5 March 19:07:53 GMT
To: john smith <appledogstime@yahoo.co.uk>
Subject: Re: How can I forget you
You don't give up do you. You just keep trying..
You're very persistent like my ex
That's why he may still stand a chance… M x
From: john smith <appledogstime@yahoo.co.uk>
Date: 8 March 09:10:47 GMT
To: monika_nw3@yahoo.co.uk
Subject: Why should I give up

If I do that I stand no chance to reach any shore and I drown. Cut to the chase I like everything I see about you. I want to stay in the race.
love john

From: john smith <appledogstime@yahoo.co.uk>
Date: 8 March 21:45:58 GMT
To: monika < monika_nw3@yahoo.co.uk>
Subject: Lets walk and talk

Wed night at the office it's nearly ten o'clock and I'm looking at your picture. I'm wondering where you live? Must be close. It feels close. You may go for a walk one evening and I may go for a walk the same evening and then we bump into each other (big smile on my face) how sweet and nice would that be. I could chat and say what a nice night it is and you can either agree or disagree. Tell me what street and I will walk it till we meet naturally love x john

March

From: <appledogstime@yahoo.co.uk>
Date: 11 March 12:30:16 GMT
To: monika < monika_nw3@yahoo.co.uk >
Subject: Real love god, how some things are meant to be. Life, who are we who doubt the things we see.

Hi special lady.
Hope you are good or feeling that way. Sat morning and I'm in the office working hard. New British shares up for grabs, lots of money to be made...if I can get them and move them on at a good price. How is your life? I heard from my ex today, (she was moving out just as I found you) she wants to talk and be good friends as well as go out sometimes. I'm all for that. After all we spent a lot of time together and I still find her sexy and would still like TOO sometimes. We were good together in that way and we both miss it but we can never get back as a proper love. Her family and my family hate each other. She's Jewish and I'm from the way way back old English and Polish background. Yes that's it R.C. (Roman Catholic) and all that jazz. But her family are very strict and because of that we were always fighting. Anyway, I'm glad in some ways it's over as I would have never of found you. I'd be really glad if we get to meet this year sometime and I hope we do. You know so much of me what about you??? Yes your beautiful, the world can see that. I tell the chaps at work that you are my girlfriend...they asked me when they saw your picture on my desk. I said I met you when I went out walking one evening. Do you have a job Monika? Are you happy? You must have lots of men running after you. Young and Old. Wish I could catch you some time..Or are you a student or something? May not be living in nw3? May be a very up market part of London? If you need help with any thing let me know. Come on tell me about you, anyway a kiss for you XXXXXXXXXX Hope I get something from you soon..as its gets lonely thinking of you (and she took the dog) when she moved out.
love John xxxxxx

March

From: john smith <appledogstime@yahoo.co.uk>
Date: 11 March 13:41:15 GMT
To: monika < monika_nw3@yahoo.co.uk >
Subject: Spring

Just about to leave the office, half day today thank God! Gave your photo a kiss. I'm about to lock up and catch the train to Maida vale. Made £4000 today so good day. I sold the shares to a German company. My company gets 75% and the rest comes to me. I'm sorry if I might have upset you in my last email, hence this one. It was most unfeeling of me as you may be Jewish like my sweet little ex. If you are no bad feelings were meant. It was a family issue, completely different. Chalk and cheese etc...Are you free Sunday afternoon? Hope? Hope? I was thinking that may be you would like to come with me to the river? The river Thames is one of the nicest rivers in the world. The theatre in the park opens soon, I would love to go with you to see a play...So long as men can breath or even eyes can see. So long lives this and this gives life to thee, what love can express the flavour of her face to whom in this distress I do appeal for grace A thousand Cupids fly about your gentle eyes (The sonnets 17)
love to you John x

From: monika < monika_nw3@yahoo.co.uk >
Date: 11 March 20:01:20 GMT
To: john smith <appledogstime@yahoo.co.uk>
Subject: I live in NW3

Dear John,

Thank you for your Emails. I am still not sure who you are.. My ex is trying his hardest to get back with me, but I miss him terribly, and I miss his love and affection. Though like you and your ex, there is a lot of feeling still there. You can't help it after being with somebody for some time. We never lived together though. I do live in NW3 it is a lovely area. I have lived here for a long time and love it. Like you I have been

working today, full day though and not even time to take a break. But it was o.k. I worked all day yesterday and also the evening till 1am. Actually I am at work now until 10pm and maybe a few hours tomorrow. I should stop working these killer hours I am in a need of some time off. Not sure when that will happen. I enjoy working, but only sometimes it gets too much. I'm really sleepy now. You write about The River Thames; the views and the history connected to it are impressive but the river it self is in a very sorry state. I love the South Bank walk by and into Battersea Park. What is your bit? Where do you go when you don't work? And how do you relax? John how can you get away with telling your friends I am your new girl? Telling fibs to your work colleagues, not very nice is it. Just think you might have to come up with the goods and it isn't written anywhere that we will ever meet. Or maybe you were just being discreet about the origin of the pictures, which is very nice but in my experience if you are searching these kinds of websites there is a good chance that your work friends do the some and might find out where the pictures come from. Would not put it passed them. I should go clothes shopping tomorrow as well as everything else and I really don't fancy it. I hate clothes shopping (unlike most women) I wish somebody could bring all the clothes which are right for me to my house for me to try on so I could make the final selection and send the rest back. Instead I will have to traps over the shops full of stupid people and wait for the changing room! Too depressing to even contemplate. I will probably put it of again. How are you on shopping? You were asking whether I am Jewish. No I'm not, I am a good Catholic girl but I can imagine the problems your ex-girlfriends religion brought on. It is bad when you don't get on with the family of the person you are with. It makes it twice as hard for you and I am sorry that that was the reason for which broke you two up. Do you have visiting rights for your dog?
I should go. I feel mellow with tiredness and there's another two hours to go. Have a lovely Sunday.
Love Me

March

From: john smith <appledogstime@yahoo.co.uk>
Date: 13 March 17:17:07 GMT
To: monika < monika_nw3@yahoo.co.uk >
Subject: I WISH, O HOW I WISH

Dear Monika

Thank you so much for your kind and long email. I wish I were your Ex. He's a lucky man to have had you as a girlfriend. Sad to say I'm not he, unless he is thirty years old and works in the city of London and has a large flat in west nine?? Then I'm sorry and sad to say no. There were things you spoke of in your letter that delighted me and things you said that came a cross as very hard. Almost hate full. It's something I touched on in other emails as well. Some of the emails I sent you I tried to be nice and polite but your reply's were some times cutting and hard which is why I asked you before if you'd been hurt by men. My first letter to you was in early Jan, just before my birthday and I invited you to my party, which was held in my office. My girlfriend was just moving out at the time with the dog (Yes I can go see the dog any time I like). My ex and I love each other a lot and feel strong in our love for each other. Only last week she asked me to spend the night with her as she missed me so much and I missed her as well..so we did and it was nice to hold each other again and be close. It's something we may do more often in the future, I guess till one of us falls madly in love with someone else. We agreed. It's the trend these days to let each other down gently and stay real good friends as well as soul mates which we are. We both love each other very much but until we find someone new we go out together three or four times a month and sleep together when it happens (Three times so far in four months) If you and I meet and we fall in love, I would tell her the situation and that would be the end of that side of things. I like to have one woman only in my life and don't believe in sleeping around due to my Catholic upbringing. My Father was from Liverpool and worked as an Architect. My Mother was a window dresser and was Irish from Dublin. They are nice and very kind and support me when I'm down.

They live happily as two children and play and have fun. I have one sister who is twenty-six years old, her name is Fran Smith and she is a Theatre manager. Now what more can I tell you that will make you want to date me?? Well for starters my love for you got more and more when you said you were a Catholic. This was the BIG BIG problem with my ex and my self. She, her parents and her three brothers are all strict orthodox Jews. Everything was fine for two years and then she moved in with me. Then it became three years together and the topic of marriage pops up. Then the nasty started big big time. Her family wanted a Jewish wedding...my family wanted the full church thing. Then further in to the future..children..if a girl was born it had to be Jewish...my family said 'NO WAY Roman Catholic or nothing!' We could have gone on with it but we would have lost both our families. (My father is seventy-five years old) Things started to go down hill from then on wards. The invitations to her home stopped and things got bad. So here we are now. What do you work as? You work long hours. I'm in the office now, we start early and finish at four. I love nw3, nw6, west 9, west 10. They're nice parts of London. I don't blame your ex to work to get you back. I would if I were he but why so nasty to say you are glad you split if he loves you and you him? That comes across as hard. How long were you two together? I love the country and all the large London parks. My hobbies are stamps, tennis, film and theatre land. I also enjoy taking pictures. I try hard but only sometimes I get them sharp. I love to travel. I like to shop quickly when I do. Walk in find something I like and take it there and then. I only used the sex lines twice. I was in Germany down and low after the brake up and found your pictures. I don't think the chaps at work will find you. I have a gorgeous picture of you on my desk and look at you all day long. I'm looking at it as I send this to you now. I'm so glad you gave up the world you were in and put it behind you. You are too nice for it but it has left you with a touch of hardness, which I hope you can overcome. Your first emails were strong. Please don't get upset for me telling you that as that's something I would not wish in anyway to do. Be nice to your ex and yourself and love yourself. Try not to work so hard in what ever it is you do... life is short. I hope we can meet soon, you are a nice girl. It comes across in the long email you sent that your last job has left you a little bitter and hard in life. I hope you can work it out with love and kindness. I read in a book once and I'm sure it's true. "The more love and kindness you give out, the more you get back". I look forward in getting your next letter and I hope you have a nice and pleasant evening. love John x

From: monika < monika_nw3@yahoo.co.uk >
Date: 13 March 21:57:21 GMT
To: john smith <appledogstime@yahoo.co.uk>
Subject: Re: I WISH O HOW I WISH - don't wish, DO!

Dear John,

Thank you for your email. I appreciate all the honesty in it. You say my first emails to you were hard, they were. No question about it. You must appreciate that one of my rules was that I would never go out with a client and unfortunately you were just another client who was short of a girlfriend at that time. I promised myself that those two did not mix however tempting that might be. I hope you understand that. That is why I have reservations about meeting you though in some way I am glad that you know. I am not sure what to do with this one. How would you feel going out with a girl and having all this knowledge? My Ex and me - that is another story. We have been together for a very long time and didn't ever move in together because he was already living with somebody else..namely his wife. Yes I was going out with a married man. My life is complicated and has been complicated for years dear John but I am working on simplifying it as much as I can. My ex is the best man in the whole world. I love him dearly and as you said about your ex lady, he is my soul mate and he is also the sweetest kindest man who would help anyone. He has a heart so big, I can't describe it. We still see each other and go out together, but I was unfaithful to him on two occasions. I don't believe that justifies being nasty. I enjoy his company but he can be extremely overwhelming and controlling, which I would find normal in a man so disciplined in his work. I am a moody person and very very difficult to live with, as having lived on my own I am quite set in my way, which makes it easy for him to rub me up the wrong way a lot of the time. In a way I am glad that we managed to split up but I'm very sad and unhappy as I said before, he is very kind and caring...(In comparison with most men). I am not sure what and how you will be reading in to all this but one thing is for sure, deep down we are very good friends and I hope we stay good friends for the rest of our lives. I am very tired again today, you are right I should not work these long hours. I don't do it very often, last week was hectic though. I am off tomorrow. So little bit of me time. Not sure what I am going to do? Probably the unavoidable clothes shopping! You don't want to do it for me do you? How was you Sunday? Did you do anything nice?

Ps: That is a very good-looking photo of you, especially your body and your special parts. It is a great pity you did not send me a picture of your face... just your body and your most important asset. A photo is just an interpretation of a person by the photographer. It is his way of seeing you?
Love M x

March

The Sun Girl

Sometimes every day
At a certain time
The sun will play
On a window on a little house
That will open and a girl will look out
That's everything to me that I could not know
She's everything a girl could be

Sometimes every day
At a certain time
A lovely girl turns her face to mine
And as we kiss in the morning light
It dances and starts to show
That she is a woman now
And all that she can be
So much you cannot see

Look at her body now
As she stands there like a child
Sunlight in her hair
Through the window dances
Rays falling through the air
So much you could not see
But oh how beautiful for me

March

SHOPPING
14th March

I arrived at 8:30 in the morning and thought about the vision above. She was probably running around in her little white knickers trying frantically to get dressed. This was shopping day, and I was taking her to the Freedom Shopping Port in Essex, where every major shop and boutique was, but 40% cheaper than London prices. It was a strange feeling not going into the house. It was like a second nearly-perfect date. 'See you next Wednesday' she'd said and here I was. I am here, and eager.

She called me on the phone to say she would be at least another 20 minutes. Some things never change. I sat and waited playing music on the CD player in the car. She eventually materialised from the front door, a vision in a long white coat which I had chosen for her just before Christmas, and in practical shoes for walking and shopping in. I could not see what she wore underneath as the coat had covered her completely. She looked tired as she always did these days and always apprehensive. I did not know what to say. Part of me was still numb and could not feel anything. Part of me felt sad and sorry, both for her and myself.

Despite my own anger at still not being let into her inner world, and her resentment and guilt, I made up my mind even though I felt inwardly tearful, to make the best of the day. I tried to be as stoic and ambivalent of my feelings about losing her as I could. It was not the kind of end that either of us, in a more mature, from her side situation would have desired. She still carried with her, an enormous amount of guilt and with it, the accompanying anger that the frustration had brought.

The sun came out and off we set.

We drove for nearly two hours and then pulled in to a motorway diner. I had a phone call on the way from some stupid girl complaining about her photographs and the way I had taken them, and the fact that she had told me about her relationship with her boyfriend, and I told her that when she became a famous actress in London that her relationship would probably disintegrate. So suddenly in the diner, I had some stupid girl's father telling me that I have upset his daughter! When I explained the real situation, he calmed down and said that he would definitely have a strong word in his daughter's ear.

Back to us. We were both on our best behaviour, staying off all controversial subjects and keeping the atmosphere jokey and happy. After a hearty breakfast we set off down the road again and as usual nothing had changed over the years. She decided to wind me up again, trying to get me angry, so she insisted on putting on Gloria Gaynor's 'I Will Survive' on the CD player, which was played at least three times. Also, as a remembrance of her previous black lover, she insisted on playing 'I'm not in love, so don't forget it, it's just a silly phase I'm goin' through.' (which was not guaranteed to put me in the best of moods).

We carried on with an average speed of 70 miles per hour.

At 12:30 noon, we reached Freedom Shopping Port. Surrounded by thousands of beautiful shops, she was like a kid in a candy store, overly excited and running around choosing clothes everywhere.

It was tiring, but I tried to be as kind as possible and choosing items with my vast knowledge I had gained from my 30 years of being a fashion photographer. (Me and my big ego!) I selected clothes at random, trying to make it look easy and saying in a definitive tone, 'This one… and this one will look fantastic…'. I chose a beautiful gypsy dress I absolutely adored, and a little white cotton blouse with puff sleeves to go with it, which I have to say she looked adorable in. She also seemed delighted with the choice I had made.

She took the items I had picked out for her, as well as the numerous others she had grabbed off the rails into the changing room. I sat outside on an uncomfortable bench waiting for her to come out.

Finally emerging wearing the pretty gypsy dress, holding a couple of other tops in one arm, she was a vision of absolute perfection.

'You are so beautiful.' I gazed at her bare legs that seemed to go on forever. She teased me and curtseyed.

'Thank you kind sir.'

Then, as she turned to change into her next outfit, she dropped the items she had over her arm. Looking a little embarrassed, she bent over to pick them up, and as she did so, and of course it was intentionally, I caught a glimpse of her tight little pink thong with the words 'SEXY' emblazoned across the front in diamonte. My eyes took on the sight intently and she knew I was getting excited, though I tried to hide my emotions as best I could. I could tell that even though she was embarrassed at being looked at half naked in the changing room, the attention I gave her also excited her. I could barely control myself to keep my hands off her and she could sense it. We hadn't been together for nearly three months now.

She smiled at me and told me to wait while she tried the rest of the clothes on.

We ended up with an armful of shopping bags filled with tops and dresses, one of which I purchased for her. I even took out a Freedom Shopping Port credit card which I intended to use if we should ever come here again.

We made our way to the car loaded with goodies with her chatting like an excited child about all the nice things that she had bought. Which ones she preferred, which one came second in the pecking order, down to the one she liked least. I find it incredible as a man, how the female of the species, when shopping, can analyse all her purchases so critically, after having just purchased them. I have never found a man who has ever gone through such a strange procedure.

Having loaded the bags into the boot of the car, we made our way to a very nice little restaurant with a big log fire. As it was starting to rain quite heavily it was a very welcome sight. The meal was excellent and can you imagine apart from her choice in music, we did not have one single row and the atmosphere was almost starting to get intimate.

In the car, driving back to London, she was very affectionate, rubbing my back and apologising profusely for the fact that she could not drive and therefore she realised that I was getting extremely tired. She also thanked me over and over again for the pretty dress that I had bought, and after 14 hours of each others 'company we finally got to her house.

She sat in the car and hesitated four or five times, pondering whether she should invite me in and not quite sure what to do. In the end she lost her courage and said, 'Next time I promise I will try the dresses on for you in the bedroom and give you a catwalk show… then you can see how I look in them with a little privacy…' She collected everything from the boot and with a wave, was gone.

I made my way home, rather sad but still pleased that we had had such a nice day.

March

As sex takes a rest in a relationship
Between a man and a woman
Wisdom and knowledge sometimes takes over
Friendship, true friendship
Can be the most beautiful thing in the world
If we can find it
We should treasure it for as long as we can sustain it
No other lips can smile the same
They drive me so wild
I'm a child
When you come near
No other lips taste just like yours
And when they've been kissed
They beg for more
So tenderly
When I look deeply into your eyes
I drown in your sorrows
I live with your sighs
Your body sways
No other lips
No other smile
No other eyes
Tonight

March

From: monika < monika_nw3@yahoo.co.uk >
Date: 15 March 22:34:47 GMT
To: john smith <appledogstime@yahoo.co.uk>
Subject: we went shopping

Dearest John

I have to admit that maybe some of your theories of friendship, friends as lovers and buddies may well be true. Billy and I have a wonderful day shopping and we did not have one single hard word or nasty. Without thinking, (typical me!) I did wind him up a bit with some of my choice of music. I also wound him up in the changing rooms enormously... at least that's how it looked from where I was standing! But I can assure you it was quite unintentional. He bought me a pretty dress and altogether the day was the best we'd had. Thinking about how sweet he was on the way back, I became very affectionate and I did want his arms around me but was frightened about what it might lead to, knowing that I could get carried away too... We finally got to my house and I was really tempted to let him in. You may not believe this, but I'm not completely devoid of feelings, and his kindness and sweetness had made me feel affectionate and sexy towards him. In the end I found the strength to leave, but the thought of him making love to me again did excite me, and I almost had a few seconds of fantasy sitting inside his car. Please John, don't tell me off! I know... don't tell me how much of an idiot I am anymore. The choice is down to me. But next time I may not be able to resist. Hope you're being a good boy, still keeping Ruth happy.

Big kiss Natasha xxx
From: john smith <appledogstime@yahoo.co.uk>
Date: 15 March 07:24:41 GMT
To: monika < monika_nw3@yahoo.co.uk >
Subject: my ex, you me and the future

Dear Monika
I could not send you an email back last night and the night

before because I spent those nights with my ex (don't worry you are still my big new love). It was hot and the best sex ever! We even found new things about each other in bed. I told her about you and she was happy that I have found someone that might bring happiness to my life. Will write a long reply to your long letter later. I just got in to the office so must start, we start at seven. Speak later.

P.S. I did not send you a photograph of me. Someone else must have sent you one by mistake. I only sent you a picture of my hard cock.

love and closeness x x x john

From: <appledogstime@yahoo.co.uk>
Date: 15 March 15:09:30 GMT
To: monika < monika_nw3@yahoo.co.uk >
Subject: As promised, all of me, my thoughts, my feelings, my everything...

Dearest Monika

Thank you so much for your email, it gave a very good insight explaining the hardness in your earlier emails to me. I'm sorry to criticize you or cause you any sort of hurt if I have. In case you and I take off (who knows people have walked on the moon) I think its better to have a truly honest and frank beginning so we know who we both were and are. Yes I agree with you if I had ever been a client or paid you a relationship like that would never work. I know that two of my colleagues at work have met girls, fell in love with them and after a few months they broke up in bad ways. As I know that men cannot forget how they met a girl and what she has done which leads them too becoming tormented souls. They wonder how they compared etc with other men. They guys even threw it back at the girls once they saw their relationship going down hill (As they usually do in those circumstances). The failure rate must be very high. 'Pretty Woman' was a dream, and all must remember that. Thank god I was never your client. As you said you gave it up a long time ago even before I met you. Every man and woman you meet must have skeletons in their cupboards. Your past is your past, as mine is and that part of your life is a closed door and I hope as you said closed forever. You had your reasons at the time. Maybe one of those reasons was to try to get on the property market? I can understand that, as it must be impossible for most young girls. A lifetime of saving just to get a deposit to put down.

Any way well done if you ended up with a flat in NW3 as well as now having a steady job. Your trying to make something of your life and I respect you for that and that you had the strength to give it all up. That's the most important and most applaud able part, having the strength to put all your ex clients behind you and forgetting about them all for ever. My work friends tell me some of the girls do it till they are 50 years old. Sad, so sad and some of the poor girls still see their clients due to loneliness. The men don't even pay them any more, they just take them out for a drink and they know that it will never go anywhere but the girls get close to their clients. A very sad situation. Money only gets hitched to money and not to a working girl and the type of men that use them. I know that from my office no one would never marry them, they would just string them a long for years. But enough of all this, its dead and over so let me tell you of me...Well you know a lot already but I know very little of you. In fact nothing but I hope we can always be honest and truthful with each other so that if and when we do meet it will be wonderful and we can be ourselves. I know I can love you for the little you have told me already about you and you are really beautiful. You say pictures can fib but in your case..no way! You have a beautiful mouth, beautiful eyes, bone structure and tenderly slim. My mother and father are both catholic from Irish decent. My mother is Irish and my father is half polish from his mum's side and half English from his dad's side. They worked very hard and sent my sister Fran and me to a private catholic school in bath. It's a beautiful town. My farther is 25 years older then my mother. He met my mother when she was eighteen and I was born when she was twenty years old. My mother was pregnant when she walked up the isle of the church by four months at Liverpool cathedral. It was a very grand catholic wedding which had 200 guests and a lot of Guinness was drank on that night. My mother is fifty now and my father is seventy-five but they're still like a couple of kids and have a lot of fun. You wouldn't be able to spot the age gap. Very young at heart. My family home is in Liverpool. I have two degrees, one in philosophy and one in psychology and now as you know work as a city trader after starting as a junior stockbroker. Ruth is my fifth serious girlfriend and my biggest relationship so far. We were together for five years and three months in total. I had my first girlfriend when I was 16 and we lasted for two years. The next girl I went out with was when I was at university and that lasted for four years. She moved to the USA. Then along comes a French student, she finished her course and left after a year. After that I had lots of nothings, just casual, which I did not enjoy at all. I hate one-night stands and would rather not sleep with some one until I'm sure I love and respect them. The girl I dated for a year and a half was from Finland. That lasted a year and a half and then love at first site Ruth...I got into the office at seven today. I was worried because I hadn't been in touch with you for a couple of days. This is my first serious love letter to you. Now let me elaborate on my previous email from this morning. My ex and I slept together for the last two nights, but no future. Still big problems with families. We both agreed that we could never over come them. She asked me to come over as she had a rather silly one-night stand two nights ago and was upset about it. It didn't go too well and wanted me to be with her as she needed someone around her who she could trust. It was nice and different as well as quite exciting. You tend to look and feel very different after not making love for a long time. She said she had been silly to go with this man but was feeling lonely. Any way she paid me a nice compliment and said that she'll never sleep with a stranger again. She won't now until she feels real love. She said size certainly dose matter so I felt quite good when I went in to the office this morning. I told her all about you, she was happy for me and hopes it works out in the future. She is a lovely sweet girl. So now you tell me about you. You say your ex is married, did he ever try or would he ever try to get a divorce and marry you? I say this because you still feel a great deal of love for each other or is it because he's got young kids or something? You say you were together for a long time but can that be possible as the web site says you are 24 years old and you certainly look that age or younger and yet you write as someone much older and mature. Where are you from? Your English is very good and I can't remember too much of what was on the site apart from your breath taking pictures. (((wow you take my breath a way))) You must be English or some beautiful mixture. If a long time is for example six or seven years he must have met you when you were sixteen or seventeen, so tell me to mind my own business or tell all now. Where did you meet him? Does he love you as much as you say you love him? He must be very sophisticated, mature and intelligent in his thinking to have let you done the work you have, as well as having to understand and help you to cope. I can understand your deep feelings for him. You have to study philosophy and psychology as I have at university to know the background for you to open a way of thinking of the oldest profession in the world. It dates all the way back to JESUS and Mary Magdalene. The great cortisones that litter history and became more famous then the people they slept with... so I may be making a real fool of myself here, but to let you do that while still in love with you, shows a great deal of care and love for you. He seems to have a great deal of knowledge about the world we live in and in history. Did he take your virginity? Is it that you want to try other men? Because he was your only man beside clients. So don't take offence in these questions, just want to get to know you. I suspect like my father and mother who have a very success full marriage he was an older man? Well that's all I can manage now Monika as work is calling big time. Will try to write again tomorrow. Stay well and don't work to hard. Stay beautiful inside and out until I get a chance to write again. I hope the shopping went well. I hit my car a week after I broke up and had to go to hospital. I felt so bad at the loss of her, I was thinking of her and not the road.

Looking at your picture on my screen saver as with love I say goodbye x

John x

P.S. Hope you put my cock picture on your screen saver xxxxx

From: monika <monika_nw3@yahoo.co.uk >
Date: 15 March 20:36:21 GMT
To: john smith <appledogstime@yahoo.co.uk>
Subject: Re: As promised, all of me, my thoughts, my feelings, my everything...

Dearest John,

Where shall I start? There is so much to know about me. The site you saw me on is an illusion created to only one purpose. As you know, most of the stuff on the site (apart from the pictures) is not true. The pictures are me I suspect, I am quiet certain that they are me. I am not 24, even though most people think I am much younger than my real age. I got a nice compliment paid by a patient today, he thought that I was exactly that age. I am the same age as you, well a few months younger than you. I will be thirty, and written like this it looks better, July 3rd. As I said my life is complicated and sometimes very complicated. My ex is 35 years older than me. Two of his children are grown up and almost the same age as me. We were together for the past nine years. My family didn't really like the set up so we never really went to my hometown together, though he met my mum and then my dad but on separate occasions. My parents are divorced but they lived together for a long time after the divorce and finally split up last February. It was all highly traumatic and still is as you can imagine. I split up with my ex before last Christmas and it was extremely stressful and traumatic. I found that it was nasty, uncivilised, brutal and horrid. We are now working on staying good friends. I don't like and appreciate stress and disagreement, I will try to work things out by talking and arguing my point but it is difficult with somebody who doesn't want to see it. We are both strong-minded and it sparks sometimes. So when you started writing to me I was in the thick of it, which might explain why you were not very popular. Anyway he came shopping with me but as a fashion adviser only and we had a really nice day. And do you know what - I really enjoyed it. He was on his best behaviour and so was I. Apart from getting a few tops I got a beautiful dress for the summer. I can't wait for the right occasion so I can wear it. I also bought some useless bits. My ex took those photographs of me you saw. He is a fashion and advertising photographer but we met in a hospital where I was as a patient. He was visiting a friend with his wife. You were right, he is larger than life. I was never bored with him. It went wrong somewhere and now we can at least enjoy being friends. I wasn't sure about telling you what I have just now but as you are being so honest with me about you and your ex, maybe I should as well. I feel a bit peculiar about it as we have never met and these are very private and intimate things but what the hell, you are right, and I agree 100% we should be honest with each other. No lies or half truths, what ever it might be. I don't sleep with my ex anymore and haven't since we split up. If we did it would put the relationship on a different footing and I can't face that. I am enjoying my body for my self (and not the way you think) the feeling that I don't have to share it with anybody is good. I miss the closeness of somebody's arms around me and the gentle moments we had. If I allowed my self to go back to him I'd be and am worried about the fact that it may mess with my head. Something that would not be at all good for him in his current state of mind. Some doors are better closed forever. Though as my mum says never say never...I am having a little bit of me time. I feel lonely at times and very wonderful other times. I don't have many friends as I spend most of my time with my ex. He was my whole life. I studied business administration, computer technology and English. English isn't my first language. When I came to this country I couldn't speak more than twenty words, I would never again go to a country where I didn't know the lingo. It wasn't fun at all. I did tell him about you yesterday and he was pleased, he said that you sounded nice. He especially liked the bit about you being RC, as his dear mother was Irish too. Religion is important to him. He goes to church, he attends only the big days. Mixing religions only brings problems in the long run which is very sad, especially in the case of your ex lady and you. My name is not Monika, surprise surprise, it is Natasha Nemcova. The girl on those pictures is part me part Monika. I would love to go back to studying, as my ex said I am an eternal student. I love it. I want to study dietetics and nutrition. Maybe one day I will. I have to run I am starving! Been writing since I came from work. Do you enjoy cooking? That's an important question on which I would like you to elaborate on. Not what you cook but how much you enjoy it on a scale of one to ten? Love and kisses

Me xx

From: Natasha <natasha_nw3@yahoo.co.uk>
Date: 15 March 20:38:33 GMT
To: john smith <appledogstime@yahoo.co.uk>
Subject: Re: As promised, all of me, my thoughts, my feelings, my everything... P.S. from now on I will write from my personal email address xxx

I don't want to walk on the moon, the country side will do.
Love Me xx

From: Natasha <natasha_nw3@yahoo.co.uk>
Date: 16 March 09:23:20 GMT
To: john smith <appledogstime@yahoo.co.uk>
Subject: Re: I'm falling asleep here it's so late and have so much to do the last ten lines are missing from my letter to you

Hi John,
I am sorry that you have to work so late. I don't think that I got all the Email. What I did get is not much nor does it make much sense. I guess the late working hours might explain

that. My ex didn't take my virginity. I had a relationship, which lasted three years before him. I'm not sure why this is so important? But I'm sure you have your reasons. Do tell...
Love Me xx

From: john smith <appledogstime@yahoo.co.uk>
Date: 16 March 16:34:03 GMT
To: Natasha <natasha_nw3@yahoo.co.uk>
Subject: To the sweetest girl

Dearest Natasha,

Well what a lot of information, you are certainly one hell of a lady. Your wonderful, stunning, crazy as well as beautiful but mixed up. I hope to be your future friend, lover, soul mate and future psychologist too. There is such a lot to sort out and I don't know where to begin. Let me start at the beginning. According to Carl Gustaff Jung, there is no such thing as a peaceful brake up if two people are in love. If you have no feelings and no love for each other then you just get up in the morning, pack your bags and walk but the deeper the love, the stronger the feelings, lead to a more dramatic, hard and horrible brake up. This is natural and normal. Pain, blackmail, torture and even physical abuse is normal. 99% is excessive jealousy...all normal. If you feel love you feel hate. If you can't get your own way you feel frustration and then follows the anger. The brake up of your parents may have contributed to the brake up of your relationship. Much more then you know or care to think about or face. Even if I kick myself in the face here I would not give up on your ex just yet, I would leave the door open as I would like the best for you and he. You may or may not have been told this by others beside me, but four months is not long, and where as my relationship is hopeless, your one has some promise. He sounds one hell of a nice man and very intelligent and caring. LETS TALK OF ME, SO YOU CAN SEE YOU. When Ruth and I parted she moved out and we went through hell! I followed her everywhere, thinking there might be someone else, thinking our families were just an excuse for the brake up. I crashed my brand new Porsche

Boxter twice and during a row I picked her up and threw her a cross the bedroom. She hit her head against the bed headboard and had to have three stitches but as a doctorate of psychology (yes big head me) I can rationalise my actions but still can't stop them or my feelings, as this is human nature. We are not robots and if we love somebody or something we don't want to let go of it. Nine years is one hell of a long time. It includes all the hard work, love, caring and compromises you make when in love and to throw away just like that is incredibly hard. There's one thing that you haven't come back to me with (which may hold the answer) did your ex seek or want a divorce? If the answers no then ok, there is no way forward but if he agreed to leave her for you(his wife that is) then you have to look at your self more closely and say "hey what's wrong with me? Is this brake up my fault more then his and why I am acting like this" there is a lot you have not told me here. I can understand you might not want to. Is it time for that walk in the park together? You also seem to be punishing your self very badly and him even more. It's almost as if your a teacher and he's a naughty boy. Why I wonder? Are you blaming your father for the brake up of your parents? Then punishing your EX for it?! Are you now trying to make him your segregate father? Punishing him as you can't get to or hurt your father as he wont let you? So your taking it out on you ex lover as well as holding sex from each other and from your self (another form of punishment). This is all deep hurt as a child. You are the same age as me or will be soon. Ruth and I enjoy sex together twice a month. It shows deep love and respect for each other. We care so we give. Now we are best friends, it's even better sex with out the commitment. Two people whom no each other and their bodies. No pain no horrible one-night stands and no unwelcome surprises. It has helped to make our friendship deeper. Good sex is always good as it's emotionally satisfying and physically exciting because of the change in the status of the relationship. So stop punishing your self and him and using sex as a weapon and a whip. He wont let you down or destroy you. After nine years he has proved his love and loyalty to you in many ways more then most men in what you have told me but with the strict understanding to him that if you both do enjoy your bodies and hug each other it's between you two only and no one else. Until you meet and fall in love with someone new. Obviously it stops then. Ruth told me the word is buddies. Why not help each other in these difficult Times? Love and cuddles is the best way to make your friendship even deeper... and now for the rest. My sister Fran has just broken up with her partner and I have to help her through it all so I've got a lot on my plate as well as all this. You still haven't told me here your hometown is? What country you are from? What your mother and father do for work? You have a lot of real charm in the way you write and express your English. You make men fall in love with you. It's a rare combination of that and flirty sex. Please take care of this little girl. Very clever. I spent my whole life with Ruth. I work for a large city trading house who are part of Goldman's in the city. I get up at 5am every morning, I spend 25mins on the excise bike, I then shower, have breakfast, walk ten mins to where I park my Porsche boxter and then drive in to the office. I have to be at my desk at seven, work till five with out much of a break. Reach home at 18.30 have another shower to wash the dirt of the city out of me, then one hour of research on stocks then out to eat somewhere. I would rate my cooking a 2 out if 10. Mum and Ruth wouldn't mind if they had to wash up or dry if I knew how to cook. I could learn how to cook if I had the time but at this time in my life why? I'm earning great money I can eat at the best restaurants in London, Paris, Germany, so why when i'm on my own. I would have no one to cook for apart from my polish cleaner who comes in three times a week. She even took the dog. Ruth cooks because she starts at ten every day and finishes at five so she has plenty of time to cook and shop and all the girly things. I knew your ex was a good man. You tell me he is R.C so I can understand a lot of things. Maybe the reluctances to divorce, which is not approved by the church. You have not told me about that. Great pictures he took of you by the way. He's a genius as well as everything else. You are a lucky girl and even luckier as you met me. There is always the possibility that he does not want you back but I think not, some how I'm sure you are his life. Glad he approves of me just like Ruth approves of you. Maybe we should all be modern and meet for dinner soon? Anyway, I'm in love with you already silly me. Stay well and don't work so hard. What do you work as???

X's john

From: john smith <appledogstime@yahoo.co.uk>
Date: 16 March 18:44:49 GMT
To: Natasha <natasha_nw3@yahoo.co.uk>
Subject: In bed now wish you were in my arms my lap top on my bed

Fed up of working so hard, its just not on as well as having to spend so much time on my own. I'm off to Germany tomorrow, back Sunday so will write to you
Sunday morning. It's driving me silly that you are so close to me. Your just up the road! I want to reach out for you. I'm flying from Heathrow, have an early flight. Attached is a photo of Ruth. You may decide (as you call the shots) that the best way forward is to meet up for dinner and then we can all get to know each other.

Love to you, xxx john

From: john smith <appledogstime@yahoo.co.uk>
Date: 16 March 18:57:39 GMT
To: Natasha <natasha_nw3@yahoo.co.uk>
Subject: I wont go on to any sex sites as I will only think of you..

By the way Ruth is thirty on Nov 20 this year. Whilst I'm away I will think of you and her as my friend all the time. x john

March

From: john smith <appledogstime@yahoo.co.uk>
Date: 17 March 10:55:49 GMT
To: Natasha <natasha_nw3@yahoo.co.uk>
Subject: I can't get up from my desk.

It's cold here and even colder without you. I'm in Frankfurt but the office is close to Essen, a short drive from the city. I was dreaming about you last night. I'm looking at your pictures now on my screen saver. I'm finding it very difficult to think about work it's all you. I can't get up from my desk because people would notice. Sorry to tell you this but yes I do want you in every way, your letters drive me wild to meet you. I have to try to think work but I'm still waiting for a reply from you to the last email I sent you to which I notice has not come from you as of yet. Come on drive me over the top of my desk. Tell me more about your life and what
you like and don't like? Do you want kids and how many? I will keep checking my mail. Is it getting hot in here? Have they turned the central heating up? NO it's you, you witch and your dammed pictures! I can never get too much of them wish you were here with me. I have a wonderful five star hotel to spend the night in...would love to take you on my next four day trip with me in may to the states. You can meet all the chaps I work with and we can have a great time. Well till I return save yourself for me, back on Sunday. Ok the ex is allowed. as I do with my ex. No one else. only me or him will hit my computer on Sunday . Be kind to your ex and most of all you.
love lots john x

From: john smith <appledogstime@yahoo.co.uk>
Date: 17 March 16:02:31 GMT
To: Natasha <natasha_nw3@yahoo.co.uk>
Subject: Cannot stop thinking of you (my little spice girl)

Hi my little spice girl. Wanna be be my lover, wannabe my friend I will tell you what I want..what I really really want, what I really, really, really, really want is you. I have had it today! I can't work cant do anything except think about you. Next time

I make love to Ruth I will think of you (she wont mind she is a sexy lady) she may get hot on it. If you make love to your old man then think of me and he will wonder what has made you so crazy..A little bit more of me. Well Ruth and I really love sex and I would say that part was well ok. We do our best to please each other all the time. Some more facts about me..I am 6ft2inc in height, chest 40, waist 34, shoe 10 and collar 16inc. There you go that's me and Ruth says I'm big in the love department. Give me a box number or something (if you don't want me to know where you live) and I will get you some nice underwear as I'm out here. I can even think about you wearing it. I'll send it to you or you can put it on for me when we first meet? I'll run off some colour zerox's for you to look at when I'm in my bed at the hotel tonight. So I'm keeping my promise only you and Ruth but I'll be looking at you. God this is madness but everything you have told me about your life, the older boy friend, being a mistress. Everything just makes me think you are so perfect for me. My Mum and Dad will be so pleased if it all happens. A good R.C. girl but also much more than just that. Looking at you all the time. The chaps and me are going to a German pub tonight and will drink Irish. Wish you were coming with me. St Patrick please help me get this girl. I want her I really, really, really want her. Be nice to your ex and to yourself. Don't get to drunk with him, as I know he will be celebrating tonight. I hope for his sake he ends up in bed with you. Lucky man.
Kiss x John

From: Natasha <natasha_nw3@yahoo.co.uk>
Date: 17 March 16:12:11 GMT
To: john smith <appledogstime@yahoo.co.uk>
Subject: Re: Cannot stop thinking of you (my little spice girl)

Dear John,
You are reviving my waning libido, I was shocked to find my knickers very wet after reading your endless supply of e-mails… Yes, I am getting off on them and wondering what new exciting sex thing you're intending to do with my poor sick body to drive it crazy. I've started to pleasure myself

while daydreaming about you in the shower, and brought myself to a really big orgasm with the warm water. Why I'm telling you this I don't know… Anyway thank you. Have to see Billy tomorrow. Love me, Natasha x

From: john smith <appledogstime@yahoo.co.uk>
Date: 17 March 16:32:25 GMT
To: Natasha <natasha_nw3@yahoo.co.uk>
Subject: Sorry but my hips

Are 36 in size. I need your size for the knickers and bra I wanna get you.
love x john

From: Natasha <natasha_nw3@yahoo.co.uk>
Date: 17 March 18:09:49 GMT
To: john smith <appledogstime@yahoo.co.uk>
Subject: Re: Cannot stop thinking of you (my little spice girl)

You are a case!
I will write a reply to your Email when I am at work tonight, if I get a minute that is which I should if not it will have to be Sunday as I work all day Saturday. My ex will not be with me this evening, he is going to stay with his daughter in Essex. So no happy loving for me tonight. Hope you have a good evening.
N xx

March

18th March

She rang me in the morning and said she would love to go out with me. I picked her up at 9:30 pm and took her to the Café Rouge at Belsize Park. She was working hard and her illness was making her tired and depressed, but still she was trying to make the friendship work.

We had a delectable meal. I had spaghetti Bolognese and she had pasta primavera. For a while she was distracted by a large group at the table next to us who were having some kind of work celebration, and I studied her. I noticed the little things that a lover sees: the variation in her hairline, the mouth that always gave her thoughts away, the slight elevation of one of her eyes as compared to the other, the way her left earring caught the light of the candles, the diamond throwing a small rainbow on to her neck at exactly the point that made it feel extremely sexy. When I kissed her, she moaned a little bit.

Even a routine dinner on an ordinary night in our own neighbourhood had such a quality about it, gave me so much pleasure, it took even me by surprise. After all, I had been on hundreds of extravagant dates with glamorous women in exotic locations all over the world. Yet here, on Haverstock Hill, on a chilly March evening, with rubbish blowing along the pavement outside in the late winter wind, I knew that I wouldn't want to be anywhere else with anyone else, even if I'd had every option in the whole world to choose from.

After we finished eating and the waiter cleared our plates away, she gave me a probing look.

'I've been writing to John,' she said, 'He's a really nice, intelligent man.' Here it came; she was going to talk to me about him. 'And?' I said, trying my best to sound disinterested. 'He knows about money and love,' she said.

'Is that right?' This time I raised an eyebrow. Hmm, I thought, as if I don't know so much more than any 30-year-old man could about these things.

'Oh yes,' she said with a little smile. 'He says he uses a cushion under a girl's bum, like you do.' 'Well, any man who knows anything about a girl's body and how to please her, does that. He probably read about it in some man's mag.' I said, wanting to put him down, trying my best to sound like I did not really care. But yes, I did care, and I could feel a terrible pain slowly spreading along my rib cage, inch by inch creeping towards my heart.

I felt a compulsion to say, ‘Some City traders earn a lot of money, with bonuses of over a million a year’. Why did I bring this up? I wondered. I was complicit with her in causing myself hurt. I was making this man look even better to her in comparison to me. I was also taunting her greed, feeding her desire for this man who was nearly half my age and worth maybe five times as much as I was, maybe 20 times as much.

She looked at me sharply with a flash in her eyes that seemed to indicate that she intended to wound me, to punish me for something. ‘I think he’s falling in love with me,’ she said. I sighed. ‘How can he? He has not even met you.’ ‘So what!’ She gave me a defensive look. I didn’t say anything more. The pain was squeezing my heart at that moment, and I didn’t trust my voice not to break a little if I said something. After an uncomfortable silence, she looked up at me and said, ‘I’m tired… let’s go. Let’s walk for a while.’

And so we did. She took my arm gently and it felt so good to have her by my side like this again. We strolled down Haverstock Hill, along Howitt Road, then around and back again to where the car was parked. I was happy in this moment. I thought to myself that all I wanted was but another year with her. I loved her so much, so very much, and come what may, I always would. I knew that, and I accepted her, all the bad, the good, and even the horrible.

We got back in the car, where she started to get a little grumpy. Yet she swivelled her head around and gave me a lopsided smile, as if to say, ‘I’m glad you’re still here for me.’ We got to her house and she gave me the smallest of kisses on the cheek. She jumped out and ran to her door, then turned her head and shouted, ‘Don’t try and rush things, will you?’

March

From: john smith <appledogstime@yahoo.co.uk>
Date: 18 March 20:33:35 GMT
To: Natasha <natasha_nw3@yahoo.co.uk>
Subject: I know and feel that you want to take it slow Natasha in all ways but at four tomorrow I will be only two miles away from you

I feel I've got to know you now. I can feel you, as a woman who is her own self. No hurry lets take it slow as Ruth and I still have sex and see each other. We both have time on our sides- all the time in the world. We can send letters for say two months, then go out for two months holding hands getting to know each other. Kissing you at every corner. Then if you're ready for me around your birthday...you said July 4. You get the best birthday present in the world...me in side you? Until then we can carry on and get hot and sweaty with our exs but continue dreaming and fantasising about each other. But I know you will want me before that Natasha, my sexy little minx, and I know you want me now just as bad as I do. My body is burning for you and I cant sleep with out thinking of you. I cant cum with out thinking of you. You will ask me in after a wonderful night out...your little dress fits like a glove, you have been getting looks from other men all night but all you want is me now. As we get in to your flat its dark. You go to turn on the light but I take your hand and stop you, pulling you towards me. I start kissing your sexy neck and nose and then gently, slowly moving towards the corner of your mouth. I take it really slow, and really gentle. My hand climbs up your bare thighs, up and up, and I see that you have black stockings on. I start to undo the buttons on your dress with one hand, kissing and teasing you with my mouth and hot breath on your neck and feeling you with my hands all over. My finger's starting to get wet as your pussy weeps. It's starting to excite you. You feel the wetness inside your silk white knickers spreading all over and the hardness of my cock inside my trousers pressing hard against your body. You know I fucking want you. I want to fuck your brains out. You feel it throbbing large and hard... so very large and very hard, and you know it's still growing bigger for you and you are feeling faint at the very thought of it. You know this is going to be the biggest cock you have ever taken, and my god woman are you going to feel it! The sensations will overwhelm you. You are so excited that your legs are starting to become weak. This has been a long time, four months. My hand reaches your stockings and reaches round to stroke your curvy buttocks. My fingers play on them. I slide your woolen dress off you and it drops on to the carpet. You are beautiful before me in your knickers and white silk bra and black stockings. You are so bloody hot now, I'm burning myself on you. So hot your sexy face is on fire. You arch your back and push hard up to me, so the hardness of my cock is pressing where it should be. Your arms are around my neck, your hands playing with my hair, and we are in a sort of slow sexy dance. Your moans are soft as it rubs up and down on the silk of your knickers. Your hands reach down... your body gives a great shudder of excitement. It's massive.15cm round and 22cm long. I move your panties aside and lightly touch your shaven-wet pussy again. You're so much wetter than you were a few minutes ago. My finger lingers for two minutes and plays with your juicy, sexy, red hot lips. Your pussy lips are now more swollen than ever. I then bring them up to your mouth and you suck and taste your self on my fingers and I carry on playing for 30 mins. It's time you were in my arms. So I pick you up and carry you to the bed. You moan softly. It's been so long. I slip your high heels off and stroke your pretty little feet, take you by the ankles and spread your legs wide apart before me... then my tongue and nose bury deep into your pussy. I start to suck and tease on your clitoris, and you can feel my tongue is rough and tender at the same time as it edges its way in. My fingers are also busy fucking you with increasing force and with the small and bigger flicks of my tongue it climbs and sucks and teases and stops and starts again reaching it's target over and over again, screaming out my name over and over again. You are screaming and screaming and screaming. John, your body shudders and jerks as you come to orgasm filling my mouth with you and all your beautiful, creamy juices… You want to make me cum...You pull me up and on top of you but you are

not to have him yet. I will keep you waiting while he grows hard with anticipation. The bed is wet with you, your wetness is everywhere- my mouth, my face, my body is all wet and I get even harder as now I smell of you. I pull your panties down your legs as you hold my hand tight on your pussy. You spread your legs further out again and I reach for one of your pillows to put under you, so when you arch your back and move your beautiful bottom again (as I catch the beat of your body) you won't wear yourself out too much. We both know it's going to be a long night a head of us. The time has come...first the head goes in, you shudder violently and let out a rapturous gasp. You are so very hot your face is burning up- you're red-hot. In your gorgeous eyes, I see fear and excitement together. I take your hips with my hands and lift you up from the pillow, your legs are wide apart and I start to fuck you deeper and harder. You can't see how I can get it all in... shaking, shaking. You push your pussy up to take it. You are terrified but we both know your body wants it so badly. It overwhelms you. My hand goes to your neck, and I hold it tight because I know it makes you feel kinky as it's linked to your sexual parts, and as a doctor I know that I need to grip it tight as you submit to me. Now I start to fuck you slow and deep, but you feel like you are being split into two halves with the size that's in you. You have never felt so full but you are wet and you take it easy as I fuck you over and over and over on and on and the feelings are building up inside you for maybe the first time ever. The feelings are so, so strong and you know its going to happen..you know it..you know it. You know and are happy that this is the man you
are going to spend the rest of your life with. You are now thinking of your ex and you know I am thinking of Ruth but we are so excited for us. I am fucking you now, really fucking you on and on! That cock is in you and it wont stop, it's not going to stop, it's fucking you so hard. You are now as well moving your hips and body with the same movement and beat, holding on to me tightly feeling our skin burning up against each other. It's been nearly two hours of sizzling hot teasing sex. Your body is crying out for the madness and torture to stop, but you still want more. I change my movement, I push

low and upwards sliding my hand on to your bum, separating it from the pillow. I am now really thrusting in to you, groping your arse tighter and you start to scream like you've never screamed before, shouting my name over and over! John! John! John!!! at the top of your voice. You have lost complete control for the first time ever, you are hot and cold you are shaking over and over. You have acted this lots of times before but this isn't an act. It's never been like this. You know it too as you take in deep, slow breaths, getting quicker as you're coming closer. You feel it from your anus, to your pussy, and back again to your anus again, and again I'm driving you mad. You are screaming and crying again. Moaning and gasping for breath. Your g-spot is on fire, hot and inflamed all the way up your cervix. The rhythm is so mad now I'm still plunging in and out going deeper and deeper in you. You scream and scream and I as well as we both cum together everywhere. There's dripping wet cum all over the place. You stare at me with your eyes wide open and then you whimper beside me and have this deep feeling that you never felt that before. We fall asleep together holding each other like darling babies. This is our first night for the rest of our lives... But we are big babies, but did we make a baby? Are all my sperms rushing to find your egg at this moment as you lay there exhausted with your eyes shut, perspiration covering you? Not even bothering to shower, too tired, too sleepy, and knowing that in less than an hour I will take you again. So why bother? You are so sexy when you are sleeping, he keeps getting hard for you in the night even though you are asleep.... kiss x john

From: Natasha <natasha_nw3@yahoo.co.uk>
Date: 18 March 20:37:51 GMT
To: john smith <appledogstime@yahoo.co.uk>
Subject: Letter on its way!
Dear John,
I have a letter started for you but have to stop now and meet the ex. Will finish it when I come back and will read your long letter as well.Kiss Nxx By the way, I'm talking about Billy (the real ex)

March

Poem from Natasha to Billy

Could we find love
And want it all the time?
All you need's a someone
Who's your hero in the end
Everybody wants my body
But I also want a friend
Beautiful, beautiful, beautiful man
Good friendship never ends
So happy that you're mine
I want it all the time
Want it, want it, want it, want it
All the time
Please turn out the light
I think I'm falling in love

March

MOGAMBO

I phoned her early, I'm a real film buff. I feel that film is part of my craft as a still photographer. I absolutely adored the cinema, and I could be quite obsessive about it. I loved everything about film and everything associated with it. Having worked as a stills photographer on some of the Bond films, and for quite a few leading directors, and spent part of my life photographing some of the most beautiful women in the world, it was like a drug, I could not get enough of it.

I decided to take her to see the amazing film "Mogambo' which starred Ava Gardner and Clark Gable, one of the last great white hunters. Ava Gardner, to my mind was probably in my mind, one of the most beautiful women to have ever lived. She actually played herself in most of the films she starred in. She also complimented my other hobby, which was music, as she was married for some years to Frank Sinatra.

When I say she is one of the most beautiful women, I do mean besides Natasha.

She came running down the stairs towards the car and I gave her a large bunch of flowers and some After Eight chocolates. Rather than take them upstairs straight away, she said 'Let's take them with us and have some in the car!'

It always took ages to find a parking space along the South Bank by the big wheel. But after half an hour of driving around, we found a free space in front of a pub. The car parks in this part of London are extortionate, so by the time you have had a nice meal and gone to the cinema, it can cost as much as £30 for a night out.

We went to a gorgeous little Italian restaurant overlooking the Thames. I loved the buzz and excitement of the Thames. It was always like a large party. As spring was on the way, girls start to wear their sexy little mini dresses, and the men are prancing around in t-shirt. Music plays, buskers, people shopping up til 10 o clock, the big wheel keeps on turning, and Big Ben keeps a watchful eye on everyone, letting them know the time on the hour every hour.

Tonight it felt like a carnival weekend. Yes, we were happy tonight. Happier than I thought we ever could be. She laughed and looked at the Thames. The tide was out so we could look down on the mud and sand on the banks. Look at the old boots, bits of wood, a yellow bucket, a kiddies toy and an old trunk washed up from god knows where. I love it, love it! It's like a dream. Like treasure Island, and finding Gold Bullion.

During the meal, she always talked and looked at the people. She often avoided talking about anything important though. Something that might affect her life directly, like she had a mental block on things that may make her happy. Her brain has a way of shutting down on these things. She shuts out things that she doesn't want or like. I had now not been with her for some time, when before the split, we used to see each other and talk every day.

Suddenly she came out with it. She said she thought she saw someone watching her with some binoculars from the flats opposite her. There was a window about 35 feet away from hers, almost level. I told her she should draw her blinds as soon as possible each night.

'But I don't like to do that… I feel so isolated, so closed in, so shut away. I'm on my own most of the time anyway. If I close the blinds, that shuts the whole world out. And anyway, it's nearly spring and I love the evening sun through my window.'

'Okay, but be careful.' I said, 'And if you notice him again, call the police.'

The film was magic. Many beautiful animals, and that was not including Ava Gardner. She was a wonderful actress.

Natasha cuddled up to me in the cinema, holding on to my arm, her hand on my knee, or taking my hand, laughing at the funny elephant and the beautiful leopard.

The film had put me in an amazingly good mood, and I was even happier as I had just bought the biography of Ava Gardner, and the writer was in the audience, and gave a short speech about interviewing the actress for it. He signed my copy for me.

We drove home, chatting like crazy about the nights' events. As we got to the house, she got out of the car, she grabbed her flowers and After Eights. But then I saw her start to get nervous again. I thought it was because she could not make up her mind whether to invite me or not. But it was not that.

'Look at that window opposite.' She said.

I looked but it was too late. I only saw the bottom part of him as he quickly drew his curtains, which I noticed were quite thick. He must have realised that she had spotted him.

She put her arms around me in the middle of the road and gave me a big kiss.

'Don't worry for me.' She said, 'I have you, and also Big John on the internet to look after me. I'll be okay.'

When I got home, my wife had come back from one of her many trips abroad.

'Did you enjoy the film, Billy?' she said. Yes it was wonderful I enthused. I love Ava Gardner.

'I'm off to bed,' she said. 'I'm, jetlagged.'

We had slept in separate beds for several years now, and she was ill with tummy problems and fibroids, which made sex difficult for her. She knew of Natasha, but we avoided talking about it.

As I fell asleep, I thought of what a wonderful night it had been. But the voyeur across the road was a little creepy. Her whole life had been filled with odd balls and strange people who fancied her. I tried to shut it out of my head and not think too much of it.

Now there are two to think about. John Smith and god knows who! Don't go there Billy! I thought to myself.

March

Black Plastic

Black plastic
Sing and shout
Black plastic
It's all about
Environmentally nasty
Beauty news, quality street
A touch of blues
Indestructible
Black plastic
You're down my street
I'm in your arms, only in between
Black plastic

March

Sugar Decay

Hey, let me be
Your sugar daddy
Till my teeth fall out.
Twice a week I'll visit;
Let me lie with you.
I know it costs me plenty.
Tooth decay I caught, it's true.
But my dentist says
He'll patch me up-
I might last a year or two.
Anyway I'm going blind-
My mother
Told me
I would.

March

From: Natasha <natasha_nw3@yahoo.co.uk>
Date: 18 March 23:50:35 GMT
To: john smith <appledogstime@yahoo.co.uk>
Subject: Re: know and feel that you want to take it slow in all ways but at four tomorrow I will be two miles from you only

You are a clever boy my Dear John Smith.

You press all the right buttons and you know it very well. All the aces have been drawn, the most important Information revealed. If I felt nasty (and you know that I do that very well) I would say you have done this before but I don't feel nasty anymore. You are a real person to me too now. Far too real for comfort. You made me cry this evening Dear John with the degree in psychology. Was that the effect you were after? Probably not. It was the bit about the pillow, which did it. My ex was the only man who would use that technique no other man ever did. I feel like every word I write to you is being analysed to the last letter. Well, do your analysis and do them very carefully John. Go easy on me, there is too much going on around me and in me for me to get too involved too fast. There are not enough hours in the day to think about another person yet. But as you say you have your lovely Ruth to keep you happy for now and lovely she is in a Jewish sort of a way (and I can say that as I have worked on photo and film shoots and castings) By the way, this is not, as you can see the letter I was working on but I will finish that one and send it as well.

Sleep well Nxx

From: john smith <appledogstime@yahoo.co.uk>
Date: 19 March 00:45:18 GMT
To: Natasha <natasha_nw3@yahoo.co.uk>
Subject: One thirty in the morning here in Germany and its a 2pm flight home tomorrow and you

I can't sleep..I think of you. I want you so much but first before we meet my sweet beautiful Natasha, I want to cure you of all your problems. As I'm a top doctor with the very best degree I think I can. Believe and trust me that I can, you will have to trust me. I want you to do certain things that you may not want to do. Your old ex knew a thing or two, as the pillow is what all-good lovers do for a women. It brings her pussy to the correct place to receive the cock with less strain on her when she arches her back to receive it and take it in deep, there by conserving her energy of the so called weaker sex. I know from what you have said in your email that you have never had an orgasm by penetration and even if you hate me saying it you are punishing your ex, your father and all men for the hurt that you feel. Trust me. By the time we meet you will be the hottest woman on this planet, which I'm sure, you already are in some ways. First lesson tomorrow to make you a happy fully adjusted women.

kiss x john... On a cold night in germany I admire your beauty. I looked at your pictures hard for twenty mins...and wanked hard. Can go to sleep now as you brought me off. You are such a good girl xxxxx

From: john smith <appledogstime@yahoo.co.uk>
Date: 19 March 18:16:14 GMT
To: Natasha <natasha_nw3@yahoo.co.uk>
Subject: Back in England and you..well not quite in you yet but hopefully in the not to distant future.

I'm in my office, I've been home thirty mins. My office at home has large blow ups of you all around the walls. Seven pictures of you in total. I woke up this morning in my hotel room and really believed you were in bed with me. It was so realistic I came. First time for me as you come out of a dream. This is what went on...I was in a deep sleep and I awoke to find you between my legs. You had pulled my tight tiny white pants I wear in bed down, (I wear them in case you have to go somewhere or someone comes in and needs something) you take my cock out and as you do you are fascinated by it. It's so broad, heavy, large and really taut. It looks as if it's about to explode. You take it in your hand and I grab a handful of your long blond hair and slowly pull your head down until your mouth is on my gorged cock. You try to swallow it but find it hard to get your lips around it. It's so large your throat catches on it at first and then you suck it very slowly between your closed lips. You start to really try to please him, your lips lingering on the tip. Your tongue comes and goes licking and lingering on the most sensitive spots. You concentrate on my pleasure, which you can feel rising now, faster and faster. You take it deep in your throat again then you pull it out very slowly...accentuating the pressure of your lips, you kiss and suck, kiss and suck. You can now feel and hear my breathing getting faster, you take your time then you stop when you feel my pleasure mounting and for a few seconds you slow down keeping only the end of my cock on your tongue, then holding your head I can't stand it no longer. I plunge it deep in to your throat again and again and I feel you savour and enjoy it with infinite slowness. Every inch of my most important bodily part, my life, my cock, my balls, my me you pay attention to. My hands slide down to touch the lips of your wet pussy as you kneel between my legs and as I do I feel an eruption about to take place and before I know it I explode down your throat and you swallow over and over licking my throbbing head and rubbing my balls. Guess what happens then...I wake up! It was so sad that you were not there. I was in my hotel room on my own...And now I'm in my office (in my flat) on my own and you are just up the road. God come to me Natasha. I haven't even phoned Ruth yet. I had to tell all to you first. I need you to answer all the things I asked you. Here is your first lesson to make you a happier lady in the future with no moods flying about. You'll be a sexy lady all the time, so happy that you'll want to sing. For this to happen you must do what I say and follow each word to the letter. No deviation and believe me this is not some kinky game for me, this will start to work and you will be shocked and surprised at how you start to feel as the weeks go on until you finally meet me. I want you to pick a day next week, any day, phone your ex and tell him you want him to come over. You are to invite him into your bedroom. You told me you have had no contact or sex for months. Well now you must. Lets say you invite him on Tuesday night. This lesson must be extremely accurate. Every thing must be to the minute. The same night I will go to Ruth's at the same time. This is what you say to him...you tell him that you want him to make love to you but he must do it as you say in every way and if he doesn't you will never let him touch you or go near you again. He can't do it his way...he must only follow your instructions. The instructions...He comes round and you will let him in, he must not say one word to you...this is standard Jung to help you relax, be in total submission and to forget you and relax for me so I can make you orgasm when I come to you. It will take about two months with your ex before you are ready for me. With me you submit?? With him you won't before you meet me. I want you to fuck him six or seven times of your own choosing but each time you must not submit to him, he has to totally submit to you and only you..no other man or women just you and him and me or Ruth. I will start to make love to Ruth at eight o'clock on Tuesday night. What with foreplay and everything it will be nine before I penetrate her. Now as you know this you must think of what I am up to all the time as you make him submit to your every whim. He must not say one word to you or talk in any way. You don't talk. Silence, complete silence no talking you tell him everything to do on the phone before he comes. There are no lights on. Total darkness. All the phones are off the hooks. He comes in to the dark room (I will be up to the same as you with Ruth at the same time) You pull his pants down and strip him to his t-shirt and underpants, you can both moan if you need to. You then strip to your knickers, in the dark still standing you press your self up to him hard and grind with your hips, your panties into him, rubbing against his cock, but it is so hard in his pants. You then start to kiss him. He has to let you do it all and remember you will never let him touch you again unless its done your way...you kiss him as you never done before. Crazy deep kissing and he has to follow you. You then lead him to the bed, pull his pants down, put a condom on him and sit on him... then you fuck him over and over. Holding him tight you turn him till he's on top of you and you push his head between your legs hard. You push your pussy hard in to his mouth and he has to lick and suck you off with you pushing hard. You will cum really, really big and I

promise you it will be earth shattering. You then spread your legs wide and he has to fuck you hard and deep. Use the pillow. Once he comes you tell him he has to fuck you again in ten mins. You suck him till he is hard again and this time as he fucks you (any way you want) you must try to wank. When you and him cum again it will be ten at night and I will have finished as well with Ruth. You cuddle for an hour, no talking, touching and feeling only. Then you tell him to go home..the first words you have spoken. He goes with a little kiss and you will feel more relaxed, happy and so full of life that you won't believe it. The key to this is that he must submit to you. You only submit to a man when you come to me and by that time I will give you an orgasm by penetration. Well I await your long letter my little Natasha. I will be thinking of you every second on Tuesday as we both do it, but in your case your partner will submit to you totally.
x John P.S. Thank you for the kind words of Ruth xxx

From: Natasha <natasha_nw3@yahoo.co.uk>
Date: 19 March 20:01:24 GMT
To: john smith <appledogstime@yahoo.co.uk>
Subject: Re: Back in England and you..well not quite in you yet but
hopefully in the not to distant future.

My Dear John,

I am sorry you have to work so hard, but I am sure that you derive a great deal of job satisfaction form what you do. I am sure that you don't mind me questioning your professional advice but you don't expect me to blindly follow what you say to the last letter. I don't own my own place I rent a studio flat so it is important that I don't upset all the people here. I am also a very private person and I hate doing my dirty washing (so to speak) in public. That is the worst humiliation there can be. I don't need an audience to sort my personal problems. I am sure that that part of our life is well and truly behind us. I will meet him outside and go out with him or go to his house (which I don't like doing for obvious reasons) I didn't feel well today and had a funny notion of inviting him up. We had a lovely afternoon together, but the place was in a mess and it didn't feel like a good idea. One more thing about me..I did say that I didn't feel well today, well I haven't been feeling well for the past year or two. It has been really bad for the past four months. I have been diagnosed with ulcerative colitis two years ago and don't seem to be able to control it with the drugs, which I take. The steroids, which I am on, don't do much and I have to run to the hospital every five minutes to have a fight with the doctors. I feel incredibly tired all the time and spend a lot of time at home in bed writing E-mails to some strange but endearing man who thinks he can sort my life out in two months. So until I get it under control I don't think I feel in the right frame of mind to make love to any man. I am not opposed to the DIY notion, though after all I know my body the best. You should take a better care with your writing dear John, you write well but it can be so much better. I realise that time is not on your side but you should try. I enjoyed reading about your lovely dream. Something for your analysis porto-folio. When I have these dreams (and I don't have them very often) I always wake up before the act is to take place and then I am annoyed at the fact that I woke up missing the best bit of the dream. Some sort of old inhibition, I am sure that you will have the right name and explanation for it. You always do. What is the relevance in this experiment with my ex of you and lovely Ruth being at it at the same time? Maybe you should shed some light on that as well, otherwise I will think that you have a perverted mind(which you probably do and to a certain extent there is nothing wrong with that as long as you are not hurting anybody physically or emotionally). Would you send me copy's of the pictures you have of me, so I know what you are raving about all this time. As I promised I will go and finish the E-mail from yesterday night and send it to you maybe not today as I am shattered. I think I will have something to eat, bath and go to bed. I look like death warmed up. At the end of my working day yesterday I was told by my colleague that I looked dreadful. I love when people do that, I am sure that she didn't mean it in a nasty way as she is not a nasty person. It just came out

wrong.
I saw Billy by the way. He was sweet to me... Sunday lunch at the Spaniards. It was my idea for him to see me on the Sunday. Nice walk together over Kenwood before he dropped me home at 5:30. He also bought me the newspaper, The Mail on Sunday.
Love and kisses Natasha xx

From: john smith <appledogstime@yahoo.co.uk>
Date: 20 March 19:51:34 GMT
To: Natasha <natasha_nw3@yahoo.co.uk>
Subject: Re: You cheeky monkey when we meet you will have your bottom spanked not your hand held.

Well there is a right cheeky lass for you! One who criticizes my writing, punctuation and spellings when your emails to me are littered with the same! If you wish to write me letters and vice-versa, we can do that. Give me your address and you will get beautifully handcrafted letters. But emails like yours to me..No time for that. I type as fast as I think. Unless we correspond in word (which we can do) I'm a moneyman with facts and figures. But you paint the pot black to yours (an Irish expression). We also agreed together to be 100% honest with each other, but are you? Yes I am analysing everything you say and send to me, you could not expect me to know any other way as you may be the girl that I spend the rest of my life with..as I feel that I'm falling in love with you. I have told you only one lie since I've started writing to you. Ruth was only 5ft 4ins and she would complain because she would have to wear much to high heels to come up to me, so not wanting to put you off I told you I was 5ft 11inches but as you know now I am 6ft 5 inches. That was the only lie. So come on now Natasha lets have the whole truth. Why did you break up from such a fine, intelligent and sensitive man? Did he ask his wife for a divorce for you? I suspect he did, as after nine years it was time? I am going to tell you my worries even as I confess to being in love with you...one I can't stand promiscuity or men and women who sleep around. I think if you have a partner you should stay faithful to them. As Ruth and I have done. If and when I start sleeping with you then I would stop sleeping with Ruth. Your background shows you come from a strong manipulating father and a strong stubborn mother. Therefore I can see you would have developed the problems you have. Please remember Ruth had to have stitches in her head. A brake up of two people who love each other deeply is not a light affair. It's deep and with strong ambitions. I strongly believe from everything you have written that he did seek a divorce from his wife for you, that he loves you deeply and that after he got things moving to be with you forever you did some thing very silly.. like had a one-night stand and then you changed your mind about marriage. If this is the case then you have been a very silly girl. As the man who has been loyal, the man who stuck by you through thick and thin for so many years gets that sort of appreciation from you? You wrecked his life and he destroyed his marriage for you and he is still your friend, taking you out for Sunday roast. Natasha what could you have you been thinking of? There is no real excuse for that behaviour. Could I be wrong??? From your background that is the best annalistic answer to your actions and his. If it were another, they may have killed you for what you have done. As I say I could be very wrong. But I think not, I think you took another lover and may be it was out of curiosity. You are creating your mother and fathers life over and over again in your own life. Maybe he was not the only one? May be you had two or three. Repeating your parent's scenario over and over. I doubt you would have ever have gone to see a doctor about this. After your statement of not wanting to show your dirty washing in public. No wonder you are so ill with stomach problems. The illness you describe is related directly to stress. You were deceiving and lying to your partner and if I'm right your lover on the side as well which would have caused the kind of stress needed to bring on your illness. Think back tell me if I'm not right. Natasha, were you not unfaithful, and did not all your illness start shortly after that? I am so sure I'm right? We did hundreds of cases like this during the studies for my doctorate. You are beautiful, you are strong, you have given up the old business and you have got a good job now. On another point I can't send you the pictures, as I have not got them on my system anymore. I told you I downloaded them on to my laptop in Germany after Christmas but then I wiped the pictures clean, as I did not want Ruth to get upset. I had burnt them on to a CD though so when you did respond I took the CD to the photographer and the old man who runs the shop made seven 10x8 prints and seven pocket prints which I now carry around with me. As you well know. He then tells me that he has mislaid the CD and they have been trying to find it. If you need to see the picks I have one only which I like and I still have it on my system. I can send it to you or you can phone the man in the shop or pop in and if he has found the CD tell him to let you have it, it's under my name. John Smith. By the way when he gave me the prints around 17th Feb he said he thought he knew you. He said he thought you had been in the shop before. You are a famous lady, my god the saints preserve us. Am I to go out with a famous lady at last? In the mean time why should you sleep with your ex? You know that already yourself. You should stop punishing yourself and him for crimes he has not committed. Also I don't want you to sleep with anyone else for this very important exercise of which is called body awareness. I think you must agree that you have already done enough of that in your short life. I also want you to be relaxed and calm and with someone you know and love intimately, which is your ex and you know you can trust him to do what you want. This exercise I have asked you to do heightens your sexual awareness in every way. Makes you forget yourself and helps you loose control and to start letting go of which you need to do to start enjoying really hot satisfying sex. The reason I want you to think of Ruth and me is not because it's some kinky sex thing, no, if you have something sexy to pin your thoughts on you will forget yourself completely in that dark room. No light, no sound, no talking, nothing for you to see at all. All your sensations will be touch, feel and smell and NOTHING ELSE. Your thoughts will be on something sexy not you or your ex but Ruth and me. Trust me on this one, the results will be spectacular and the feelings that you will experience will be the strongest you have ever felt. Each time you do it like this they will get stronger and stronger, then hopefully with me you'll orgasm straight away. As soon as I penetrate you? You never know. But who knows..by that time you might want to stay with your ex? It will be so good you will shock yourself, but if you still decide to move on I am waiting for you natasha....x john

From: Natasha <natasha_nw3@yahoo.co.uk>
Date: 21 March 00:20:46 GMT
To: john smith <appledogstime@yahoo.co.uk>
Subject: Re: You cheeky monkey
John,
I feel like crying I spent four hours writing a reply to your E-mail and now I have lost it all. Maybe it wasn't to be and you are not to know.
Thank you for the photograph of Ruth.
Kisses N xx I will try again tomorrow...

From: Natasha <natasha_nw3@yahoo.co.uk>
Date: 21 March 04:37:19 GMT
To: john smith <appledogstime@yahoo.co.uk>
Subject: What a night

Dear John,
I am having a horrid night. Went to bed at twelve thirty slept till three and can't sleep since. I had a stressful day at work, my boss is on another planet, he is lovable but totally bonkers. I am also really upset for loosing that e-mail I wrote for you this evening, it took a lot of effort to put in to words for the questions you were asking me. All that stuff is deeply painful and I am trying to move on from it as best as I can, and for the first time in my life I can see the light at the end of the tunnel. Good job I am off work tomorrow and on Wednesday I am seeing the clever people at the hospital. I can't go on like this. This stupid illness is running my life and is not funny anymore. I am sorry my dear John to be so depressing as you probably have enough of your own problems.

Hope you sleep better than me- Love Natasha xx

March

From: john smith <appledogstime@yahoo.co.uk>
Date: 21 March 15:33:24 GMT
To: Natasha <natasha_nw3@yahoo.co.uk>
Subject: There is always one who is stronger and one weaker in every love

There is always one who has more control and one less in every love. This is in nature, from lions to people. Nature is what it is. There fore there are no excuses. We can say he made me do that or she made me do this. It's rubbish in the end, we do what we want to do then try to blame the other party for what we have done if it goes wrong. You were 18 or 19 years old when your parents made every decision for you with a very strong father who ruled you with a glove of iron and still will if he had the chance. A strong mother with her own ideas of how your life should run and who you should be. You then you came to London and after a time of trying to swim on your own and nearly drowning you found someone else to make decisions for you to replace the two people who made them for you all the time. So you sought him out, found him and grabbed him with both hands. He was what you needed at the time and still do to a certain extent. Then 5 or 6 years down the line you can't blame him and say he made me do this or that, it's what you wanted and what you got. You want to become independent, o.k. we all do but we are never complete. Ruth relies heavily on me and I still on her. We relinquish some of the control that we have on each other as we get older but one is always weaker and the other stronger in one way or another. You found him, gave him a role to fill and he took it on. Now may be you give him another source that helps him? The help of a friend? Lover? Which he may take on as well as this makes us people. In the end it all comes back to our parents. Mine and I suspect your ex's gave me complete freedom to do what I wanted with my life and supported me with all the help they could give in every way. You did not get that. That's the card you have been dealt. You have to get on with your life now and make the most of it and the best of it. You could have been born without legs, but there is no one to blame so forget the past and make the most of your future. love yourself John x x x

March

From: Natasha <natasha_nw3@yahoo.co.uk>
Date: 22 March 12:32:46 GMT
To: john smith <appledogstime@yahoo.co.uk>
Subject: Re: There is always one who is stronger and one weaker in every love

I have just popped back from the Royal Free (hospital). The clever people decided I should go and stay in for few days so I will do as I am told. I printed your E-mail and will read it while in bed thinking of you.
Love Natasha x
Ps: I am not taking my computer in so you will have to wait for when I return, which should be early next week I hope.

From: john smith <appledogstime@yahoo.co.uk>
Date: 23 March 13:26:51 GMT
To: Natasha <natasha_nw3@yahoo.co.uk>
Subject: Hope you get better soon

You little monkey you cost me a lot of trouble as you never gave me the name of the ward you were in, so for hours and hours of hard work I found a ward in the royal free that had a Natasha in it. I sent you a get well card and a flower in a pot for you to look at everyday and watch it grow, just like one day in the not to distant future you will watch my cock grow (with your help) I'm sure as I hope you want children as much as me. You have green fingers with plants which grow, they are your children for now and I'm sure you can make me grow big and hard as soon as you're out of that hospital and back home. Ruth lives in a really nice flat in West Hamstead and just one hundred yards from her flat is a flower shop so I ordered one in a nice pot for you. I hope you like it and think of me every time you shag your ex and think of me. Ruth lives in broadhurst gardens in a big flat just down from west end lane. You may meet her one day in Sainburys, she shops there but maybe your a Tesco girl? Anyway I want to start making babies with you as soon as I meet you, if you want that too that is. Ruth and I never use condoms, we hate them which is why we are so strong on sleeping around. After we

go out a few times and you decide that you are in love with me as much as I feel I'm in love with you which leads us to shagging like rabbits...lets not use anything as there will be just us two and nobody else. I will stop with Ruth and you with your ex and if you fall pregnant lets get married straight away and have a real big wedding. My expectations for us, and your expectations of me... What do you hope for me? I have nearly in million in the bank, a £450,000 flat in Maida Vale and I have £125,000 in my hand every year after deductions. It's all yours to share with me in a love nest if we hit it off in and out of bed and fall madly in love as I think we will. My only thing is that I love to shag everyday. Once we are married with kids on the way I would take a lot more time off and spend it with you. Have amazing trips and nice holidays, so if it fits in with you (as I want to let Ruth down gently) we meet in early July and after a month or when you feel like it we go to bed. We don't use anything and we start to go out, have good times together where ever you want and yes we shag like rabbits. If you fall we marry. How is that for you?
What are your expectations of me? What would you like from me?

I told you I will penetrate you in july and you will be blown away with the orgasm I will give you when I fuck you. Forget all the bad times in your past xxx
John X

From: Natasha <natasha_nw3@yahoo.co.uk>
Date: 23 March 19:45:06 GMT
To: john smith <appledogstime@yahoo.co.uk>
Subject: Re: Hope you get better soon

Dear john,
When I told you which hospital I was in I didn't expect you to search 4 me. Thank you for the flowers but they are not allowed on the ward. You could have asked them when you found out where I was. Please don't think I am ungrateful. I am sure you know by now that they know me in that shop as well. Please don't make any more enquiries about me, I will

tell you all you need to know as I have been till now!!! I am still in but would appreciate if you didn't come to visit, it's not that I would not like to see (I know that is a first for the book) but it would make my life difficult and all I need now is time and peace. Hope you understand all that and will respect it.
Love N xx

From: john smith <appledogstime@yahoo.co.uk>
Date: 23 March 20:28:54 GMT
To: Natasha <natasha_nw3@yahoo.co.uk>
Subject: Wanted to be nice to you and love you as always. Hope you get well soon
I was just trying to be kind not nosey. Sent you flowers as I thought they would cheer you up to have a nice flower like your self. I asked you your expectations from the US..if you want it to get started. What you want and what you would like from it? Nothing is cast in stone but as you are 30 soon and as a doctor I know baby time is running out so not getting heavy in my last email, just thinking of you that's all as I want them as well and I'm sure you want a stress free birth. After 30 everything gets more stressful as time goes by. I won't write again until you get out of prison, which it must feel like and I won't come to see you. I shall wait till you say you want to meet and will wait till I get an email from you. Will not write till then. Will not try to find you. Get well soon and get home safe. Hope your ex is looking after you
love John xxxxx

From: john smith <appledogstime@yahoo.co.uk>
Date: 23 March 23:38:17 GMT
To: Natasha <natasha_nw3@yahoo.co.uk>
Subject: may be too many
I spent all night tonight to study all your text from the first till the last one tonight. I really fancy you and like you as a person. I think you have a heart of gold beneath all the damage but I worry. Your ex is a great person and has all the qualities I admire in a man and I really think he is a good man. I did speak to the man at the photo shop before I got your text tonight but I am in love with you and am thinking if you feel

the same way about spending the best part of our lives together. The reason I worry is because I think you may be hanging on to men from your past and I think there are too many men in your life. Like most men I want a girl I can trust as...((((and all my worldly goods I thee give to you till death do us part)))) can I trust you if we fall in love?? Your writing shows a strong leaning to the fact you cant let go of men who are may be no good for you. You hang on to them. I am at home looking at your pictures, can't you draw a vale on the past? Apart from your ex close the shutters on all the other men for good and with your job and your new life start a fresh. I look at all your emails and everything I learnt at college tells me to worry. Tell me about it Natasha, tell me how many are there still hoping to make love to you again? why when you have so much to look forward to? Do you do this to your self? I'm not wrong am I??? There was a nasty feel in your email tonight that spoke of guilt again??? Why? John xxxx

March

HOSPITAL

She phoned me to tell me she had had to go into hospital. I mostly blamed Chris for this, the selfish bastard. He had a girlfriend in south London and just wanted Natasha as a plaything. She practically had suffered a nervous breakdown. The guilt she was under from keeping a secret love, plus working hard in a new job and trying to satisfy a demanding boss, had been too much strain for her precarious health to bear.

She had chronic colitis, which is a stress and nerve-induced illness. Ever since her childhood she had not been physically strong, and the colitis had worsened terribly. They were going to do more tests. The doctors said that the worst that could happen was that they would need to cut her whole bowel away. I thought to myself that it could hardly get worse than that.

I observed her vacant eyes, the dark circles underneath them, the paleness of her lips. Poor thing, she was not well at all, and I was worried sick for her. I knew that if I lost her, I would be destroyed. She had been as near and dear to me, as integral a part of my world, as the sky is to the earth. I didn't tell her this, but before I went to visit her in the hospital, I went into the little church near Quex Road and said a few prayers so that she would get well soon.

They put her in a little ward which had five or six other ladies in it. But an infection developed amongst some of the patients there, and she was transferred to a private room so that she would not catch it. Her immune system was weak and open to infection, and it was one of the deadly Staphylococcus range of infections that inhabits so many British hospitals.

I was sick with worry. I wanted to take her mind off things, but I could not get my own mind off of anything else but her condition. I did not want to tax her energy too much, so I left after two hours and promised to return as soon as I could.

A flower in a pot had arrived for her with a sealed card, but the hospital would not let her have it in the ward, so I offered to take it to her house on my way home.

March

If I should lose you where could I run to?
If I should lose you how could I live?
Without you to think of, nothing would matter
Promise me darling, promise me
You won't die tomorrow
I will get you anything that money can buy
So don't die baby
Let fate spare you
If I scream for you in the night
But in the darkness you do not answer
If I can no longer turn and hold you tight
Taunted by cruel daylight who refuses to come
Heaven has too many angels already

March

From: Natasha <natasha_nw3@yahoo.co.uk>
Date: 25 March 14:24:11 GMT
To: john smith <appledogstime@yahoo.co.uk>
Subject: Re: may be two many

Dearest John,

I am still in the hospital, have the whole room to myself as the other ladies went home yesterday. Have a painful thing in my arm so sorry for the writing. I feel extremely tired and warn out from the treatment and from my life. I have no energy left for anything now but it might be the drugs and the illness. Here we are, the trust issue and you have been asking around about me. I don't need a degree to know that, you shouldn't have done so. I promised that I would be honest with you, how ever horrid and uncomfortable the truth and I mean it john. I don't sleep around and don't look for casual flings. It only leads to disappointment, stress and heartache. But I do have the experience. I will not go in to the details now, I just want you to know that I don't need it to be happy, you have to do your homework and go by your experience and instinct. I am not an easy person to get along with. I can't be the sweetest and the most loving person and I can be a real nightmare as well. As regards to us I am not sure now what I want, you are very much involved with Ruth still. The more stressed I get the worse the illness gets. As regards to children, nothing would make me happier than a loving man and a baby. I wanted one ever since I can remember but most woman my age would so there is no problem on that score. We can't go and proceed just because we fancy a child, we don't know each other at all and I am very much worried I would be just filling Ruth's shoes and that is something which terrifies me. Also there is stuff in my life and probably in yours we need to talk about. I don't like the fact that you went and did your investigations on me. But how can you have a relationship without trust? I can't live like that anymore. When I asked my ex whether he trusts me he says he doesn't know and yes there are reasons for his behaviour that is why I am trying to be truthful with you. I want to trust but I also want to be trusted. The whole saga with going out with a married man is not a very nice story, though we had lots of brilliant times together. I am not a monster john and deserve to be trusted! For once, you want to know something ask me and I will tell you. Just don't do searches and ask around about me, afford me that courtesy. My arm is really hurting now, I should go. There are computers in the staff cafeteria area so that is where I am. Not sure whether I am allowed to use them but nobody is saying anything so far. I think I will be allowed to get away with it. Love Natasha xx Hope you are fine and looking after Ruth.

I put my head in a paper bag
To shut out the world
And guess what happened?
The world shut out me!
I sat in a paper bag
In a cupboard, and waited
For the phone to ring.
The bag was like
The world
And the waiting
The loneliness you feel
The phone
It never rang
I better take this paper bag off
And get on with my life

March

STAFF CAFÉ

I went to the hospital today, and she still looked very ill and in a sorry state. The nurses were very nice and friendly and helpful though. She said she wanted a drink and something small to eat, and whether we could go down the lift to the basement where the staff café was. She told me she hadn't had any complaints so far, and no one had thrown her out, or asked her whether she was a doctor or nurse. The good thing about it was that it had a huge computer console in the middle, with internet, which was free for the staff.

When we got there the place was littered with multi-cultured, multi-coloured doctors and nurses. We had some tea and cake together, and I sat at the table at a respectful distance, so she could not accuse me of reading her e-mails and prying. She waited for a space on the console and started to write a long e-mail. I knew she was writing to John Smith. She seemed to be obsessed with him, even though she could hardly walk, but at least she was still happy in her illness. She had something to look forward to, a buzz, an energy and something to give her hope, and we were happier than ever.

She spent 40 minutes of my time and hers on the internet, and then I took her up to her room. They put some more drugs into her veins, which were very swollen. She was in a lot of pain. All the different drips and injections, but it was nice with flowers and her own telephone in her own private room. Not bad for the National Health. But she had only been moved to a private room, because of the immune suppressives, and the hospital was so full of bugs.

I spoke to her every day. She was very, very tired, and physically drained all the time. I gave her a big kiss as I left her, and I had the strangest feeling that she wanted me, happy to know I was there for her, but did not want me at the same time. I drove back home with my mind full of thoughts.

March

From: Natasha <natasha_nw3@yahoo.co.uk>
Date: 25 March 14:39:38 GMT
To: john smith <appledogstime@yahoo.co.uk>
Subject: Re: may be two many

John

I have re-read the note again and you don't know how sad it makes me to read it. Everybody was trusted apart from me. Where I am going wrong or what am I doing wrong? Suspect not much with my past and my history, I am not surprised but I am not even going to contemplate a future with anybody who can say they don't trust me. John I do like you, look forward to your e-mails and to our discussions but I will not end up in a relationship where I am not trusted ever again. So you do some sole searching your self my lovely man with the degree in people behaviour. By the way my ex has an experience of people first hand which makes for the degree it self. He is a little genius and I mean that in positive way. I wrote a lot of nasty stuff about him as we went through nasty stuff but he has my best interests at heart and really loves me. He always comes to see me, and even brought me some realistic looking iguanas. They look so real! A boy and a girl one.

love me Natasha xx

From: john smith <appledogstime@yahoo.co.uk>
Date: 26 March 11:27:48 BDT
To: Natasha <natasha_nw3@yahoo.co.uk>
Subject: Just tell me three things

Where and with who did you spend your last birthday with? Day and night. Same for the 25th and 26th of dec? Day and night. The same for new years night, with who? Get in touch when your well, happy and home.
John x

From: Natasha <natasha_nw3@yahoo.co.uk>
Date: 26 March 14:34:09 BDT
To: john smith <appledogstime@yahoo.co.uk>
Subject: Re: Just tell me three things
Dear John
I am not sure why you are asking me all that but no doubt there is a reason so this is my answer to you. I spent my birthday with my ex. Day and the night. He called it our last holiday on the third and he left early in the morning on the fourth. On the 25th and 26th of December I was at home with my parents in the czech republic.
love natx

From: john smith <appledogstime@yahoo.co.uk>
Date: 26 March 19:08:12 BDT
To: Natasha <natasha_nw3@yahoo.co.uk>
Subject: Carmen
I go for you.. I just had an urgent call from big boss so I fly to New York tomorrow morning, early back Thursday night. You did not give me an answer to the last question? Where and who did you spend new years night with and the following day. Did you spend the new year with someone who was not your ex and did you sleep with any one on that night? I still love you... desire you and want you... but until I get back on Friday I leave you with the immortal words of the famous words from the opera Carmen. 'I don't pick out a man and he doesn't pick me out. I let my crazy heart think for me. You go for me and I'm bad news and if I go for you boy that's the end of you. If you're hard to get I want you more...one man gives me a diamond ring... I would not give him a cigarette, another man treats me as if I'm dirt but all I have that man can get.' When was the last time you hugged, held or kissed your ex? That man really loves you and you say to me you are a sweet and nice person? Have we both found (((the real you))) on this journey that we have made together for these last three months. Speak to you friday night when we will be both wiser after thinking of Carmen XXXXXXXXXXX John

March

From: john smith <appledogstime@yahoo.co.uk>
Date: 28 March 13:36:06 BDT
To: Natasha <natasha_nw3@yahoo.co.uk>
Subject: pleasure unlimited you

At the Hilton hotel, New York city. Wonderful seven pictures of you laid out on the bed and you just made me a happy man for the third time in 24 hours...wish, wish, wish the real thing with you but that will have to wait. Love to have made you a happy woman. Put a smile on your face as well as hearing you shout and scream at the top of your voice with pleasure and feeling your wonderful body shudder and shake with your sexy face on fire...not forgetting the feel of your wetness and excitement all over me. Kiss my wonderful girl. x John
From: john smith <appledogstime@yahoo.co.uk>
Date: 29 March 15:51:38 BDT
To: Natasha <natasha_nw3@yahoo.co.uk>
Subject: Billy, you, me and Ruth. We have all the names.

Back in London tomorrow night sexy woman. Met friend from London out here at the Hilton Hotel selling cars in New York. H.P. cars just by chance he flies back tomorrow as well. He also tells me that you are the most sexiest girl in Swiss Cottage, he wanted you him self but he's married. Anyway we had a quick drink and everything I told you from your letters is true and your ex is called William and is truly nice man. I did not check up on you, true as god and Mary in heaven one million to one chance...we meant to be? I believe in these things. My friend goes to the USA to buy and sell cars three times a year. That's where he makes real money. Anyway love you more then ever now. x John x

From: john smith <appledogstime@yahoo.co.uk>
Date: 29 March 23:37:13 BDT
To: Natasha <natasha_nw3@yahoo.co.uk>
Subject: What a strange girl you are..Very early morning New York City after drinks with my friend... When you said you broke up with your ex boyfriend...late last year December (which is when you started to write to me) you never told me

and I never thought that he would turn out to be one of the top 50 photographers and artists in the world?! No one can ever take his fame away from him and he came from nothing I have been told. To give everything for art and art sake. That's a genius! x John

From: john smith <appledogstime@yahoo.co.uk>
Date: 31 March 00:52:25 BDT
To: Natasha <natasha_nw3@yahoo.co.uk>
Subject: 12.45 back in my bedroom in London. Night. You are 15min from me.
Its very early Friday morning...yes I have just seen and looked at your pictures in my tiny bedroom office. I'm in my white pants in my bedroom and yes he wants to be free from his cage. He is so hard thinking of you. He wants to burst free. I take your 7 tiny prints from my coat pocket and lay them out on the bed. Now you know and I know what I have to do. I can't stand it, the thought of you in bed so near yet so far! The head is now two inches out of my pants. I slide my pants down to my ankles and look at him proud and hard thinking of you. My hairy balls are bursting with want for you, Natasha, natasha, natasha natasha, natasha come to me now for god sake. How much can a man stand? I close my eyes feel my fingers wet with your pussy, the lips open, my eyes are shut tight, I see you in my mind, I feel your clit hard on my finger tips, I'm rubbing and hurting him he's so hard the throbbing is mad Crazy! NATASHAAAAAAAAAAAAAAAAAAAA! NATASHHHHHHHHHHHHHHHAAAANASHHHHHHHHHAAAA AAAAAAAAAAAAAAAAAyesyesssssssssssssssnatashayess sssYessssssssssssssssssssssssssssssssssss!!!!!!!!!!! I have come lots, lots and lots all over my red carpet next to my bed (my poor little polish cleaner). My eyes open bed is empty..no you?...just the pictures. Empty room x John

March

From: john smith <appledogstime@yahoo.co.uk>
Date: 31 March 08:36:51 BDT
To: Natasha <natasha_nw3@yahoo.co.uk>
Subject: hard, hard, hard on!
Just woke up, big hard cock, thinking of you it's eight o'clock on a Friday morning London Maida vale. No work today and sad to say no you. What shall I do? Go visit you at the royal free and make love to you there? Pull your pyjama pants and panties down? I know you will be wet for me the min you see me. I pull the blinds round your bed as I walk in to the ward, I plunge my face between your long slender legs and my face and nose into your pussy, my tongue lingers, turns, accelerates. I trust my instincts as regards to your body as it's the first time. I push my tongue in and gently lick, it's slightly bitter, slightly acidic. I can smell your pussy in my mouth and the smell excites me so I push two fingers up inside you as well and rub and massage the top and all the inside of your pussy. You fill all my hand and fingers with your wetness, I keep sucking and licking you with the excitement that a nurse might pop her head in anytime, I have to make it happen quick, I feel the pressure of your mucous membranes on my fingers as you hold them tighter, you stretch your body, your legs open wider, you are so excited now you are shaking. My tongue can feel the heat of your body, you start to sweat, my tongue is more determined, my fingers work deeper, you dig your fingers into my hair, you cling to it bracing yourself and suddenly you scream and your orgasm overwhelms you and inflames me, my fingers are still inside you your cry's are still coming, then a moan..a last spasm. I can hear feet I pull the sheet over you stand up as the nurse pulls the curtain back. I stand up kiss you goodbye and walk out of the hospital. Our first meeting and we said no more than six words and some moans x john

March

From: Natasha <natasha_nw3@yahoo.co.uk>
Date: 31 March 17:25:48 BDT
To: john smith <appledogstime@yahoo.co.uk>
Subject: I'm sexy today

Ok, yes I am wanking to your e-mail. My hand is inside my tiny pink knickers… those ones where you came over your bed. Dirty boy (…), but you made me so horny. Please don't keep wasting it, I feel so broody, sexy and depressed because of my illness.
So yes, I came thinking of you making a baby with me, gorgeous man.
Love Natasha xxx

From: john smith <appledogstime@yahoo.co.uk>
Date: 31 March 18:47:43 BDT
To: Natasha <natasha_nw3@yahoo.co.uk>
Subject: so many letters and no answers to anything

Hope when you get home you will tell all as I have to you everyday. Will see Ruth tomorrow night. Sat on my own all day, thinking of you. Drove by the royal free on my way to Hampstead to have a lunchtime drink, (Old bull and bush) looked up at the windows and wondered where my sweet Natasha was? Hope you wont blame bill for anything when you send me a long letter. The past is the past it's over now. Be nice, make yourself well in doing it and stop punishing him. You chose him, you wanted him, you got him, he gave everything up for you so he deserves better treatment. Whatever mistakes he made... you should be eternally grateful as he did his best and you said over and over you still loved him so stop the punishment. x John

April

From: Natasha <natasha_nw3@yahoo.co.uk>
Date: 1 April 21:13:02 BDT
To: john smith <appledogstime@yahoo.co.uk>
Subject: I am home

Dearest john,

I have discharged my self from the hospital this morning as they can't do anymore for me and I can take pills myself at home. No point staying there over the weekend as the doctor suggested. I do feel much better now, but I don't believe that the drugs work as I expected they would but I am happy enough for now. I have never been so ill with this thing before this was the first time and it was not good. When I was diagnosed two years ago it was almost non-existent. Last august it affected 20cm now it is almost everywhere. I am a bit if a masochist (no I don't trust the doctor). I watched the investigation on the screen and it didn't look good apart form the formations and the lovely colours. I am going back to see the doctors on Wednesday to get some other drugs. There is a lot you have written to me over the past few days and even more I would love to write back in response. I haven't written because the pills make me feel and think funny and I end up writing something I later don't like the look of. I start feeling human again in the evening, I'm out in the morning. Answer to your last question where did I spend new years eve...I had two invitations both form married girlfriends so I spent the evening with one of the couples. We went to a restaurant where my friends husband works (so she can be with him while he works). No other men that night or any other night, just the three of us. How very important is that. So you have a friend from Swiss Cottage. That is a first one for the books! I am sure that he has supplied you with some of his secret pictures of me he that he is keeping in the bottom cupboard. I heard he was a fan of mine but I didn't believed it. I believe he would have given you a lot of information on my lovely Billy (as he now has a name). Billy is an artist and a person and not an easy one. He wouldn't have made it otherwise. You are right he was in the hospital every day doing his best as always and driving me mad in the process. He doesn't do things by half. I am trying my best to be good and nice to him as the doctor suggested. The baby substitute is sitting happily on my table looking nice joining the rest of them. I am over run by plants I love them. Will have to reduce most of them or find a good home for them but I don't give my babies away, what sort of mother would I be. I buy the ones which need rescuing and than I care for them. I would keep my heating on just because of the plants so they would not die. But I don't do it anymore, I adopted a philosophy of natural selection. The strongest will survive at the flat, though warm but it is too dark for the most delicate plants to grow so now only the hearty will make it and the rest if it doesn't grow has to go. Hope you are feeling fine and happy dear John Love Me xx

From: Natasha <natasha_nw3@yahoo.co.uk>
Date: 1 April 22:03:26 BDT
To: john smith <appledogstime@yahoo.co.uk>
Subject: Re: time table for real love forever. You are the one, I know it.

April the first,
No doesn't look as an April fool's day joke but it can easily be though. I have a funny feeling that you are serious. You are very good at planning and I feel that you are another man who is planning my life dear John. I worry about you a bit, how can you almost propose to a girl you have not met, heard or seen in the flesh? It all sounds lovely John but I don't think that I could deal with another heart break few months down the line if it went wrong. I can see my self getting attached too much too soon to you (and I don't know YOU). My life is even more up side down now than it was ten days ago. I am not sure what will happen with my work, my health with the whole thing. I am cutting all unnecessary stress out of my life or trying to and this could turn out...(well you are right, it can turn out all right as well). Don't put pressure and time scales on me unless you are running out of time. Have a fun evening, I am in bed will go to have a bath and then sleep.
Love nat

April

The little mermaid wept with joy
The ugly duckling was your delight
The real princess slept on her pea
How many birdseye wrappers around your bed?
To bring you such happiness and joy
Each day may see you better than the day before
Thumbelina loved her tin soldier
The tinderbox, the red, red shoes
The days filled with night
And the nights filled with love
Were all born to set you free
For all the joy you gave
To a man who loved you

April

Saturday 1st April

April fools Day, and I was taking her home. She couldn't take any more as she was just getting more and more unhappy. Anyway they needed the beds at the hospital.

When I arrived, she was pale and drawn, and her arm, both arms, had swollen where they had had the catheters in. Pale, drawn and very weak, but she was going home, and they would now treat her with modern drugs and poisons as I am into alternative medicines. But she wanted to give these terrible mixtures that they were injecting into her body a try, so there was not much I could do about it. She is very strong and stubborn,

It was self-help time for her now. She was not going back to work. She was going to try to get lots of rest, and I would do my best to give her lots of love and no stress. Her boss wanted her back as he needed to go away somewhere, but he winds her up more than anybody, so he could go stuff himself, I thought. She could not even walk down the stairs without getting worn out.

The plant that she received looked nice on her table. It looked like a cock, long with a big red head.

Oh well, she was happy to be home even if she was sick.

I left her to go home after three hours.

Faded Photographs

Faded photographs, you and me
Night-time shadows disappear
Old love letters I can't bear to read
Music I can no longer hear
Is it too late, or has she died?
Have not heard now, for over a year
Should we both hide away? Sometimes love, will just not stay

April

From: john smith <appledogstime@yahoo.co.uk>
Date: 2 April 01:46:54 BDT
To: Natasha <natasha_nw3@yahoo.co.uk>
Subject: Re: Time table for real love forever. You are the one, I know it.

Billy has excellent feel for beautiful women how after what you have written. Could not any man love you and keep loving you forever and want to take care of you? I hope so much that you continue to gain strength and get better. I'm off to Ruth's for sat and sun night will try to write you a long letter from work on Monday. Thank you, glad to know your home and looking after my baby as you will look after my real baby one day xxx So glad Billy took care of you...as I knew he would. Hope you were real nice to him, he deserves it. That man would die for you. Will write Monday x john

From: john smith <appledogstime@yahoo.co.uk>
Date: 2 April 10:19:46 BDT
To: Natasha <natasha_nw3@yahoo.co.uk>
Subject: Re: I am home

I Am at Ruth's house she is cooking breakfast for us both. We had a good hot night of sex, she wore me out. The drink she had at the party made her wild and all the idiots there (most of them jewish) feeling her up when they could. He does his best for you, goes to the hospital, gives you lots of love and attention and you grumble. Think if you had no one or he was not there. He fights for you so shut it, your spoilt be grateful as Ruth says your a lucky girl. She looked at his pictures and the painting of him looks like a self portrait he is really sexy, intelligent, caring, helpful and he must be able to fuck.(Ruth's Words not mine) with his history. What do you want? Superman? Anyway we shagged and shagged, she thought of your Billy an older mature lover and I of you she said it was a great fantasy and brought her off twice. I just cant wait to get my hands on you. Would love to take you to New York in late July, early August. Anyway be positive, get rid of a life time of abuse of your body by others and your family as well as things you inherited. Get well and become the lovely, sensitive and beautiful woman you are..as she is now looking over my shoulder. For the first, last and only time. Love from Ruth and me John x Ha Ha Ha!!! She has vanished into kitchen again. Quick word before she comes back..I think she fancies you her self a little johnx

From: john smith <appledogstime@yahoo.co.uk>
Date: 2 April 10:48:23 BDT
To: Natasha <natasha_nw3@yahoo.co.uk>
Subject: Exhibition
Ruth and I are looking at his show on line. Fuck, fuck, fuck! What a turn on! You are so fucking sexy and horny that has got to be you running up the flight of stairs at the start. Fuck now I can see you walk and run naked. Where else can I find you till we meet? Just your voice is missing x John

From: Natasha <natasha_nw3@yahoo.co.uk>
Date: 2 April 21:22:14 BDT
To: john smith <appledogstime@yahoo.co.uk>
Subject: Re: Exhibition
Dear John
What a language!
You can find me if you looked close enough. But I strongly suggest you don't do it. I work not far from where your lovely Ruth lives and when I go to work I pass her house on the way, some days. But I don't work now. I now worry about going shopping as you said she shops in Sainsbury's. Have been there today and couldn't think about meeting you and her there. I am sure that she looks like the pics you sent me. You might have a job recognising me in the street. Did you have a good day with Ruth? Let me know what you did apart form surfing Billy's sites. What does she think about this obsession of yours? And how much did you tell her about me?

Ps: Yes some people do say I am sexy but I can't see it myself but I will not argue. (Billy is my biggest fan and he thinks I am absolutely gorgeous. So if I have a big head about

myself, it's because he tells me this everyday) But apart from the outer body which will go one day I am not a bad person either but you can't see that from a picture. Probably a very different one from the one you have in your mind of me.
Keep well Love natasha xx

From: john smith <appledogstime@yahoo.co.uk>
Date: 2 April 22:14:45 BDT
To: Natasha <natasha_nw3@yahoo.co.uk>
Subject: sex

I just admire talent, nothing wrong with that. If I see you (and not until you give me a nod) I will walk by you as instructed. Me and Ruth talked about how sad it will be when we stop shagging and let go...but it has to happen when I start with you? She loves the fantasy of you and me fucking you hard. She likes beautiful women but has never had the guts to kiss or go with one but she said she had some great fantasies when I was fucking her today. She has made her self off to bed early tonight, I will join her when I finish this to you. We fucked and talked and fucked all day. It's as if she can't get or has to get as much as she can before it all stops. Sex has got better since we split up its more thoughtful towards each other and more hot as it will be with you when you shag Billy's brains out in a dark room. You will see it will blow your mind. No I am not over the top and neither is Ruth. Just love someone who has worked and perfected their talent to perfection. Real intelligence in his work, he thinks about everything he makes you see that. He has a thinking brain if you know what I mean. In
other words he is clever. I know what you are like, your words tell me everything and Ruth knows everything. I told her. She thinks it's normal. A new person is always exciting...and even if we have not met to touch we have met..and began to know each other...what about sex??? What do you like? Do you like to kiss deep? To play? Ruth likes it from behind. Always 80% dog way she comes always that way and she can fantasize face down. A pillow or two under her belly, bottom up in the air. Oh yes. She likes to feel like a little girl. Pull her panties

up tight between her legs, give her a smack or two and then penetrate her hard. We foreplay face to face first, she loves that sometimes but not always. I leave her panties on her, pull them a side from the back as she wanks at the same time. Her hand down the front of her panties as I shag her hard. I love fucking her and fucking her so sexy hard that she comes whilst my cock is inside her and I feel her hot cum dripping off my cock. She blows me real hard after that. You say I write like your bill? I'm sure I don't and I am not like him. He is more arty and poetry type than me. I can be a little crude sometimes, a real hard money man but I go with the flow. What ever the woman likes I go with...but i try to teach them to fuck. Now she always comes when I penetrate her. We sometimes come together. Well better go to bed as she is waiting half asleep for me but she can't sack me for not making her happy x john

From: Natasha <natasha_nw3@yahoo.co.uk>
Date: 3 April 23:13:13 BDT
To: john smith <appledogstime@yahoo.co.uk>
Subject: Sex rules the world No just Johns and Ruths lives
Hi John,
I feel almost human now. I feel like a cosmonaut floating in mid air my thoughts all over the place not being able to still think straight. No there is nothing with admiring talent. I am glad that you and Ruth are getting on so well, it is like you have given your selves permission to be nice to each other again. I have sure been given something of that sort my self. I had a nice day with my ex cooked us some lunch for the first time in four months and we went for a short walk in the park it was lovely. I find the honesty in your letters a bit much sometimes to be truthful but I can picture you both giving it your best and enjoying every second of it. When you have been with somebody for so long you reach a state of perfection, when you know exactly what you both like and that is worth working towards and that is from personal experience of me and Billy. He is the best lover ever. I didn't mean that you are the same as Billy, he is him and you are you but he is also a hot blooded man and I know what I am saying. I have

been with him for years you haven't. He is as crude as you if not more, our billy can be very, very crude how ever difficult you might find it. The same sort of sex talk as you my friend it is unbelievable. I wasn't talking about your obsession with Billy dear John I was talking about your obsession with me, what does Ruth think about that and did you tell her about the origin of my pictures? I have not felt like making love to anybody at all for the past few days, but after four months of self inflicted starving sex diet it will be explosive when I do. There was one moment in the hospital when you made me feel wet after reading your two e-mails from NY. One was from your trip and the other one from your home. I don't envy your little polish cleaners job cleaning up after you. By the way tell Ruth that she has still lots of time left with you and not to wear you out, the way she is going you will be no good to me. You two are sex mad! I have days when I can take it or leave it and would make love mostly to please the other person but I can get grumpy if it is too often. Days when I feel it would not be a bad idea and days (and very, very few of those) when I can't think about anything else but that. Those are worth waiting for. I love all the sensual stuff, kissing and touching for hours. Foreplay taking over, slow lovemaking with my man or me on the top. I do like to be on top having the power over my man being able to control what is happening. But I also love to be fucked hard into total submission possessed and told what to do. I don't keep my panties on as they get in the way. My body is totally naked (after all you took ages to undress me). I feel naked most of the time I write to you, as I am aware that every word I write is analysed to the last letter. One more thing John I don't write letters, e-mail people for precisely this reason. As they can be reared again and again. You are a very big exception. I suppose I don't mind you re-reading my e-mails. If or when we meet and we do get to make love I promise you the best blow job (for luck of the other phrase) you have ever had in your life. If we ever do it, it will be better than the best.. Love and kisses x Keep well and don't let Ruth make you in to a sex slave (only if you enjoy it) Natasha xx

April

From: john smith <appledogstime@yahoo.co.uk>
Date: 4 April 00:36:01 BDT
To: Natasha <natasha_nw3@yahoo.co.uk>
Subject: Oh my god! Oh my god, that's it! You have done it for me girl!

O god you gave me such a hard cock! It grew so big and heavy that I fell over when I got home late from work. I came three times! A record for me in two hours. My god you really got me on the go with that letter. I work so hard that I don't mind to only make love two you three or four times a month when your on heat like a bitch. If that's how you do it and describe it. That's something else. I'm so worn out with reading your printed out email and wanking to your pictures. I have to leave at six tomorrow, give me a few days to draft a reply. Get your body ready for me. Your orgasm will blow your mind you will pass out. God please God I so want you just ten lines of words and you blew me away! It's true in this world if you want the best go for it. There is no substitute for experience, it's the only thing. Little Ruth is good but she can't match up to you. She had eight men in her whole life and three of them were one night stands. You must have had and made happy over a hundred men? The way you write it shows that you're an experienced lover. God that Billy knew a thing or two when he grabbed you. One day I would like to shake him by the hand for helping to create an angel. A women, a girl, a venis de millo, a women who knows how to make a man happy after he comes home from a hard days and nights work. Why does he work? To give her a good and happy life with everything she ever needs to make her happy. Worn out but worth every min to find you waiting for me. Oh god please soon. Counting the days and mins. Bless you xxxxjohn

April

From: john smith <appledogstime@yahoo.co.uk>
Date: 4 April 17:33:30 BDT
To: Natasha <natasha_nw3@yahoo.co.uk>
Subject: Liberation- freedom from guilt- freedom

You know what you're expected to do. You know that we are meeting in August and that I plan to take you to New York, so you haven't got long. The room will be absolute black. There will be no sound. If it's not dark enough then you should wear one of those little eye-masks that you have worn in aeroplanes to block out the light. Better that you don't see him at all. There should be no sound, no sight, so that your sense of feel, touch and smell will be heightened, but you could perhaps have some music if you like. You leave the door of your flat open, he phones you and gives your phone four or five rings, to let you know that he is outside. Remember this is the man who you have made love to many thousands of times before, but after a long gap of some five months, he is a new man and you are a new woman and nothing after this will ever be the same between you again. Even though you have blindfolded yourself you hear the door open and you know he is in the room with you. You can sense his presence and you can sense that he wants you. You have chosen your underwear very carefully. You decided on white as the room is dark, almost black, so he will just still see your white underwear through the shadows and it will turn him on. You wear your favourite knickers for sex. You've worn them hundred of times before, and hundred of men have pulled them off you, as you want him to. You feel his fingers around your waist as he pulls you closer to him, drawing near to his face you have his lips grazed you without kissing though. He is being so teasing, and you feel so naughty. You inhale his scent and listen to his breathing. You put your arms around his neck, pulling his face towards you and devour his lips, sucking and biting them. Your tongue met his and his was hot and soft. It caressed your mouth gently like a feather, making you tremble with excitement. You don't remember him ever kissing you like that before, but because of the unusual circumstances of the situation, the kiss has started to turn into a red hot dirty encounter. When we make sex exotic, and do something more naughty, like doing it in the back of car, with people watching, or with a blindfold on, the sensation can be much, much better for a woman and a man.. He started to touch you and caress you. His fingers running lightly under the little dress you were wearing and starting to play like a piano with the outside of your tiny white panties. He caressed the top of your bare legs above the black stockings that you look so hot in. Then he increased the pressure after almost half an hour of playing. His hands slid between your legs and he started to play harder, his fingers touching you ever so lightly. It makes you want it harder, but it makes you so very wet. You knew what he wanted and even though you were standing, you pushed his head down between your legs. His tongue caressed and flicked your pussy and clitoris, which was as soft as a newborn baby's cheek, because you shave and cream it so carefully for him. Slowly and gently, the pleasure you started to experienced became continuous. The pleasure is relentless, dense, sweet and fragile at the same time. You knew you were starting to melt in his warmth. You have made love to this man so many times before, but this time it is a different sensation completely. He rose from between your legs and his tongue flicks over your lips and you tasted your own pussy honey juice on his mouth and for the first time that you can remember, it tasted sweet and delicious. He started to moan with pleasure about to say something, but you put your finger on his lips to remind him that he must not speak, though he can moan with pleasure as much as he likes. Your dress was on the floor now around your ankles and you stood there in the dark, in your tiny white panties, bra, black stockings and high heels. He was wearing just a pair of jeans and a T-shirt, which you could not see, but your sensitive hands recognised the texture of his clothes as well as him throbbing and hard for you inside his trousers. As your hands brushed against them, you felt the hard strong shape of his member, which you had felt so many times before, but this time it was rock-hard and meaty beneath his jeans. You unbutton them and slid your hands down to grasp it. You felt the velvet tip, smooth and soft, and move your hands around his arse bringing your arms round him, willing him like crazy to fuck you. He too wanted it so desperately and you heard his breathing grow stronger and stronger, more and more aggresive and wild. He picked you up and carried you three feet to the bed and you immediately went down onto him, your serpentine tongue wrapping around him and driving him crazy like every snake that nature could imagine. He was so excited now and after four months, so were you. You knew that in the darkness he was gazing at you and taking every detail of your body in, going mad for your sexy, naked figure. His hands felt their way under your back to release the bra and your breasts. Then he started to kiss all the way down your body pulling your tiny white panties down your thighs until they were dangling just on one ankle. Your legs parted, ready for him- you could not wait anymore. Even though you usually like to spend one or two hours in foreplay this was something completely different. The sensation was too much. You had to know what it felt like again, right now. You felt the wetness pouring from you onto your bedspread. Suddenly he thrusts into you and you give a slow long moan of ascent positioning your body for the next one. It is so tantalising in the dark, when you don't know when it's coming next. You gazed in the position you knew his face must be, imploring with your lips on the outside of his mouth, wanting to feel him again. He paused for a few minutes with it inside you knowing that this would make you more crazy and intensify your pleasures. Now it was your turn, as instructed, to make him submit to you. In the dark, you felt around and took off your high heels and black stockings, so that every cell, every inch of skin on both of your heaving bodies would touch and share these exciting new sensations. You straddled him and began to ride him sensuously, alternating between gentle rhythmic thrusts to ones that were hard and abrupt, grinding your hips against him. You licked and kissed him and you heard his moans and the sound of his moans were killing you. For the first time you started to lose control. This was different. You had become like an animal. You were an animal. Moaning and groaning, getting crazy and hot. You had never made love to him before like this. You felt the burning heat in your face and neck and in your pussy, and you started to grind and thrust harder, and embrace, seize the very pleasure that you thought no man could ever give you, the pleasure that you alone could never even create for yourself. Although you knew it was not the full orgasm that I would give you, you felt hot, warm spasms everywhere throughout your whole body, in your legs, in your pussy, in your arms, even on your face. You removed his black sweater and rubbed your nipples against the hairs on his chest and because of the darkness and sensuous feelings that were building up inside you, the prickly sensations became a marvellous discovery for you. He now started with some help from you and your wild movements, to shag you back, hard and relentlessly, over and over and over. You felt for his face and with your fingers could tell that even though in the dark room you could see nothing, his eyes were closed. You rolled off him and your tongue and mouth, after removing the condom, swept over him and even though you could not remember it, you had swallowed the most sperm you had ever tasted. His tasted slightly salty with a touch of sulphur tonight. When you are excited and your sexual senses are peaked, you always swallow harder and more. You could not see, but you knew he was still staring at you in the darkness. Men are never satisfied with your body, even when they have it over and over again, beyond caressing it, kissing it and fucking it. You lay there and felt for your panties that were still on one ankle, yet they don't simply belong to you. Even though they are the panties that most men have fucked you in, they are part of your body, you have worn them so often when men have made love to you. Imagine your body wearing nothing but these tiny white panties. Your sensuality and the inner sexual beast in you are unleashed when they drop round your ankles. You were born to fuck and you will spend the rest of your life fucking men. Whoever the lucky man is that takes your panties down will not only see your sensuality, but your whole soul. This time is the first time that anyone has possessed nearly all of you. You never gave all of yourself to any man, because when you give that other part of yourself, that very small, tiny part that is buried deep within you, you escape to a whole new universe of senses. You are in new un-chartered territory. Out of your depth, knowing that the only one you could possibly trust is your ex that you can never forget about, but then the day will come and may come sooner when the jailer arrives offering you the keys to release all of your spirits, and not be afraid that you no longer have that stable rock figure to cling to. To release your sensuality, you love and your deep inner self and for you to let it take wing, to make you feel good about yourself, free and satisfied, so that your mind and body no longer ask, as it has always done, since you were fourteen, young and eager, for something more. Men need no longer torment you with their endless requests. The tender secrets that are freed by hands that finally know how to caress you how you want to be touched. Know how to make you throb and glow and grow hot at the thought of that hand. Now you ask him to smell that milky part of you between your legs, in the centre of your body, between love and sensuality. It is your soul, heart and mind which seeps through your panties with those thick, white fluids. I am so, so right, when I told you that you were born to screw and fuck hard. As you see his soul wishes to be desired as much as yours, as he smells as you give off your scent, the female smell. Perhaps the hands, which free your spirits, may beat me to it. In the sexual sense, this will give you the opportunity to find things about him you never knew or tried to find because of all the rubbish we have to struggle through when in a relationship, but now you are both free one way or the other. Your curiosity may still reach out for me, even if he achieves and finds your ultimate secrets, but maybe you feel you must do it, because at least in the future, you wont ever regret not doing something and losing an opportunity before grasping it. His thing is as hard as a rock still grinding, pushing and throbbing inside you. You can hear the loud, wet noise of your pussy and his cock, like a door that needs to be oiled, or a drumstick beating on a drum. In the darkness and the silence, the noise with your erotic gasps and his grunts, is deafening when he is with you and you are in his arms. Your chance of freedom, you must take it as I have told you because the horrendous and unjust wall of time,

guilt, grudges, pain, past hatreds, past accusations must pass and be cleansed from your own life, slowly to fast for the new life that lies ahead of you. A series of figures and past memories that you have kept at arms length. I hope you are mathematical, sophisticated and now a woman of intelligence as well as sensuality, because this insight might offer you some hints on how to solve this terrible equation. Billy is fucking you hard now and you know that you finally might reach orgasm with him. You can feel it coming, your breath is gasping and hot in the dark and as he shoots and shudders into you as part of you cries out. The feeling has to be shared with another male. It's now up to you to decide whether to bring about for the last experiences with him, an important change in your relationship, whether to make it for the first time, more sensuous and more spiritual or more profound even. I put my trust in you, you sweet, sensitive, sexy lady and I know that you will make the right decision for yourself.
John X

From: Natasha <natasha_nw3@yahoo.co.uk>
Date: 4 April 21:34:47 BDT
To: john smith <appledogstime@yahoo.co.uk>
Subject: Re: Liberation- freedom from guilt- freedom
Dearest john I have printed your E-mail and will read it in bed before I go to sleep. You must be careful my friend or you will get in to trouble because of me. Make sure that even though you do erase the mail from the computer it can't be retrieved by your clever support people. I don't want you making your life difficult unnecessarily. You work hard enough. I am going to the hospital again tomorrow and even though I am very positive, I am apprehensive about it. The steroids are working but not hundred percent so the doc said that I need to go on something called Azathioprine. As he says there is no other option. Well I will have to just see what he says when I get there. I am off to read your long mail. Love N xx Ps: don't get caught by the company spies, naughty boy!

April

From: john smith <appledogstime@yahoo.co.uk>
Date: 6 April 02:00:37 BDT
To: Natasha <natasha_nw3@yahoo.co.uk>
Subject: My hot bits for you to get pleasure from
This is called tease. There will be four pictures of me in total one every three weeks till we meet in august..my torso, bum, back and yes we save the best bit till last. Kiss my darling until all of this is on top of you and the bit below this is moving like a wild dog deep and hard in to you, wonderfuly horny sexy woman xxxxxxJohn

From: Natasha <natasha_nw3@yahoo.co.uk>
Date: 6 April 10:01:34 BDT
To: john smith <appledogstime@yahoo.co.uk>
Subject: Re: My hot bits for you to get pleasure from
My dear John, Those are killer hours you are working. Almost un-human or superhuman. I have to admit that I think about you when I wake up only because I am still asleep when you are already busy working. I feel like I have been working your hours. I will write you again in the evening when I recover. I think I over did it yesterday a bit. I went to Hampstead heath for a walk with Billy after the hospital and it was glorious the weather is so lovely and you are shut in an office all day. I am sure that you enjoy your work. Today is my anniversary. I arrived to England on April 6th ten years ago I don't know where the time went I was nineteen years old. Don't work too hard my lovely John keep well natasha x

April

THE RED LETTER DAY
6th April

Sex again at last, and I can tell you it was extremely unexpected. Not what I thought would start the day, nor did she. In fact afterwards, when we reminisced, we could not believe it had actually happened. We went to the hospital for one of her regular visits after I had a cup of tea at her place. Yes! Miracle of miracles, with her strange old fashioned, quaint ideas and ways, when she has an argument with a male she is involved with, you have to go right to the beginning. So yes, I am back at the flat again, even though it has been 9 nine years of being with her. Everything goes back to square one. We're allowed to cuddle standing up, and sometimes to play on the bed. I'm allowed to touch her body, her legs, her bum, her arms, but nothing else. No pussy or bum hole but some times she weakens and I can play with and suck her tits

It was a bit like a slow torture for a man in some Japanese concentration camp. I am allowed to run my finger along the little cracks on the cheek of her bum. I am allowed as close as one millimetre of heaven, but I am not allowed to lay a finger on the temple of delight.

After the hospital, we had a nice meal together in a little Italian restaurant of which I had known the owner for some years. We then went for a long walk over Hampstead Heath. She got very tired and worn out very quickly with her illness, but we talked a lot and got very close, and she hung onto my arm with grim death. The sun was shining and she confided in me that it was the anniversary of the day she had first arrived in England 10 years ago. April 6th.

She started talking again about this John Smith. He is getting to be very important to her. Apparently she wrote to him most nights and him to her, getting rather intimate. She practically talked about him all the time, at least when she was talking to me. Even more sometimes about his wonderful girlfriend Ruth who she and seen pictures of. I thought she was in love with Ruth. She had always toyed with the idea of making love with another woman. She played with the idea and teased herself, but never actually did anything about her feelings. There were a couple of women who got her excited.

She was quite intoxicated about a little French girl who

lived in the flat opposite her. Also, one of her close girlfriends she tried very hard to seduce, but it didn't work out. I am sure that if she had had a serious come on from either of them, she would have gone the whole way.

Anyway, after the walk, we finally got back to our little Pied de Terre, and she invited me in for some hot chicken soup, which was homemade and wonderful. She always used to get the bones from her local butcher free of charge, and she served it up with a good helping of lentils, with those little black pepper corns that blow your head off if you happen to crunch into one by mistake.

After we had chicken lentils and rice, she washed up the dishes and then we both went to lie on the bed together. She really surprised me as it had been four months since anything had happened between us, but she took her jeans and top off and lay on the bed in white cotton knickers, a tiny white vest and no bra.

She asked me to give her a cuddle. I started to play with her and she moaned about my hands always straying near the naughty bits. In the end I played with her bottom, legs, creases, her back, pulling her vest up to the top of her neck, but never letting my fingers get closer than a millimetre from her pussy. I even pulled her panties up between the crack in her bum so that I could play with her creases more. She got quite emotional and cuddled me and kissed me as it was her anniversary. But she would still not let me put my finger inside.

I was laying on my side in my black pants and black t-shirt. Her nipples had stiffened and my cock was getting rock hard. She knew it and she could see it, and she was getting excited. Her libido had completely vanished over the past four months, but in spite of all the barriers and problems, she was getting hot. It had been a long time for her as well as me, without any real sex.

I held her close, her body pressed up against me, my hands everywhere, as I did not know when I would get the opportunity again. Suddenly, in the spur of the moment, she was holding, rubbing and playing with my balls.

'No!' she said, 'You can't fuck me.' But you've been a good boy today, so she said, and she looked at me with that look in her eyes, 'I'm going to reward you a little bit.'

Her stomach was noisy and fizzy, and she was nervous, but obviously excited. My fingers were twanging and playing with her damp knickers. She wanted to say 'Yes! Yes!' so much but she was strong when she put her mind to it, and my balls were aching and she knew it.

She was rubbing him faster and faster now, and she had that really horny, sexy look in her eyes. She was staring at me intently. She knew that this was a special moment she was creating. She was one of those special girls. When one of the things that she'd really like to do, but only when she was really in the mood for it, was to suck cock, and when she sucked cock, she really loved it. She could feel every twitch as my penis got hard and more and more excited, with me desperately trying not to come.

One of the beautiful moments between a man and a woman, is when you want each other so much, you are aching so much. You want the aching to last forever. I let my cock slide in and out of her mouth the way she wanted it to. Her tongue circling over and over the head. Then she started to deep throat me, and her tongue went up and down over the shaft, from the tip and all around my balls, which were now overheated, swollen and ready to burst. I could see she was really wet as well.

'I really want to fuck you…' I said. 'I really want to.'

She looked deep into my eyes. 'No,' she said, 'Not yet, it's too soon.' She massaged the head of my cock again, her tongue swirling relentlessly. My arousal after four months was certainly a sight to see. She was driving me mad. I could not stand it anymore so I took her hair and her head in my two hands and then started to fuck her mouth, and within seconds I ejaculated over and over and over. There was so much of it, her mouth was full of it, and she gave me a nervous little laugh as she swallowed the lot.

'I just thought I'd reward you,' she said laughing. 'But don't think because of that you could weedle your way back in again.' She said waving a finger at me. She laid breathing deeply with her head on my chest. It felt like old times again. I played with her back and her hot little bottom and then she said, looking seriously into my eyes, 'The reason I did not let you fuck me, is because we have a very special exercise we have to do soon.' Oh yeah? I said. 'It will make us better sexually together, closer together, and get rid of much of my bitterness and anger that I had pent up inside me. The sex will be so good. John told me all about it,' she said, 'it's a deep psychological exercise to get rid of feelings of repression, hatred and anger that people bottle up.'

I hated the way she used his first name in the familiar. It was as if she had known him for years.

'I want you to come here' she said.

'Next Friday the 21st of April. You have to do exactly as I say. I will leave the doors open for you, and when you come in, you are not allowed to talk at all. There will be music, and I will be completely in charge. You will follow my lead exactly. Absolutely no talking. If you talk or break any of the rules, I will ask you to leave. It has to be done my way. Is that okay?'

'Okay…' I murmured. My long wait was coming to an end. I was eager and nervous at the same time, and a little worried as she was falling again, with a deep infatuation for this new man. But she ran him down all the time, always saying that he told her off for this, or for that, or he said she wasn't doing this and that properly. She even said to me, 'He's worse than my bloody father. He's such a control freak. You had better go now, she said, I'm very tired, It's been a very long day.

I stood up and dressed and she hugged me tight In her little white cotton knickers.

I drove home in a daze, wondering what the Friday would bring. I almost crashed the car thinking of her the way home. That final hug and kiss felt very awkward. Much more so than the first time I held her today. After so long it was like we were strangers having sex together in some strange fantasy dream or fairytale.

I slept like a log that night, passing out the moment my head hit the pillow. At least my love wand between my legs was happy and contented. I wondered what would happen to our relationship after the date we had fixed for the exercise.

'Oh well,' I said to myself. At least we were moving forward. And I fell into a deep sleep.

April

Tell me all about you
What's really in your head?
'Cos sex gets in the way
I want to know your mind
What you really feel for me
'Cos tears, passion and kisses
Really make my blind
Can we wrap up close in a blanket of dreams?
And let our love keep us warm?
Can't let you go,
My woman of the night
My friend in the day
My secret delight
My hope for the future
My pain of the past
Please oh please
Make our love last
Tell me about you
What troubles me
We stay in our blankets
Our tears will set us free

April

From: john smith <appledogstime@yahoo.co.uk>
Date: 6 April 21:23:23 BDT
To: Natasha <natasha_nw3@yahoo.co.uk>
Subject: Our last holiday in the Maldives. Xmas 2005. 2nd Jan she moved out

As she moved out in the early part of Jan we decided to take one last shag every day holiday together so for xmas we went to the Maldives and did just that. We swam, ate our selves silly, she loves her food and shagged every day and night. I decided next time after five wasted years I would go for something different, then I saw you and fell in love. Now here is the good news, she has fantasized so much now that when I start with you she really would..if you don't mind and I told her I don't mind...shag Billy's brains out maybe two times. When I'm with you as she has never been with an older mature lover. I give her orgasms and she is sure Billy will as well on penetration. If your happy we both are. It will help Billy and Ruth's broken hearts and minds(who knows they may fall in love he may drive her mad with desire) while we carry on with engagements, babies and our future. Mean while I sit here in my office waiting on something from you to cheer me up and excite me and drive
me more wild with desire xxxxxxxxx my wonderful Natasha xxxxxxJohn

From: Natasha <natasha_nw3@yahoo.co.uk>
Date: 6 April 22:52:53 BDT
To: john smith <appledogstime@yahoo.co.uk>
Subject: The E-mail

Dear John
I got the big E-mail you sent me, I have read it and thought about it but I am not sure whether or when I will act upon it. The decision will have to ultimately be mine and I will have to feel comfortable with what I am doing. I believe I can see the logic behind it but this would put the whole relationship on a different footing. Billy when he wants something he will go after it at any cost and that is a fact. I could tell from the way

he got excited today when we were having a little play around. He won't take no for an answer and that is what I am worried about, also all the stuff around it but I have not dismissed the exercise completely. In fact, I mentioned it to Billy today. We'll see what happens. I want to do it… I really want to with Billy, for myself and any future lover I might take. I really would like to get rid of all the hatred and anger that I feel inside myself.
Love natx

From: Natasha <natasha_nw3@yahoo.co.uk>
Date: 6 April 23:05:51 BDT
To: john smith <appledogstime@yahoo.co.uk>
Subject: Re: Our last holiday in the Maldives. Xmas 2005.

2nd Jan she moved out
OH DEAR that is a WOMAN. I give you that and I as you said something very different you are not kidding my friend. I am so skinny compared to the lovely Ruth you might...well I am skinny always have been and always will be. She has a body on her that girl. Your Ruth and my Billy are on the some wave length as he came with the same idea. I can see us all ending up in bed one day. Or maybe that would be a bit much. So Ruth and Billy and you will have all the fun there is and I will end up with the stretch marks big veins and childbirth pains. I like the sharing spirit..on the other hand what would not I do for you my dearest darling John. Anyway the doctor said that I should not get excited and I should keep calm and stress free so I should stop thinking about babies and Billy shagging Ruth and you shagging me and go to bed. I am not going to promise you a story to cheer you up but you just might get one tomorrow. I might dream of the womanly body your Ruth has! Kiss natx

April

From: john smith <appledogstime@yahoo.co.uk>
Date: 6 April 23:26:30 BDT
To: Natasha <natasha_nw3@yahoo.co.uk>
Subject: I don't believe that...

He will let go of you now even if you shag his brains out every single night till we meet he will let go of you he will fight up to the last min but because you are giving him every thing and I mean everything he every wanted your soul, your arms your body your kisses everything
and you are doing it in a special way. The reason he treated you the way he did was because you treated him so badly but he was your choice so you made that decision. When you can let him go your rock when you can forgive him every thing when you can give him every thing no holding back everything then you will be free of every thing. Guilt, pain, your old self, anger and so will he the worry for the new man on the scene. At medical school we watched this happen. Out of twenty chosen couples who did this experiment, it always worked. The woman starts to orgasm and both parties feel free. After 17 of them grew closer together and instead of taking what was on offer actually went back to their ex's, thrilled at the new closeness and sexiness of the whole thing..as i said you might change your mind about everything when it happens. The first time will be way out and special, after that it will become explosive and you will love it! Even Ruth and I are 60% better now and I'm a doctor but what it will do for you and me will be magical. I don't want you with all that baggage and guilt so stop running away from growing up and stop running. This is not your dad, this is a man who loves you still and you are both adults xxxxxx John

From: john smith <appledogstime@yahoo.co.uk>
Date: 7 April 00:06:12 BDT
To: Natasha <natasha_nw3@yahoo.co.uk>
Subject: my darling Natasha, dearest girl and woman

There you go again. You are running away from freeing your self of anger and guilt and now you making yourself inferior and small as regards to ruth. Your dad certainly worked on you as a young girl stop it nat now. your beautiful and mature and experienced. Ruth would cut off her hand to have been to bed with the men you have been to bed with and she is keen to learn a few tricks that I can't teach her from your Billy. Who in this world says you will fall straight away...we could do it for two years before you get pregnant..so lots of time to have fun and games and believe me we will. You will be having enormous orgasms and you will be over the stars and the moon and me I hope. Crazy! Stop punishing him, can't you still see it? Your still clinging on to the past, unless he truly loved you would he be there still? No he would not. You deceived him, cheated and then used what ever he had done, how ever bad as an excuse for that infidelity and then blamed him again from what I have heard. He is divorcing his wife and you still punish him. For god sake nat grow up. I love you and I will fall in love with you ..but please don't blind your self though the real truth..people kill each other when they our together for all sorts of reasons and do the most terrible things but still love each other and then find reasons to drop their knickers or pants to someone else...but the only real reason was they wanted to. It's because they can't face the guilt blame there partner. time to stop running nat, he has faced up to the truth so must you forget the past everything. Fuck his brains out, take a chance. Swim you don't need the rocks and then when you have enjoyed it, loved it, gone crazy on it and thought about it...Come to me or stay with him. Yes she has a woman's body but she is a little girl,,, you are slim but you are a woman a..women..a women a 100%! Ask billy as you said he's the best lover ever and he has 100% red hot blood in his veins who would he rather be with you and has over nine years. Stop it nat. Stop putting yourself down. Your a woman be proud of it and strong. Make the strong decision don't be a coward and run any more. Love him, enjoy him and watch the change in him and yourself. Watch him respect you and want to make you happy in what ever you do in the future. My friend told me that his friend said that all his ex's love him and admire him and some would like him back. What can you read from that? His pretty oriental wife would forgive him anything. Think Natasha. What it tells you is that they all respect him. Now nothing about your upbringing or your roll models. I told you at the start what you give out you get back. Give love, forgiveness and respect and you will get it back. Now go to bed you bad girl or john will spank you when he gets his hands on you xxxxxxxxx john x Be kind to Billy and yourself...???? and mean it not act it xxxxxxxxxxxxxxx

From: Natasha <natasha_nw3@yahoo.co.uk>
Date: 7 April 10:18:31 BDT
To: john smith <appledogstime@yahoo.co.uk>
Subject: Re: I don't believe that I have him pretty well thought out
Dear John,
You have hit it in one. Mean it, not act it. That is what I would hate to do, act it as Billy is the only man I have never and I mean never acted anything. John I am sorry to say that you don't know the whole story about me and Billy the infidelity wasn't only from my side. So you understand it clearly I wasn't the only one who was unfaithful and I don't hate the wife. Especially you. About the lovely Ruth. I wasn't putting my self down at all. My body is what it is and I am very happy with it and have been for a very long time I wish it wouldn't fall a part but that is a different story. I abused it and this is the result. I was merely commenting on the contrast between our body shapes that is all. She looks a very happy and jolly person. I believe that my body is beautiful, most woman would give their right arm for what I have so I thank God every day for what he gave me I don't complain about it, far from it. And Yes we will give him credit for that as well - if you are told every day hundred times that you are a goddess after a while you don't doubt it. You write that I am clinging to the past - yes that is true my past is the only certain thing in my life for now. But I am also trying to move on form the past and I have been together with Billy and my father. Maybe not as fast as you would like me to but hay who is counting. I am not in a rush like you seem to be. I have came a long way and do have problems but for the first time in my life I am prepared to tackle them head on and not run away form them. And I am

admitting it in writing. So give me a break John. I had a call from my father last night as I was writing you an E-mail. And we seem to be getting on OK. but my dad and I that is another can of worms as you know only too well. I will not go in to it now. These decisions are mine to make and I am pleased about it in the past I would have been scared witless to make even the simplest decision. Not any more after all I will have to live with them after I make them without having somebody to blame that they made the wrong decisions for me. Don't work too hard Lovely John Nat x

From: john smith <appledogstime@yahoo.co.uk>
Date: 7 April 11:30:08 BDT
To: Natasha <natasha_nw3@yahoo.co.uk>
Subject: Ruth also says…

Hey met Ruth and we talked of you. From today till Tuesday I'm working till 12 midnight everyday. She says she will be in Sainsbury's on sat at two thirty shopping. Yes she said same as me... it's not Billy it's yourself you are running from. If you want to be with Billy or me what your friends or family or anyone thinks is not their business. Tell them to fuck off. It's what you feel and you must get rid of all that guilt and baggage or you will carry it with you the rest of your life into every love you have and destroy them all .you must erase the past now. Mean while I will be so bored and lonely with out you come on girly help a man out. Seduce me one night and tell me where and how is it inside or out in a car or a bed. Where? How? You will drive me insane thinking all day of you John xxx

From: john smith <appledogstime@yahoo.co.uk>
Date: 7 April 11:55:17 BDT
To: Natasha <natasha_nw3@yahoo.co.uk>
Subject: We both really hope you get yourself together soon...

We also hope that Billy really likes ruth. Ruth said that when I go off with you she may never marry. So billy would make a good lover so she really hopes he fancies her and starts to lust. Since the holiday she got quite big as she was so desperately unhappy. She lost 20 pounds, 12 kilos. These were taken on ruths new camera top of the range to impress billy. She went and spent a lot of money on it. We set it up on a tripod. I can't wait to go out with you..hold your hand take you every where with me just want to start again now. Sad but that's life. Tell billy she will make him happy, she is so sweet but he may have to teach her a few things. I have agreed with her. I won't jump the gun or even though I dream of you every night and think of you all the time and wake up with a big hard on for you. Ruth has come to terms with it now but if you will let her have billy she says it wont be so bad. We can meet up some times say twice a month all of us. I'm keeping my promise..but sorry a lot of people no you both. Any way hope billy likes ruth and you the latest of me xxx John

From: john smith <appledogstime@yahoo.co.uk>
Date: 8 April 02:29:05 BDT
To: Natasha <natasha_nw3@yahoo.co.uk>
Subject: I am so sorry but I have to express my feelings for you...
Two in the morning have to leave home at six what can I do..what shall we both do...out of my mind. By the way its not circumcised it just came out like that with the skin pulled back tight. Darling Natasha my love, my life, my everything what shall I do I want you so much. I promised Ruth so can't let her down but as I lay on this bed you are fifteen mins away. God I want to come to you. This will be the longest three months of my life. I borrowed her super new camera. Still hopeless but looking at you makes me even bigger. No woman has got me as hot as you ever 22 cm long X 15 cm round. But I know you can take it, I will have to be sweet and gentle with you at first and get you very excited and then you will take it easy my darling sweet Nat it's killing me from my bed in st johns wood, Maida Vale to you my wonderful girl...o goddddddddddddddddddddddddddddd give me you wonderful pussy and lips and belly I want my mouth on your tits.

April

From: Natasha <natasha_nw3@yahoo.co.uk>
Date: 8 April 09:23:16 BDT
To: john smith <appledogstime@yahoo.co.uk>
Subject: No one is to blame so that is nonsense
Dear John
Here I go again writing to you after I have take my daily allowance of pills. I feel like a very different person. I also enjoyed the photo of you. You have the perfect body my lovely John, I have been looking at male models for a very long time and you are a perfectionist. Do me one big favour John when you get home form work at two o'clock in the morning please go straight to bed don't write me E-mails. I don't want you to have an accident at work or out of work because you are so tired. I am not going to comment on the last picture you have sent me (maybe I am - glad you are intact as I have not got a clue what to do with cut willies and that is even after all the men I have been with) You are a big and impressive boy but this is like unwrapping a Christmas present in October. You didn't think I was going to be easy did you? And do what I am told straight away without kicking up fuss. I will but it takes me a bit of time. So don't get shifty with me or I will have to make a complaint about you doctor, and you will get your hand slapped.
Hope you are OK my dear over worked John Kiss Nxx

From: john smith <appledogstime@yahoo.co.uk>
Date: 8 April 11:54:38 BDT
To: Natasha <natasha_nw3@yahoo.co.uk>
Subject: Thank you
Dearest Natasha thank you for nice things you say yes sorry about last pick ..but you do drive a man wild and yes I am normal in every way ha ha! Not like ruths lot. Sorry about the drugs and the low libido. I understand hope you get well soon and feel better. The letters may be a bit not to often for the next few days its crazy here till wed and then Thursday I go to my parents for a few days. So you to wonderful woman will miss out on my love and lust. Sorry as it's Easter my parents are quite good at the church bit and go say once a month. Anyway they believe as deep inside I do as well. What else is

there? The thought of nothing is not to much fun like the idea of spending 50 years with you and then eternity as angels. May be a bit over the top but what the hell it's better then nothing. Anyway you get well soon. Get billy to take good care of you and ruth as well if he wants to pop round to broadhurst mansions broadhurst gardens, west hampstead. She would love to see you both as she and the family don't celebrate easter. Naturally as they put him up there...not easy all this. Not a good time for Christians and Jews. O by the way my life, already my life, yes there won't be a charge to you my beauty as you said of billy. Goddesses get every thing free XXX love, Please take care of yourself, lots of care... John x

From: john smith <appledogstime@yahoo.co.uk>
Date: 8 April 18:07:04 BDT
To: Natasha <natasha_nw3@yahoo.co.uk>
Subject: Just a note to say

Yes you can make love to Billy the normal way and every thing will be fine. You can go on holiday together all those things… .but you must do the heightened awareness exercise first to get rid of all guilt and bad feeling as well as to increase your body to tactile sensitivity and
to clear out old blockages mental and body wise. Your body will then give you 100 times more pleasure. You will enjoy sex much more and you will start to get for the fist time deep virginal orgasms. 1. Three hours of foreplay and deep sex. 2 Dark, dark room and your self blindfold or mask so you see nothing. 3. No talking. 4. Everything touch and feel and smell. 5. Billy must make love to you each time twice. Billy must not stay the night for the ten times. You must be left alone with your body feelings to get used to. You must phone billy before he visits you to tell him what's expected of him. Be discreet if you need to. Tell him it's something you want to do and have been thinking about a long time. He must not talk. He can see you but in a perfect world you should not see him...door of bedroom left open for him to get in...he will enter and close door, black dark room and you dressed sexy to turn him on.

April

Men are more visual then women. White panties, bra black, stockings, high heels, tiny mini dress he slowly comes in to the room, you stand to greet him and start foreplay. Feel. Touch etc etc. He removes your dress..say 15 mins then bra ten mins then panties down. still standing kissing, touching etc....he goes down to you. You still have stockings and heels on. Then he picks you up. If he forgets you prompt him. No talking. Just arms around his neck..carries you to bed then spread your legs wide in the dark. He can see, you can't but not much as it's dark...then if he can bring you off...then he shags you hard, deep and slow with pillow etc. He comes then one hour of touching, playing, kissing feeling. You then go down to him now, make him hard and you can sit on him, suck him off but he has to shag you a little for a second time. Important... first time as well you. Sit on him first.. you must control everything..for all the ten times and he must submit to your wants and follow you.each time you must make him come twice if you can.... then one last hour of cuddles touch, hold play. Then send him home. Each time you do the exercise the feelings in your body and pussy will get stronger and the feelings of
guilt and hate and anger will go as well. What will be left will be deep love for your self and billy. You can change the sinario a little each time but don't rush it take your times both of you. You can do everything and anything, nothing is taboo. If you feel ok for it and even if you can't see anything still set the pace. Direct him by touch..bottom up in the air etc. On your back legs over his arms etc. He must submit to you, do what you want in the darkness. Good luck darling Natasha. My next break 12 tonight for thirty mins then home at one thirty..... XXXXXXX John

From: john smith <appledogstime@yahoo.co.uk>
Date: 8 April 19:44:18 BDT
To: Natasha <natasha_nw3@yahoo.co.uk>
Subject: Love...
I love you because you are intelligent as well as beautiful, clever and smart. Everything I ever wanted in a woman I can't say any more then that to you and a bonus. Yes you really

turn me on, your long slim legs, you have a sexy body, your great face and the bottom out of this world and your clever. I worked as a male model for six months when I left Uni. Joined a London agency for a short time, it was fun. You are also so sweet, the things you say. You were meant for me. Yes, yes we will have a long and happy life and you have some good friends..billy etc and you will meet all my friends and family. I just know we were meant for each other. O.k. said it now that's it? xxxx John

From: Natasha <natasha_nw3@yahoo.co.uk>
Date: 8 April 20:46:02 BDT
To: john smith <appledogstime@yahoo.co.uk>
Subject: Re: Some things are meant to be.....

Dear John
Yes you sound lovely too. Suppose you are most of the things I would look for in a man, from what I know of you from your writing. You sound that you know what you want, you are kind, honest, hard working and very lovable. Probably a bit impatient which might prove a problem as I am very, very spoilt and normally get away with murder with Billy. Actually after I split up from Billy I looked forward to my freedom which I never had in my life. Billy spoils me rotten, but I do not shag around as you might think but just to do what I wanted, go where I wanted and meet who ever I wanted, get home at what ever time and not be answerable to anybody just my self and not to be questioned about everything. Had it not been for my illness now I don't think we would get as close as we are now ever again. Though I am glad we did in a funny sort of way he is, my best friend, and my best lover ever, no doubt. John you told Ruth that we met on a chat line and to your colleagues at work that we met out walking… how do you propose those two stories go together? I have not told anybody for this reason so you had better tell me what you want to do about it? People do talk and if the stories don't match they will ask. My friends know that I wouldn't be seen dead on a chat line but I can't really tell them that I already met you because that is not true. I don't really like telling lies

but we will have to be careful about this. And for the first time I am dying to tell somebody about you, not just Billy. But I have kept him up to date so far. If only to stop my friends arranging blind dates for me with their male unmarried friends. Two of them have been very persistent since Christmas though now I am not well & it works as a perfect excuse. What is the breed of your dog I don't want to know the name though please. Maybe you should reserve your judgement whether you want to spend the rest of your life with me after you meet me. You might have some very annoying habits like wanking over the bed and the floor in my absence which I will not like and that means I would not be able to be with you. You're putting too much pressure on everything unnecessarily. I can't believe this is happening and probably won't until we meet later in the year.
Love Natasha xx

From: john smith <appledogstime@yahoo.co.uk>
Date: 8 April 23:03:19 BDT
To: Natasha <natasha_nw3@yahoo.co.uk>
Subject: Re: Some things are meant to be.....

Easy. We both did meet on a chat line and it was both our first time. I told you I walk every morning on primrose hill and one day I saw you and you saw me. I asked you if you were Natasha and you said yes and I said I was John and we went from there ..start telling all your friends about me..I don't want any of them lining up any boys for you or any one else except billy. I told you that at the start..your mine and I am going to make you mine and I always get what I go after. I also don't blame bill keeping you on a tight leash. Sorry I would too, I'm very hot with the women I love. Want to be with her and love her and that means yes the green goddess..Jealousy..yes i am very sorry hope you can forgive my one big fault..but if you really love somebody you feel it strongly. If you don't feel it you don't love them end of story. So you might finish with me now before we meet but I promised you to be always truthful. So yes I am jealous..did you expect anything else if a man loves you and wants you? So well done billy? So to put it

in the most polite terms tell your friends as regards to matchmaking... fuck off!! I am in love with you and the min we hit the end of july or august your in my arms. God billy has had to watch his back. If your friends start lining up new partners for you the min he has walked out the door after nine years how nice is that of them? Thank god Ruth likes him. I would not do that to any man and not a fellow Irish man. Yes us Irish look after our women in every way and we don't take to kindly to other men chatting them up. Normal, if you love. I can see a few men might have a black eye or two before I get you in to church my pretty one..Mean while it's eleven and I won't to go home to sleep...where is my story of how I get your knickers down and you seduce me and get my kit off and jump all over me? I'm desperate for you and to hear the words from you sexy mouth telling me what you will do to me in detail my treasure. My own dear sweet girly Natasha kisssssssss hot
xxxJohn

From: john smith <appledogstime@yahoo.co.uk>
Date: 8 April 23:15:15 BDT
To: Natasha <natasha_nw3@yahoo.co.uk>
Subject: Not rushing your own time scale, three to four months.

You said it darling
Sorry he is a full grown Afghan hound, standing nearly three feet high on his legs. His name is apple..as we both love him to bits and both want to munch him. By the way my friend at works sister had your problem...and her libido went for three months but the national health gave her an implant. Took ten mins only and she got really horny and better at the same time..you should consider it. Ask your consultant, tell him your boyfriend is suffering xxxx John X As you said your really missing it now.

April

From: Natasha <natasha_nw3@yahoo.co.uk>
Date: 8 April 23:38:21 BDT
To: john smith <appledogstime@yahoo.co.uk>
Subject: Re: Not rushing your own time scale, three to four months.You said it darling

Darling John Boy,
So he is a big boy like his daddy is, who I have heard some strange stories about. Big dogs and little girls like Ruth. But with you around, I don't think that's needed. Yes, with all this talk from you it is starting to make my libido work, and I'm getting quite horny.
Also, it is spring. Billy is very loving and romantic. Flowers, chocolate, etc... and tells me he loves me ten times a day. Too much of a good thing, but still nice. I have been doing a lot of D-I-Y. Very nice N xxxxxx
From: Natasha <natasha_nw3@yahoo.co.uk>
Date: 9 April 00:32:45 BDT
To: john smith <appledogstime@yahoo.co.uk>
Subject: I have thought long and hard about your last three e-mails

Darling boy,
John, I have thought a long time and have now finally plucked up the courage to set the date for the exercise on the 21st of April. I am very apprehensive and nervous at putting the relationship on this basis again. We have been playing a lot lately, kissing, touching... and that was nice. I have to admit, my womanly bits do miss the loving and don't get me wrong. Billy is a wonderful lover when he is on form, and we have had some of the best sex ever together. I do love him so very much... but I don't know what the future holds for us both.
Hope you are not working too hard. Don't be too hard on little Ruth.
Natasha xxx

April

From: john smith <appledogstime@yahoo.co.uk>
Date: 9 April 01:17:14 BDT
To: Natasha <natasha_nw3@yahoo.co.uk>
Subject: Home worn out up at six
Hard night..you make your self hard to be loved . I love you already. I try to be a good person and be kind and fair to everyone so I have a lot of friends .I fell in love with you. I did not want to fall for anybody as I split from Ruth then I saw you my heart skip ten beats. Some of the things you say are very hard still. Natasha my darling you have to get rid of all the hatred you have in you. I don't know what sort of life you will have otherwise... and you don't seem to see it in yourself and all these men round the honey pot still. After coming out of nine years with somebody it's not healthy. Like I said before, you're not desperate to love your self. I want you to meet my sister and family in September...but I take one step forward and two back... Hope this is not a game for you… I'm very serious. Tell me to fuck off and I wont write again??? May I ask who the other fellows are? Hope you are being truthful now x John

From: Natasha <natasha_nw3@yahoo.co.uk>
Date: 9 April 08:56:20 BDT
To: john smith <appledogstime@yahoo.co.uk>
Subject: Friends and introductions

Darling John,
They are friends of my friends who I have been putting off meeting for ages and haven't met as yet. I have no desire to meet them let alone go out with them never have and never will, you and billy are very safe. So please don't make a big thing of it as it is highly insignificant. Billy knows all about it and knows that I have no interest in these people in any imaginable way. Contrary to popular believe I do tell him everything. If this helps: both my girlfriends were told while I was in the hospital exactly that. That I have no intention of meeting or going out with their male friends and I can't believe that I am writing this to you. Would I be making such a big thing of meeting you If I wanted to go out with somebody? I

don't want to go out with A Man my girly friends think will be good for me - I want to go out with the right man one day but for now I am happy the way I am with you writing to me and with Billy here. I hope this is sufficient as an explanation. You will have to start trusting me dear John this works both ways I know that my past is not the best but you will have to take a chance or get out. I will not be doing this too many times. Trying to explain my self I value fidelity as highly as you but we can't separate ourselves from the world and my well meaning girlfriends. There is just two of them, unless you and me live on a deserted island or you lock me up. Billy tried that and it didn't work. I am difficult to love, I will go with that. I am a difficult person to love but Billy works on it really hard and I work very hard to make myself more loveable, affectionate and warm. But I think you know I am a difficult person, but you know that by now. If you don't you better wise up quickly! But I am working on it…
Love Natasha xx

From: john smith <appledogstime@yahoo.co.uk>
Date: 9 April 10:41:51 BDT
To: Natasha <natasha_nw3@yahoo.co.uk>
Subject: At my office desk ten forty one

Dearest darling Natasha my sweet little girl which you still are in some ways. Very mature in one way, a girl in another. Yes I went to a special school till I was ten years old in Liverpool. I was dyslexic so yes it's strange, weird and yet normal. He may be as well. He is part Irish and lots of Irish kids are. He is an Artist, I understand that Sir Richard Branson is also but I don't know how bad he has it. It only happens with me when I write very fast. The picture and you are just stunning, out of this world. Would he photograph Ruth for me? I would pay him handsomely for it. You are truly beautiful, a wonderful girl, much better then in the nude photographs from the old site which we will not think about...it's forgotten. That world is left far behind. In this picture billy has achieved that, he has made you into a dream girl. Something beyond flesh and blood. A wonderful dream that all men want and desire. He has brought out all the best and sweetest part of you in one click of the shutter. God the man is a true artist in every way. People will talk of his work when we are all dead and in a better world then this but they will talk of you as well. He has immortalised you for posterity. You look wonderful. I will get a print made and put it on my desk and hang it in my flat. Two large prints as it will go. You should get the implant, as it will bring about normality to you life. Everything balanced. My friend is next to me now at work and he thinks it's important. Ruth would love a picture like that! She would hang it in her nail bar and beauty saloon that she runs on the finchley rd. She has five girls who work for her....very busy my darling drop you a line soon. Till then X john X love yourself X

From: john smith <appledogstime@yahoo.co.uk>
Date: 9 April 19:02:00 BDT
To: Natasha <natasha_nw3@yahoo.co.uk>
Subject: Re: At my office desk ten forty one

Hi darling, nice to hear from you. Sorry you wont hear so much from me till after Easter. Working so hard but love you and want you very much to hold, touch and make happy. Get the print made by all means but save it for me to be framed. Give it two me the morning after I give you your first big orgasm. No gain with out strain. Every reward I
believe should be worked for, so I will work hard to give you the big O and you present me with the picture. These will go up to 6x4 easy just right for my desk at work and my bedside table. I have long gaps tonight on the Tokyo exchange... I will book air tickets for New York for the two of us for sat 10th October. No work people, just you and me so as there is no pressure on you darling as you are still a little fragile. Get better soon, bye kissessss x John
P.S. Mean while I come in to your bedroom, I'm naked apart from my jeans and calvins. You are in a tiny white G string, panties, bra, stockings and heels. You greet me, it's a hot, hot august night...What happens then ???

April

From: Natasha <natasha_nw3@yahoo.co.uk>
Date: 9 April 23:49:35 BDT
To: john smith <appledogstime@yahoo.co.uk>
Subject: Re: At my office desk ten forty one

Dearest John,

I am sorry there are no tangible rewards for you giving me my first orgasm, the only reward will be a warm feeling next to your big heart and the knowledge that I have been waiting for that day for a very long time, knowing that it just needs the right time, right place and the right man. Will you be as magic as you are promising to be? Will we live up to each other's expectations? Well let's just see. So no pressure there.
I know that I do go on a bit about it but your schedules do make apprehensive and this year is to contain as little stress as possible for me (I promised myself) in theory that was the general idea at the beginning. That if anything does causes stress I will get rid of it ASAP. I have been trying to please too many people far too longer time without any consideration for my self as long as the world around me was happy. This probably sounds selfish and somewhat self obsessed but I can no longer do that.
There has to be balance which I struggle to find. My last year was one of the worst and I believe I am now paying for it with my health. Having said all that I do want to meet you my dear John, I am just not sure if I can keep to your plan, sure as anything I will not be providing an
alternative one either. I am probably just not very good with timetables. Good job you are because somebody has to make them. I had a feeling that there was something not right about the exercise, how did you call it? Body awareness? Glad you have consulted the clever books. Do
I tell him where the idea for this exercise originated and the reason for it, because sure as anything he will ask. I will tell you my worries about all this, as I said, after the break up I did push him away until the time he took me home from the hospital. Since then he has been here every day and was with me when I was in the hospital. He would come over whether I

wanted or not and he would not take no for an answer. Please do not think that I am a little ungrateful...I do appreciate what he is doing for me, am aware of the time and effort put into. I will get close to him again and that scares me beyond belief, and that is the healthy bit of me. I love him - I can't live with him but I am afraid that I can't live without him either.. which is nonsense as I clearly can live without him. I am probably too tired and boring you to death with all this but these are my worries about the whole thing. I can't imagine how you must be feeling working for so long. How often do you work these hours? Is there a schedule of long and short hours you follow or is it random? I couldn't do that if I don't sleep, I don't function properly. Hope you are Ok
Kiss Natasha xx

From: Natasha <natasha_nw3@yahoo.co.uk>
Date: 10 April 00:24:28 BDT
To: john smith <appledogstime@yahoo.co.uk>
Subject: Re: Thinking of you it's 23.17. I'm on my own in the office at my computer looking at your computer

My darling john I did feel the cold desk under my bum, the cold air from the air-conditioning on my legs as I spread them wide for you, will anybody come in? Will we be caught? After all this is your office. My skirt is around my waist your hand caresses my thighs, the ends of my stocking slowly moves to where my panties are supposed to be. Instead your fingers feel the warmth of my sweet thick cream, you spread my pussy lips gently with your finger feeling from my hard love mount. You look so smart in your black work suit but you are so excited by now your trousers are about to burst. I stroke them at the highest point, you are so hard I release the button then the zip, black pants extending even further in to the mid air, I reach inside..it is so hot, your heart beats as fast as mine, you are hard and silky soft I am slow and taking my time caressing your hard cock and soft but tightening balls. You are so perfect the shape the length. Suddenly you interrupt me, the feelings are too strong to bare and you do want to fuck me here and now. You are in me, it happened so

fast, I am full of you so wet so excited I wanted you so much. You are moving fast, the feeling is getting stronger, I feel you getting bigger and harder and one more thrust and you are there - you shoot your load. You have done it so many times before... I am not as dead as I thought I was, I did feel you moving inside me when I read it. I do wish you were here I feel. I am wet and excited, my pussy is tingling with excitement for the past twenty minutes. It has been such a long time I just need a tender touch...
Natasha xxxxxxxxxxxxxxxxxxxxxxxxxxxxx

From: Natasha <natasha_nw3@yahoo.co.uk>
Date: 10 April 00:35:43 BDT
To: john smith <appledogstime@yahoo.co.uk>
Subject: Re: I'm on my own in my bedroom feeling horny for you

Just thought I tell you again..I am so so wet you have done it my friend. Wet war, slippery, tingly and taste sweet and delicious. Oh I do wish you were doing the tasting with me. Your mouth is what I need just now, the tender warm touch...Just thought you might like to know that my man.

Nxx

From: john smith <appledogstime@yahoo.co.uk>
Date: 10 April 08:55:39 BDT
To: Natasha <natasha_nw3@yahoo.co.uk>
Subject: Wonderful summer days and very hot summer nights walks the woods

My darling nat you worry to much. Do you think life is any different for me? Do I live somewhere else... no. Life is about growing and maturing, braking up and getting back on a stronger and healthier footing. With Ruth and myself it's the same. I lost my mind, drunk every night, crashed the car, went mad with bitter, bitter loneliness. But here we both are three months down the road making love once a week but good, good friends and always will be and you really don't

know if you can live with billy. People change all the time learn from their mistakes and if it works out between us and I want it to, you will leave his arms for mine and hopefully in a perfect world he will leave yours for little girl Ruth's. She is resigned to it and has no one else but is making the most of the moments. I'm sure deep down he is too. Think... he has had a lot of beautiful women in his life, he has been through it before and look what a man he has grown into. Breaking up and moving on makes you grow up, so let's be truthful and grow up. You might want to stay with him and the exercise to free yourself can only help whether you do it or not for someone else. You might hate me when you meet me. My god almighty have I really been here. For three hours already, nine already seems like a life time. Forget the past, give yourself to him total and enjoy your life till we become lovers. Which I long for more and more each day..walks in the woods in the summer, sun shining, holding your hand..the sunlight in your long blond hair, a pretty summer dress, a blanket in the corn fields, a basket of food and wine. A hot summers night..we make love in the corn field and we go home to dream of where we made the baby and if she is a little girl who is as pretty as her mother. Kiss my darling, free yourself my baby. Love from all that rubbish when you do it. Have fun, enjoy it, throw yourself into it as I do with Ruth. Lets not waist our lives in regret. Love the one you are with and when we are together love me and hope forever. Yes it's a time table but I want to have SOME summer with you darling so get your act and your little knickers together and make a start.
Kiss x John..Fuck back to work I'm late for the New York call!
Thinking of you xxxxx

From: john smith <appledogstime@yahoo.co.uk>
Date: 10 April 09:31:23 BDT
To: Natasha <natasha_nw3@yahoo.co.uk>
Subject: O my god!!

O my darling that's it! I am so much in lust and love for you. Fuck you finished me darling that was the most sexy letter I ever had in my life. God I want you! Want, want want you so

much. Love you, adore you, I had to go to the toilet fifteen mins ago after opening your email. Can't
work! What have you done to me? You are driving me mad!! God send me one a week till we meet you wonder crazy girl. I love you so much. Girl of my dreams. I have to send you a picture sorry but have to remember the moment with you for the rest of our lives .when you sent me our first fantasy together. Will think of you when I fuck Ruth till we meet. Came in ten mins, fastest ever for me with your print out on Ruth's camera. Darling Natasha that was truly wonderful. See you can be a sexy lady when you want to be. I am a sexy man and now I know deep down you are one hell of a sexy woman when you want to be. Will take your email to Liverpool with me darling. Love you lots and lots. I will remember that wank and you for the rest of my life. That would have made you a lot of babies if that had been in you darling and soon it will..four months will fly by. You will see..kiss my darling. The first shot is before I opened it in the toilet, the second as I started to read it. After that I had to forget the camera and think of you. One million kisses darling X John

From: Natasha <natasha_nw3@yahoo.co.uk>
Date: 10 April 09:51:15 BDT
To: john smith <appledogstime@yahoo.co.uk>
Subject: john sex and me

Dearest sex obsessed John

Well that was a pretty mediocre letter I sent you last night at least by my standards. But I am glad that it had the desired effect. You sure are an impressive boy and rightly proud of it if your employers just knew what you get up to. I am sure that they see right through you. My eyes water just looking at you and you tell me that you can last as well (though I never doubted your powers). I am worried my walking abilities will be seriously affected after a passionate night with you.

Love Natasha xx

April

From: john smith <appledogstime@yahoo.co.uk>
Date: 10 April 09:52:02 BDT
To: Natasha <natasha_nw3@yahoo.co.uk>
Subject: Natasha

I wish you were mine my sweet girly woman everything. Darling don't be frustrated. Darling please enjoy it with him for me, yourself and him..I can not lie to you, I have great sex with Ruth. I would be crazy to tell you otherwise. You go have great great sex with him. Love him, enjoy him, have fun with him and if it works out with us darling have a good, good friend for life. God I'm reading it again..this has cost me £2000 in lost shares all ready but your worth every penny. Have to go toilet again, that's not bad even if I say so myself. 30mins with your help and he is up again, thinking of you. Your name is on my cock in pen biro, wrote it on there last night. Here I go again for another quick one on you..then back to boring work. Kiss x I want you sweet loving, kind, hot and horny for me..you can't be horny enough for me. I want it to last till we are both old like my mum and dad xxx john

From: Natasha <natasha_nw3@yahoo.co.uk>
Date: 10 April 09:53:36 BDT
To: john smith <appledogstime@yahoo.co.uk>
Subject: Re: Goldmans toilets, you and me, our first fantasy

Yes John
I did get the pictures the first time, only in the opposite order. Too much of a good thing..you know what they say ... they were all cock and body shots. Have still not got a picture of your face.
Natasha xx

From: Natasha <natasha_nw3@yahoo.co.uk>
Date: 10 April 10:01:54 BDT
To: john smith <appledogstime@yahoo.co.uk>
Subject: Get down to work man!
I am not sending you any more E-mails. Get down to some work and stop thinking of me. You will get the sack and

this is the wrong kind of sack. Meaning you will loose your job if you carry on like this. So no more trips to the gents and work Mr Smith for you..while I go back to bed. Sorry about that but at least one of us has to work to keep the babies in nappies.
Kisses and hugs Natasha xx

From: Natasha <natasha_nw3@yahoo.co.uk>
Date: 10 April 10:23:34 BDT
To: john smith <appledogstime@yahoo.co.uk>
Subject: you are a healthy male of thirty!
There is no point regretting. If I do or when I do I will try my best. I believe in doing things properly not just half way so there is no problem there. No more letters for you till the evening my sweet boy.
Love Natasha xx

Poem from Natasha, thinking of John and Billy at the same time

What a combination
That would make for me
Two strong men
For all the world to see
One young and handsome
The other as crazy as can be
Eyes of blue
That show me all I want to see
Hope my love is strong enough
To keep you both happy all the time
But I know that you must see
All the things you mean to me
Darlings
You're both the closest thing to love, I ever knew
A day apart, you miss me too
Funny
I didn't write or phone you- Am I still in love?

April

Monday 10th April

It was 12:30 in the morning when I got the call from her. Everything suddenly sounded very different. She said to me, 'I feel good! I feel great! Can you come over and spend some time with me? I'd like you to stay late if you could... don't leave before 11 o clock if you don't have to. I need to be held. That's all I need to say...'

I got to her house at 2:30. She had just finished her morning job. She opened the front door and ran up the stairs before me. When we got into the bedroom, she had already made some soup and lentils, which she served up in two big bowls. She was in an exceptionally good mood, and more than a little frisky. She was even flirting with me. As I entered her bedroom, come kitchen, come sitting room all in one, everything was neat and beautifully arranged. She kept her room absolutely spotless. She was warm, very cosy, relaxed, and very satisfied with herself. She looked like she had fallen madly in love, and it felt that way too, but obviously not with me! Maybe somebody on the internet...

There was a framed painting on the wall that I had done for her. A pencil and charcoal sketch, and as you entered the room there was a beautiful picture of her in front of you. I had turned her into the Mona Lisa. It was a masterpiece

Her blinds were down and a lamp on the bedside chest of drawers lit the room with a yellow tinge. She kept her pills in the top draw, her little bras, and sexy little knickers in the middle drawer, her condoms and anything to do with sex in the bottom drawer.

The bed was covered in a beautiful handmade patchwork quilt, with matching pillows, which I had given her a couple of years before, from a photo shoot I had done. To the right of the bed was her huge wardrobe filled with all her clothes, all neatly folded like the shelves in an upmarket woman's clothes shop, and after that as you looked round, three large windows, with pure white Venetian blinds.

She flirted and teased with me. She was in a very strange mood.

'You're not fucking me yet.' She said, 'I need to keep my

sanity. But you may join me on the bed when you take off you jeans which are covered in cat hairs. And if you are a good boy, I will let you take me for a long walk after.'

'After what?' I said.

'Whatever!' she said, mimicking the hideous Vicky Pollard from the television program, Little Britain.

I threw my jeans in the corner of the room and I was wearing me real tight black pants, and the bulge in them was getting enormous by expectation, and they could hardly contain the excitement I felt.

'Well' she said with a cheeky look on her face. 'You look fine in the black pants inside and out.'

Under extreme pressure they were starting to look like a tent. She reached her hand out and ran a finger around the thick circumference and shape of the bulge. The other hand she pushed up the front my black t-shirt. She does not do that very often as she hates to see my little tummy.

'Wow! And another wow! Something has got her really hot for the first time in ages. She loves to be in control. She was starting to drive me crazy, with the beautiful captivating feelings that her soft touch gave me. I held my breath. This was all so unexpected. After the cold feeling that had existed over the last 4 months, and I was worried that it was still not too far away.

The fingers of one hand drifted up to my face, and the other hand started to play with my nipples and chest hairs. She was using both hands to caress my body now. She mimicked some sort of film star, or some little girl from a show and said, 'You know? You would be a really nice man, if you weren't so silly, jealous and possessive. I could make love to you and enjoy it much more often. But you get to silly and uptight all the time. If I just go to visit a man-friend, what's wrong with that? You meet beautiful women every day!'

I mumbled under my breath. 'Yes but that's my work! But all the men you meet want to fuck you! In fact every man you seem to meet wants to fuck you.'

'Yes but that doesn't mean I will let them.' She whispered, 'I don't need my head done in anymore, I was so ill after the last time. You silly man. Come here…' she said as she started to remove her jeans. She laid on the bed in tiny pink thong knickers with the word 'KISS' low down on the front. She wore just a light blue skimpy top.

I fixed my eyes on her nipples that were rock hard underneath. It felt strange being on the bed like this at 3 o clock in the afternoon, and the strange way she was acting today. Was she going to let the raging animal inside my pants escape? His head was peaking over the top of them now, and was starting to push the elastic to one side.

I was on the bed. I pushed her ankles apart with my foot, and run my hands down her slinky bottom, squeezing them roughly.

'Hey!' she shouted, 'Slow down!' as she gave m e a long lingering kiss.

What the fuck has got into her? I thought to myself. I let my eyes devour the banquet of her beautiful body. I was so greedy for her, she always managed to excite me so much since the first time I saw her. I ran my fingers down her curves of her waist, her hips and then up over her tits, and this time she let me.

She is so fucking hot, I really don't know what to touch first. I was so excited I tried to devour her. I felt so much passion. My tongue lashed the inside of her mouth, as she pushed herself hard up against me for a deep thrusting kiss. I felt her body pressing harder and harder, her hands squeezing my cock on the outside of my pants. Her other hand was holding my bottom.

I could feel the muscles in my ass wanting to pump her. She moaned and groaned as my fingers reach her clit which is wet and slippery. She touched her own breasts and looked at me with large eyes.

'No fuck!' She says, she is really aroused now. My fingers are playing and teasing with her and she is doing the same with me

She has this wonderful trick which she has perfected, where she pulls a man's balls them in a very special way. It is really clever and really beautiful and sexually stimulating at the same time.

She is really working on my cock now. She makes him think, and he is beginning to think that he is 25 years old again. Our fingers and hands are paying with each other, and her other hand is working like mad to try to make me come, and I could feel she was getting excited as well and almost on the edge.

My cock is brick hard as it is caught between her thigh and

her hand that is holding me. I am completely captivated, addicted and unstoppable. My sperms were running a marathon inside my balls, itching to get out, and she cannot contain her excitement either. She was starting to shout now and crying out as my fingers were still pushing. Tap, tap, push, push, on her wet clit. As I start to work on her tummy and tits, her tiny tank top pulled up to her neck.

I was covered in her as well. We both looked into each others' eyes as we came together, and it was one of the largest we'd ever had. To used an old expression, the Earth certainly did move today.

Her eyes bore into me, she seemed to be searching my soul.

'That was wonderful that was well worth waiting for… I will run a bath for both of us.'

And she did, and it was really nice, all soapy suds, right up to the top. We were both squeezed into the tiny bath together. She delighted and enjoyed soaping my hard cock in the bath. It was one of her favourite delights, and delightful it was. I soaped her tits as well, and her nipples, and I was starting to get hard again. Sometimes in the past, my cock all full of soap, and her pussy too, we would slip into each other and fuck in the bath, and when we got out the bath would be empty, and the soapy water all over the floor.

Anyway this time she was in a real special mood and brought me off again, and then we dried off and had some of her chick soup, and I had to keep my promise of a long walk. She took my arm, and we walked all the way to Belsize Village.

'This has been a really nice day,' she said, as we came full circle back to her place. I looked at her closely. So many secrets inside her head always.

Why? I said to myself, why? She read my thoughts as usual.

'Oh my internet friend got me horny,' she said, 'He really got me turned on.'

'Did you think of him when I was wanking you?' I asked

'Too much information,' she said, 'Too much. That's for me and myself to know. But I will write to him as soon as you've gone.' She was getting one of her grand obsessions again. Some things never change, but at least we were making love again, if not completely. But things were slowly crawling their way like two snails up the garden path, getting better between us. She gave me a long lingering kiss, and it was 10:15 and dark now.

That was a first for a long time I thought, as she shot into the house and her front door. Another tease.

She had a slightly cruel streak in her. She called out as my car pulled out of the drive, 'Don't phone me for two hours, I'm going on the internet!'

April

April days are here again
And love starts to show itself everywhere.
The tiny spider weaves his web
On his silken thread
In our dilapidated shed.
He's made a castle there
Like lovers wish to do
But sad to say
That each new night
He spins a shroud
Upon the dead.

The day has been so hot
As April sometimes is
Planting flowers and pulling weeds
Tending roses, sowing seeds
Crickets, bees and butterflies.

The roundness of your womanly curves
Are but a realm
Of castles, kingdoms,
Beautiful halls
Where I would like to dwell.
And then you wake with a smile
Upon your face

April

Our Love Reborn As The Butterfly Takes Wing

The butterfly takes wing
My heart begins to sing
Knowing you the way I do
Each and every night our love renew
A cocoon we will form to
Keep each other warm
The butterfly takes wing
Our love will bring the spring
The warmth will hatch us out
Our mating will begin
We have but just one day
To flutter wings of sin
To make each other sigh
Laugh or kiss or cry
The sun will dry our wings
The sand the sea the air
A field of corn, or wheat
No longer at our feet
We fly up to the sky
A day we have to live
So much to say and do
And so much more to give
The butterfly takes wing
The sun it starts to set, and we at last must die
But we have no regrets
For we have loved so much
In just one single day
And showed the world our love
In every single way

April

From: Natasha <natasha_nw3@yahoo.co.uk>
Date: 10 April 21:33:07 BDT
To: john smith <appledogstime@yahoo.co.uk>
Subject: What you can I can do...

Dearest Darling John,
First of three pictures for you to take to your Easter holiday with you. Talking about unwrapping Christmas presents in October. I have been invited for a Saturday lunch by my godson's parents. Looking forward to it already, his mum is expecting another one in June.
Love Natasha xx

From: john smith <appledogstime@yahoo.co.uk>
Date: 10 April 22:19:17 BDT
To: Natasha <natasha_nw3@yahoo.co.uk>
Subject: I want to marry you

Dearest darling anything I can do, you can do better to be truthful. I have only had or went to bed with 60 girls in my life....but she is the most beautiful pussy I have ever seen in my life..my eyes have looked at heaven and have seen what its like. God you are the girl who has got everything. What you have sent me I will treasure under my pillow and keep with me forever. She is the most beautiful, wonderful, munchable, kissable and I could lick her for hours. God what an amazing pussy you have. She is out of this world your mum and dad got something right, they created a masterpiece.

I swear to God now, as Him as my witness. I will love her, suck her, play with her, eat her, and fuck her at the exclusion of all others. I will never look or go with another as long as I live and give myself to her. I will protect her and always be there for her, Natasha's pussy. The most beautiful pussy on this planet and this Natasha, I swear to you now.
I want to spend my life inside her I want to spend my time to give her pleasure and do my best always at the exclusion of my own pleasure if need be. I want to make babies in her and treasure her till the day I go to heaven and leave my heaven

behind me (my Natasha pussy) the lips are so sweet and her wet nectar is like honey. I have tears of happiness in my eyes for what you have sent me such a wonderful Easter present and to think if you grant me the right to take care of her and be hers only. Thank you darling so much for such a wonderful gift xxxx I will go to church and hope that the months go quickly till I can enjoy her with you my special one xxxx John Take care and love yourself lots X

From: john smith <appledogstime@yahoo.co.uk>
Date: 11 April 00:29:30 BDT
To: Natasha <natasha_nw3@yahoo.co.uk>
Subject: Just home now, undressed, ready for bed and looking at your wonderful pussy
Want to bite and suck your tits, leave tiny bite marks on them. Really turn on your nipples, lick all that honey from your pussy. Wish you were here in the flat on the bed now with me and we had a night of cuddles, playing, feeling, sucking, fucking and then I leave you to sleep it off in my bed and then go to work. Want you looking in to my eyes as you ride me to your own orgasm and I suck your nipples play with your back..soon, soon darling you will be mine we will be together. You will get the best sex you ever had. Have to sleep and wank to you darling. Night Night darling x John X Take care of you love yourself
From: john smith <appledogstime@yahoo.co.uk>
Date: 11 April 00:53:18 BDT
To: Natasha <natasha_nw3@yahoo.co.uk>
Subject: In bed now and your with me

I want you so bad!! I want you so much Nat, this is torture!! I want you! I thought I was strong but I'm crazy for you! I want you so bad!!! I won't tell Ruth that you are speeding things up. I knwo you want me as well, I know you fancy me burning hot face, jelly legs and butterflies and from my side permanent hard cock and your in my mind all day long xxxxxxx john...I want you! I want you!! I want you! I want you!!!
Darling, I want you so much I can't even sleep... My head has gone. x John

April

From: Natasha <natasha_nw3@yahoo.co.uk>
Date: 11 April 09:00:40 BDT
To: john smith <appledogstime@yahoo.co.uk>
Subject: Thank you!
Dearest John
You write such nice things about declarations of love for me and my pussy, joy to read. I am sorry I keep you awake at night, I am sorry I make your head go round and I am sorry you can't work. It must be the combination of spring blossoms, warm air and the promise of us meeting at the most beautiful time of the year. I thank you for all the tender words you write everyday and for the crude ones too, they make me feel better by the hour. I was so ill (never realising it), so tired of life so worn out. You keep me going and regain my strength again. Thank you for all that. Love Natasha xx
From: john smith <appledogstime@yahoo.co.uk>
Date: 11 April 10:56:18 BDT
To: Natasha <natasha_nw3@yahoo.co.uk>
Subject: Thank you why? I should be down on my knees thanking you for letting me fall in love with you

Why sorry? I felt so bad, so utterly retched with everything that happened with Ruth. So down that I made such a fool of myself. Did crazy things when I felt her slipping away again from me. It was for good this time, so frustrated, nothing I could do. Something I could not
grasp or fight in any way. Then I saw your picture and fell madly and crazily in love. First I thought I would book you, see you every week and then try to get you to become my girlfriend and then ask you to give up the business. That was in my head but such great joy (you already had) then having found the girl of my dreams you were off. Don't need an explanation, you have told me everything. After five years which I loved (it's true) but it got me nowhere. I always wanted a permanent woman in my life who I could call my own...not a lot to ask from this world. Someone who would always be there for me and yes someone I could have the most wonderful fun and games with at no cost. Good fun and hot sex. Someone I could share my life and fun with then I

found you my wonderful Natasha who now I also find beside all the good things she already has but also has a beautiful pussy as well. God has really smiled on me this year and Ruth is still there for now ..and always will be as a friend .. So don't be sorry, you are giving me the greatest happiness. It's a nice feeling to be in love and I know you already love and want me very much. My sweet little girl nat. Yes I want to care for you loads, love you, fuck and make love to you forever and ever. Yes, you have a lot of problems, some deep rooted but I told you how to get rid of a lot of them. You have four months to concentrate hard and work on them. Give him all your time and 100% attention. I will get on with my work and you will come to me a new and free woman. Ready to relish and throw yourself into the full bloom of full womanhood, as you have never done before. A real beautiful lady when we are out together, a wonderful cook in the kitchen, a wonderful mother one day.... and a real dirty sexy slut when you want in the bedroom. To make you're man happy and content always. So he wants to spoil you rotten. Thank you my baby for saving me from total self destruction. Love you so much and yes it's true as it always is the first three years or four. Yes I want you so much!! I want to shag you silly over and over... but we will cool down together over the years and when you get pregnant. So my darling dear thank you kiss

X John

April

WHERE IS HER HEART
11th April

Her calls always made me jump. These days I was just not used to her calling me, but I knew it was her. I jumped out of the bath and rushed to the phone. She wanted to come at around 11 O 'clock to do something nice together, perhaps look at the spring flowers in Kenwood Park.

And so we went, and had some soup and bread at a nice little café when we got there. It was a warm and comfortable afternoon, which put us both in a good mood, and went for a long, romantic walk.

I was elated, and even put a job deadline back to Wednesday so that I could spend more time with her. Even after all those words, years and love, I could not say no to her. She was the air I breathed, my everything. She made me walk on water.

We did everything together. It was spring! We lay on the grass in the park, we joked and had fun. Such beautiful moments.

I was in love again, and she was joining me in the spirit and enthusiasm of the thing, or at least she acted and fooled me into believing she was falling in love again. Even so, I did not care, as I have found that all women act or pretend at one time or another, even though they swear that they are not.

I could not sleep. How could I sleep when love had come along again? I was a song; an endless melody of love.

We went back to her place. I had not even asked if I could come. She made me a cup of tea and as I sat on her bed with the mug in my hand, she took off her little white trainers, then her jeans and cardigan. She stood in front of me in her white knickers and blue tank top. She was still wearing her thick white socks too.

She put her arms around me and hugged me tight as I hugged her back, and fell backwards on to the bed. My hands groped towards her knickers, and I slid my fingers effortlessly inside of her. Her hands were now also all over me, and the cosy afternoon had moved on to one of hot, hot sex.

I knew someone was stalking her, and I knew she was thinking of someone else as we embraced, but I could not help but lose myself in the mad passion.

My fingers brought her off again, and this time she let me know with an earth-shattering moan and shudder. My pants were down to my knees now, but as I moved to climb on top of her she gave me a saucy look and said, 'No no no… Not yet. We still have the exercise to do.' She started to wank me with her hand harder and harder, and I could feel that unstoppable tingle that let me know it was going to happen.

Then her mouth was all over me, sucking and swallowing like mad, and I was lost, screaming at the top of my lungs.

'Shhh!' she let go and pressed her finger to her lips, 'The neighbours will hear!'

I looked into her eyes as she was with me body and soul. But her heart… where was that? Someone else was in her dreams. Future lovers, watch out, you are walking on a minefield of tears, promises and broken dreams.

She had so many secrets inside, each with their own separate compartment, each with its own little key.

As I drove away, I thought to myself, where is her real heart? She has one, but who will she finally give it to?

April

Morning

The city is in mourning
And it is morning
Our energies spent
You rest your head on me
The lights go out
Will we go out too?
God, what should I do?
Can any man ever know
What's inside a woman's head
I think me not
Until I'm dead

April

Where Is Your Heart?

Do you dream of someone,
Someone, not me?
Do you think of what may
Or may not be?
Does your heart hold a dream,
Am I soon to be missed?
You kiss someone new,
In the pale London mist.
Darling, where is your heart?
Are you going away?
Not a word, a goodbye?
Will you still think of me,
When you're starting to fly?
Can you keep friends,
Who are no longer of use?
Or do they die off,
When you feel their untruths?
You wear on your finger
My mum's wedding band
Your lips say: Don't worry.
Darling, where is your heart?
If I send you this poem,
A song of love,
Tell me it's true,
You'll always be there.
Let me find flowers,
For your pretty hair,
I look in your eyes:
Darling, where is your heart?

April

From: <appledogstime@yahoo.co.uk>
Date: 11 April 18:51:39 BDT
To: Natasha <natasha_nw3@yahoo.co.uk>
Subject: Re: A little something to keep you happy over the holiday.
A Little Something To Keep You Happy Over The Holiday.
Its been a week since we last saw each other and I am visiting your flat for the first time. Your first visit and the beginning of our sexual adventure together was at my flat in St.Johns Wood. I left you at six o clock in the morning, in my bed and that was the last time we saw each other. I ring the bell to your front door and I find myself in a reasonably spacious flat with a really cute little kitchen and flowers in pots everywhere. The room is dark and there is either, and I'm not quite sure..a Frank Sinatra CD playing or something similar. There's a small candle burning beside your bed, which is giving the room a really nice musky smell of vanilla and spices. It's late August and very, very hot, the temperature is over thirty, so after we kissed and held each other, I took my black T-shirt off. I saw your eyes wander over me and examine my gym-trained body almost immediately and as I am over six foot two, you ran to me, slid your arms around my waist and rested your face against my chest. You look up at my enormous, ravenous blue eyes, feasting upon the view that is you and my broad lips and you catch a glimpse of my pearly white teeth smiling at you as I look at you. You are wearing a tiny, tiny, black summer dress and sheer stockings with three-inch high heels. I place my finger on your more than perfect lips and trace a circle around them. Your lips are moist and you draw even closer to me, your face gazing up at me and your eyes brighten, sparkling with your smile. I am absolutely calm and quiet as I look down into your beautiful brown eyes. I push two of my fingers deeply into your mouth, which you lubricate with your saliva. Your dress falls around your ankle and you step out of it. You're wearing no bra leaving your full breasts completely exposed to me. Your nipples are so stiff from excitement and you are wearing tiny, silky white panties and black stay-up stockings. Your nipples become even harder as you feel my gaze upon them. My lips

nuzzle your tits, kissing and nibbling them. You throw your head back in pleasure, but keep your soft breasts remain pressed against my chest, my hairs teasing your nipples, still you yielding only to my body and my demands. My hand slides down your tummy over your navel in to the top of your tiny panties and my long fingers feel into your damp, wet, pussy as you pull me towards you. You unzip my jeans while I am rubbing more and more frantically against your clitoris and your pussy. You slide your hands into my jeans and pull them down so they drop to my ankles. I step out of them. But then suddenly you burst out laughing. You cannot believe what you see. I am wearing a tiny black pair of g-string panties, which you had left and forgotten, under my bed at my flat. But they were never designed to hold or contain what they are trying to now. The enormous bulge is unbelievable to you as my erect penis, which is getting harder and harder, is imprisoned in the fragile silk. I caress your back and you irresistibly shiver, thrusting your hips up to me close wanting me nearer. Wanting more of what I gave you last time. Wanting me to fuck you til you're sore. And then the feeling of soreness, and the remembrance that the pain brings you of the pleasure of the day before, getting you wet again and again, every time you walk, and your sore pussy lips rub together. I can stand it no longer. I take him out of his prison and slide your panties to one side, at the same time, taking you by the waist and lifting you up. Your hands go around my neck and I hold you tightly under your bottom and you wrap your long endless legs around me. I penetrate you quickly, with one strong thrust, as you equally push your hips into me and I slide into you so effortlessly through your wet. I swing you around, looking for a place to sit your pert little bottom on. I see a small dining-room table, with a vase full of flowers on it. In my passion to have you, I shove the flowers and the water and the vase to one side, spilling the water onto the carpet and breaking the vase, but you are already lost in passion and you do not even notice the loud crashing noise. Your mouth on mine, your tongue entering my mouth, biting, sucking, kissing deeply and incessantly. I pause for a moment and look down at you. This is our second sexual encounter and whether we part or stay together forever depends on two conditions. You should not ever feel imprisoned by me or my love or my affection. You are a beautiful angel who must fly free. You must never allow me or anyone else to be the sole purpose of your life. You must be free for yourself. Giving you five or six very hard thrusts, deep into you quickly and rapidly, you start to orgasm, screaming and shouting, your nails digging into my shoulders, neck and back, as you lay across the tiny table with me across you. I love you and I will love you even if our paths should divide. Your body twists and turns on the end of my cock, which is still rock hard and growing for you. You are still pushing and thrashing holding me tight towards you with both your legs and your arms, trying for a second orgasm pushing your pussy on to me hard and I start to thrust harder and deeper, seeking my own fulfilment in the most perfect happiness with the marvellous, magical creature which you are. If you turn to find me not there, it will only be because I have gone to get you breakfast in bed. You shiver and a feverish white hot heat runs through your whole body. You abandon yourself to my arms and I hold you more tightly than ever. Kissing you with an unbelievable passion, that is not just a primitive sexual desire and longing for your body, but a forever-lasting love and longing to be part of you so that we become as one. You are starting to cry and tears of joy and happiness are wetting your cheeks as your pussy is also wetting your cheeks… but different cheeks. You can feel what I'm feeling too. I'm thrusting harder into you now... harder and harder, and your eyes are imploring me, pleading me to end this madness, but now I am going to tease you a bit more. I withdraw from you for just a few seconds, turn you around quickly placing your feet on the floor and bending you over the table, entering you quickly from behind, while my hand plays with your clitoris at the same time. You feel the walls of your vagina catching fire and red hot- I have been shagging you hard for over an hour. My hands are holding the love handles of your hips and now I am really taking you deep and hard with constant thrusts every two seconds. This is why you make me lose my head and my mind. You are such a mature, intelligent and beautiful woman and the burning passion inside you is utterly boundless. You push your body and your bottom up to take me and I start to come and as I do, you orgasm again for the second time, screaming and gasping at the top of your voice with pleasure. Your pussy, your face, your body are all red hot, and far warmer than the August night. Your pussy is erupting around my hard cock, like a giant, juicy, erupting volcanic. Warm hot and creamy love juices, pouring down your thighs, like hot lava pouring down the sides of the volcano. I have just released into you all of my thick milky sperm. The smell of sex is in the air and you collapse over the little table with exhaustion and I collapse over the top of you wrapping my arms around you. Our hearts beating so fast together, we can hear them in the quiet of the room, the CD has long finished playing. I pick you up in my arms and your body is limp, yielding and submissive and I carry you to the bed to lay you down upon it. Your body is shaking, over and over, your eyes are glazed and closed, still feeling the intensified enormous pleasure of the past few fantastic moments. Every cell, every part of the skin of our bodies have touched. You lay there quietly now, still shaking slightly, with the enormous feelings you have just felt still vibrating through your spine, your breath still coming quickly, your body shaking with a mixture of satisfaction and fear that you might ever lose me one day, now you have found me, found this together. Fear of even greater bliss to come. Can your body stand such constant ecstasy? Your body is full of such pleasure, but it would surely burst. Sensations of utter bliss are still singing in your brain as well as every rock song you ever heard. You have learned, for the first time perhaps, that letting yourself go completely with someone you like and love, someone who overwhelms your senses, is a sacred thing and something that makes us feel so grateful to be alive. It's then and only then, in those moments, that sex ceases to be merely sex and begins to be what we call love. You sniff the scented aftershave on my skin as well as your pussy juice, covering my chest and neck, caressing my strong shoulders and smoothing my hair and I look down at you and your long lashes which are closed. You have a beautiful, angelic smile my angel and you have fallen asleep.. John X

April

From: john smith <appledogstime@yahoo.co.uk>
Date: 11 April 20:55:09 BDT
To: Natasha <natasha_nw3@yahoo.co.uk>
Subject: Billy and Ruth when and how

I really need Billy to get hot for her and want to bed her bad. So that the transition from you to her takes place easy, have you a hot sexy picture I can show her of Billy? and can you show bill this one of her which i took? Almost cut her out of the picture, I'm no good with
Cameras. Same time she did me in my Calvin's. Want him to want her bad so the pain of your loss is not so bad. She has already told me she will fuck him as she is a very sexy woman and has no one and I told her I don't mind and encouraged her every time I see her. She is already fantasizing about him all the time (ex lover and husband etc miss world). Back on my own computer, place swarming with security tonight. I have now taken a week off to take you to New York. Put this in your book, ask your boss for a week off so we fly out together on Sat 7th of October, if we are good together which we will be. Love you so much. We have our first meeting together and I don't know about you but I feel I know you so well already so we may if you want end up in bed at my flat on the first night..Tuesday the 29th Aug at eight thirty. I will pick you up at your place. First put the date in your book. Let's hope Tuesday will be our good news day. Just in case no pressure. Bring clean knickers in your bag and your nightwear..which will be nothing and I will destroy the knickers you are wearing for the date. That's the way I feel at this moment in time. Want and love you so much sweet Natasha. Love our chats, picture swapping and sexy talks everyday. Hope you a hot holiday Billy, all my kisesssssssssssssssssssssss X X X
Johnssssssssssssssssssssssssssssssssssssss X X X

April

From: Natasha <natasha_nw3@yahoo.co.uk>
Date: 11 April 22:50:44 BDT
To: john smith <appledogstime@yahoo.co.uk>
Subject: Re: Final Instructions

My darling John
I have just printed your E-mail out and will read it in bed, sorry I have not written this evening. I am going to bed as i am very tired and tomorrow I am going to see the clever people in the Royal Free. I spoke to the doctor in St Johns and Elizabeth's you have suggested to my GP and I will speak to the doctors in the hospital tomorrow. So you no longer can say I am not a woman who does not get things done. I have become an action woman.
Love and all my kisses to you Nxx

From: Natasha <natasha_nw3@yahoo.co.uk>
Date: 12 April 00:21:46 BDT
To: john smith <appledogstime@yahoo.co.uk>
Subject: What a lovely letter

John
I have just finished reading your E-mail in bed and I had to get up and write to you. You said you are just a moneyman, well I strongly disagree with that. You are an artist in your own right and one, which is very skilled. This was such warm, gentle and sensitive writing if I didn't know you better I would say you are head over heals with some girl. I can't find the right words to describe it, I just feel it. Yes, I love our letters too as I am still not working and it gets a bit lonely up here in my tiny flat. I do have Billy visiting everyday though and I had a friend come over today so I feel totally finished. Listen to me complaining again you are the one working. Billy is probably as keen as Ruth for them to meet. I will try to find a nice picture of him to send you so you can show her. I am sure that they will hit it of. He can talk to anybody. And that Ruth is a sexy minx, well he read yours and hers horoscope and it fits. Your one and hers fit well. So Billy knows that she is a sexy lady. She looks so happy and relaxed in that picture. No

pressure then. I can see. I forgot to tell you not to book tickets to far away places yet. But you beat me to it. I had a feeling you might do it. I am a putter offer but you are impulsive and that can be equally bad. You are saying I will have to get out of my comfort zone and travel to an airport with you, out of lovely England and stay there for a week, eat strange food, meet strange people, sleep in a strange bed. I will have to sort out my clothes. I can feel the stress already. I might have a colitis relapse by the morning and it will be all on you. This is going to be either a lot of fun or the most horrible exercise of our lives. And your sexy Ruth is after Billy how much more? Maybe I am just over tired and should go to bed and sleep. John I am not sure whether you know what you are taking on. You said in one of your E-mails that I have problems and some deep rooted ones, I have lots of problems and many of them very deeply rooted. And I know that it all needs so much work it is scary and exciting at the some time but something needs to be done and if this exercise should help I will do what the instructions say. I am scared to death but what the hell. Can't lose much. I feel like whiney Minnie and my spelling is failing me this evening. Your letter was so beautifully written.

See you later lovely man.

Nxx

From: john smith <appledogstime@yahoo.co.uk>
Date: 12 April 11:31:04 BDT
To: Natasha <natasha_nw3@yahoo.co.uk>
Subject: Don't tell me off... I love you

Please...I had to send you something for Easter. It's silk and hand made. My friend who I work with lives in Swiss cottage and he has put it through your door. Hope you have a real happy Easter and can start to make it happen. I also hope it fits tight. Am starting to write our third date together, maybe you can write the fourth one for me. I booked the time out for New York...also the hotel but can't book the air tickets till you tell me your name...you know more about me then I do about you. You know and have seen everything. I don't know your name. Anyway looking forward to the master story to take with me tomorrow night of our fourth date together. Love you, want you so much

x john x

From: Natasha <natasha_nw3@yahoo.co.uk>
Date: 12 April 12:08:20 BDT
To: john smith <appledogstime@yahoo.co.uk>
Subject: Re: Don't tell me off... I love you

John,
Telephoning people and asking about me again, you will be whipped till your bum stings when I get my hands on you. You are a naughty man. I won't be able to show my face at the photographers again. I hope I will not see you stalking my home. Or accidentally bumping in to you on the pavement or you are in big trouble! And I am Czech as in The Czech Republic. I have to say you have very nice, agreeable handwriting and thank you for the lovely card. I will be thinking about you while you are away enjoying your time with your family.
Kisses Nxx

From: john smith <appledogstime@yahoo.co.uk>
Date: 12 April 15:56:13 BDT
To: Natasha <natasha_nw3@yahoo.co.uk>
Subject: Another promise- will you keep them?

Will you whip me? Yes please. When? O.k. so where is this long sexy letter to me of your love making with me. Can be anywhere you want, your place, mine or anywhere. I am still working on a third sexy date story with you. Will send it from Ruth's before I leave for holiday. After I shagged her. You must write the fourth date for me to get excited about and when we meet our first four dates are sorted. No Simon, don't worry. It was his wife, found a receipt from you four years

ago. Have not been in touch with him. Thank you for your address at last, No I will stick to our agreement and not come near. I might send you something nice for your birthday. Get yourself sorted. In the story you write tell me what you like to have done to you so I can enjoy it but also learn what's expected of me as well. Ruth wants me to take her to Sardinia for our last fucks, hope Billy likes her and lusts after her. I'm trying to persuade her to get all her kit off to take a nude shot to send to Billy. I think she will soon..I'm working on it..need billy to take over now..were not together. She's is wearing me out. Wants it all the time and I have to work and I want to look after you and give you attention and love. So I am worn out looking after the two of you and all the work. Love you darling Nat very much want and think of you all the time. Send me nice hot story that is real you...your desires your wants, your kinks in the bedroom. So I can get to know you and enjoy you as well xxx Take care of you.
Love, love, love youuuuuuuuuuuu Natasha x John x

From: john smith <appledogstime@yahoo.co.uk>
Date: 12 April 12:15:25 BDT
To: Natasha <natasha_nw3@yahoo.co.uk>
Subject: HA HA HA

Just read your letter again who said anything about sleep. Do you really think??? No you will get a ring on your finger, out every night and bed won't be for sleep, not our first seven days together. I will want you all the time, you no what's it's like when you first get it together. You will be a full hot blooded woman when we meet so I may want to be in you on you and all over you as you do when your crazy about a woman. All night long... all night long... but I will let you sleep in the mornings if you want..but I really think and believe you are as hungry and want it as much as me already. I think you're feeling hotter every day as I am for you, I think your wet, hot and want to shag me like the beautiful bitch you are. Wild, uptight, angry sexy bitch. Can't wait. I'm counting the days, hope we have at least six months of fun together before you get pregnant. For both our sakes.

Would you like an Au pair or girl from your country to help you with the baby? I would sell the flat and get a nice house for us both with two spare bedrooms. You like me, I like you, our pictures turn us both on. You like what I write, I like what you write..we both no it's going to happen and work and I think sex wise we will be great together. I love films, swimming and reading and travel. As well as you know what..which we both like kiss xxxx John

From: Natasha <natasha_nw3@yahoo.co.uk>
Date: 12 April 12:35:51 BDT
To: john smith <appledogstime@yahoo.co.uk>
Subject: Re: Another promise- will you keep them?

Dear John
I am glad that Ruth is keeping you happy. And I am also glad that you are going home for a week. This is all happening too fast and I can feel the dead line in site. I feel very depressed today for some reason. One of my not so happy days I couldn't sleep last night. My doctor gave me the new pills something called Mercaptopurine, said that my liver is up the creak, my blood test is not very good either, nevertheless I should start on them tomorrow as my symptoms are not getting better as fast as expected. He ordered a liver scan and lots of other blood investigations and told me to come over next wednesday. You are the little organiser I can see. All sorted in a flash. I have just spoke to him. He is coming over this afternoon - no we are not going to bed as my stomach is still hurting. I got a promise that this afternoon is going to be John and Ruth free zone. We are going for a long walk to one of Billy's favourite parks in London. Hampstead Heath and the Hilly Gardens. If I am not too finished, I will cook him a meal after that.

Hope you are happy love and all my kisses
Take care of yourself
Natasha xx

April

From: Natasha <natasha_nw3@yahoo.co.uk>
Date: 12 April 12:47:29 BDT
To: john smith <appledogstime@yahoo.co.uk>
Subject: No Czech Au-pairs please

John,
I don't want an Au-pair from my country, the last thing I want is another Czech girl living in with us. I know what these girl do, remember I was a living Au-pair when I came to England. If people just knew. I will look after our baby myself, might have somebody helping but not living in. That is the plan for now. Anyway talk to me about babies and my depression is sure to disappear. I can't wait to see my lovely spoilt Godson and his pregnant mum on Saturday.
It is all just too perfect. Natasha x

From: Natasha <natasha_nw3@yahoo.co.uk>
Date: 13 April 09:41:07 BDT
To: john smith <appledogstime@yahoo.co.uk>
Subject: Don't be horrid!

Dear John,
You should not be so horrid about Ruth. You would not make love to her if you really didn't want to. This is not very fair on her, you calling her a little girl all the time. If it is so much trouble and you can't face it anymore don't do it. She wouldn't be very happy to know that you are shagging her out of pity and guilt or your personal need. Think about it. The story will have to wait for when you come back from your holiday, as at this moment the only thing I do in bed is sleep and write Emails to you. Hope you have a good time and lots of rest. I just read what I written below. I was a living au-pair yes but I was also a live-in au-pair. I am no boss I just make the decisions and you agree to them, saying, yes darling what a splendid idea I wouldn't have done it better myself.
By the way, we had a lovely time, Billy and I yesterday. I did make love to him, and we did go for a walk, but I was too tired afterwards to cook him anything.
Love and kisses Natasha xx

April

From: Natasha <natasha_nw3@yahoo.co.uk>
Date: 13 April 11:13:03 BDT
To: john smith <appledogstime@yahoo.co.uk>
Subject: Miss high and mighty

Well miss proud, you always put things off, always. Please can you stop this crazy behaviour, or I will stop writing. I am your judge, jury and verdict. Stop procrastinating. You know what you have to do, so do it!

John xx

From: Natasha <natasha_nw3@yahoo.co.uk>
Date: 13 April 12:05:54 BDT
To: john smith <appledogstime@yahoo.co.uk>
Subject: Re: There you go again

Yes John

How can a goddess like me be judged? I am perfection and reserve the right to judge you and the world close to you whether you like it or not. I know you don't like it much when the shoe is on the other foot and I don't blame you. People dish advice all the time don't they. You had problems with Ruth, you will be swapping them for a different set with me that is all, and where is it written that you will like them any better then the ones you had with her. As you said I have trillions of my own ones. Apology dear John the word pity was inappropriately
used. I am sure that pity doesn't come in to it at all. There might be all sorts of reasons but pity is not one of them.

Love Natasha xx

April

From: <appledogstime@yahoo.co.uk>
Date: 13 April 13:16:27 BDT
To: Natasha <natasha_nw3@yahoo.co.uk>
Subject: Third Date And Sexual Encounter Together.

So yes, I've just put down the phone on you, and after not having seen you for a week I miss you so terribly. The last encounter was bliss and yes I am falling more and more deeply in love and lust with you every second that passes. I left your apartment only half a mile from here at six o' clock in the morning and you were still sleeping like an angel after the excesses that we both shared the night before. The fact that we are having so much fun together in love, in lust and in every other way. You obviously want to be punished for all the naughty things you have done in your life, as you feel incredibly guilty and whether you admit it to yourself or not my sexy young lady, I can see that you obviously need to be punished for the excessive pride you show in every aspect of your life. You are even proud of being proud, are you not? But then you were never in love before. So remember the one thing a woman cannot keep if she loves a man is her pride. Pride is a ridiculous nuisance for a woman if she ever hopes to feel anything more than pure, blissful and pleasant sensations. Pride is an emotion suitable to a man's sense of conquest, but I want to seduce you until you give up all hope, which will ultimately result in the death of your personality. Only then can you find true freedom and sexual fulfilment. Only when a man is able to take you in such a way that you lose everything and are utterly lost, including your pride and you're not conscious or aware of anything except for the strong sensations your body and pussy are giving you, then, and only then will you achieve complete and absolute freedom to orgasm. Yes, I'm desolate and immoral and you are so miserable in your quest, trying to find happiness out of your guilt and your past misdemeanours. Yes, you want to fall deeply in love with me. Yes you already want me. You know that you want my baby, the security I can give you and my body, plus my loyalty to you, so when you arrive, which you will do of course, in a cab in a few minutes, you should expect to be treated extremely harshly. But I know deep down that that is how you want to be treated. For lovemaking can never be special unless we can make an effort to make it different and out of the ordinary each time we do it, otherwise it becomes monotonous and just a physical act for sexual gratification. I have a great sense of beauty of things. It's a fragile sense and it disgusts me sometimes to see the way things are managed by the majority of people in civilisations, where everyone, all men and women, are ready and have both the equipment and the inclination, but can you picture the average couple, throughout this great continent at their love-making, him perhaps sometimes drunk, her too tired and emotionally worn out with looking after the children. It's enough to bring on instant nausea. The doorbell rang suddenly and as I opened the door, you stood there looking up at me, your large dark eyes full of anguish, insecurity and pleading for me to take you in like a homeless pup. You reached out to me, almost begging for me to give you charity. You whispered, "Let me come in". I took a quick step towards you and looked down into your face with an expression of serious brooding, sadistic but with a certain tenderness and warmth. "Are you afraid?" I asked, and as I smiled at you, you could see my gleaming white teeth through my beaming expression, and just by looking, you could feel the texture of my skin, and smell the scent of my body, and I remembered instantly, the smell of your sex on my body at our last encounter. This immediately roused a sudden unbearable longing for you to touch me with your fingertips. You closed your eyes, your head tilted slightly up to me and you whispered through your cherry lips, "I'm afraid..." you take a breath, "Because I'm in love with you." My face moved down towards you and my mouth touched yours, lightly and softly and then I spread your lips apart with my own, threatening to devour, eat you, digest you, swallow you whole, leave not even a trace of you, your soul through your mouth with convulsive greed and hot, wet, rough passion. Suddenly you started to shake repeatedly, feeling yourself become excited and overwhelmed by a vibrant energy coming from deep inside yourself, but before you could come to your senses my arms were already around your body and you were locked close to me in a tight, fiery embrace. The large hot, hard, bulge in my jeans pressed into you, wanting to be closer and closer, and you were caught and helpless. Your control over your emotions had already been snatched away from you and you already felt weak and humiliated, powerless under me. One of my arms held you fast, while my free hand moved slowly up and down your bare back, leaving a feeling of spreading electricity. We were in the electric chair together, we were dying. We were being punished, my fingers running constantly up and down your spine, which made your heart pound faster and faster. So fast you think it's going to explode and burst out of your burning chest. Your body, your face, your neck, already growing white hot and burning hotter still with an exquisite delight, as your arms went around my neck, straining to hold me closer, your head twisting and turning from side to side like an animal caught in a trap, or in the beam of the headlamp of a car, only you don't want to escape. You want to die, you want to be consumed. You want to be trapped by me. As you started to moan and groan in the warmth of my rough, wild embrace, an animal, a wolf, I slid both my hands under your dress, pulling your panties down all the way to your ankles. Lightly, easily, almost magically, my hands quickly unfastened the buttons of your dress and they fell in a heap and you stood there naked. I let you go for a minute as I hastily flung my shirt and jeans aside. My hard, thick cock, stood out proudly in front of me and my left hand went around your back again, and no longer wanting to be gentle I pressed him hard against your flesh. Taking your hair in my fingers, with a gentle but also rough touch, I drew your head backwards, pulling with a steady strength until the pain became pleasurable for you, so that you neither winced nor cried out. You stood there with my cock pressed against your belly. You spread your legs wide for me and my tongue roughly forced your lips apart, darting in and out and feeling its way around the inside of your wet, hot mouth. My hand gripped your tiny arse and my other hand let go of your hair and gripped your wrist instead, jerking it above your head so that you would push your breasts up towards me. Then I took your other hand and did the same thing and held you up against the wall just inside the front door which you had recently come through. I carried on deep kissing you and you lost your breath and began to groan, as my hard cock rubbed against your clitoris between your legs without actually entering you yet. A sensation of incredible warmth and delight flowed instantly to every single tingling part of your body, so that even your throat and your thin wrists where I held them, were turning hot and starting to burn. You knew that you were already losing yourself and you would never be able to claim yourself back again, never be able to find yourself, or want to find yourself, until I chose to free you. But you are trapped. You are my prisoner, and there is no escape for you. Alcatraz. Sing-sing. Holloway. Every prison you've ever heard of. There was for one fleeting moment in your eyes, resentment, and a passing desire to run and then you yielded yourself to me completely. You are not going anywhere, lady, until I unlock the door and let you go. When I don't want you anymore, I will leave you and vanish to a far country across the sea. But now, yes, now, you are ready to experience whatever torture was about to be inflicted upon you. I placed two, then three fingers in your wet pussy and then roughly, having let your hands go, my arm encircled your waist and I picked you off the floor, holding you through your pussy and your waist. You were gasping, shaking and shuddering, feeling violated but so delighted for it, and my fingers and hands were full of your wetness. All sense of time disappeared and your breathing came faster and faster. You felt a terrible desire from me and a feeling that you had aroused in me, a passion which you could never satisfy with only this earthly body. Now, as we both become so, so wet with your fluids, my cock entered you deeply, my hands holding you by your arse and you wrapped your legs around me and your body started to swell up and glow and seethe with sheer excitement and the sensations as I thrust deeper and deeper, harder and harder into you, gradually became greater and greater, as I rode on and on, into you, almost thrusting through you, unmercifully to unendurable excitement. I carried on fucking you harder and harder and your arms flailed as I held you tightly by your arse.

Twisting your head from side to side, your eyes and mouth opening and closing madly, pleading, begging, like a butterfly's wings. Like a fish on a hook. You lost yourself, all awareness of yourself as an individual, experiencing feelings so violent, yet so ecstatic, so hot, that it must be the end of you and everything that you believe in. We fell on the floor now, your legs still wrapped over my body as I continueed deep kissing you with my tongue, my cock penetrating you over and over again in a ceaseless, surging rhythm, and the pain, pleasure and soreness you were starting to feel in your pussy felt natural and sweet. You cannot believe how sensational and erotic such pain can be. There were no more walls between our two bodies. They have been destroyed. Our bodies are so close. You felt I was going to ride you to the brink of death, and I was, the old you will be gone forever. The new woman is here to stay. The animal that you found was never going to stop, and you could never escape. You started to scream now and struggle as I fucked you on and on. You tried to claw at my arse, leaving rake-like welts and marks upon it. Getting more excited and wild, you fastened your teeth in to my shoulder to stop yourself from screaming too much, and I fucked you harder and harder, my cock going in and out of you every second. Then your body exploded.Your ears were ringing so loudly I could almost hear them, your face and hands were burning hot, your head had fallen to one side and you lost all sense of time, totally dazed and frantic. When you returned, it was to find me still not finished with you. I turned you over, face down on to your tummy and entered you from behind and then fucked you deeper, hard and fast with forty sharp, hot thrusts. I was grunting loudly and getting faster and faster, using you for my pleasures until I could not hold it in any longer, and then you felt the hot sperm filling your pussy and running down your thighs. You felt worn out and exhausted and there was, throughout your belly, a warm and wonderful sensation of me spreading within you. You could feel the blood pulsing in your legs and hard in to your pussy. You opened your eyes for the first time in a long while and looked to find me laying on the floor next to you, smiling at you. My broad brown chest rose from my nipples to my flat hard belly and muscle tapered legs. You had been ravished and extinguished and used like a toy, a foolish little girl, fucked and discarded, but that is what you secretly wanted, and you had shared the voyage with me, to mutual orgasmic pleasure. You looked up at me with big eyes and you said "I feel like I've been dead and come back to life again." I bent down and first kissed you on your forehead and then on your mouth where you clung to mine, refusing to let it go. When you let go you said, "I was terrified for the first time in my life in making love. I thought you were going to split me in pieces. I thought you were going to hurt and destroy my body." You closed your eyes, feeling my warm breath upon your lips and I said to you, quietly, nuzzling your neck and your ear, "If a woman doesn't feel some fear, she won't feel great pleasure either". I looked at you, and you gave me a quizzical look, then closed your eyes, laying on the carpet on the cold floor and you had fallen off to sleep, your legs still wide apart, your knees bent and with the slightest trickle of your love juices and my sperm still dribbling down your thighs. When you woke up the next morning, the house was empty and I had left you there, lying naked on the carpet. It was six o'clock and for a moment you couldn't understand where you were. You looked down at your naked body and was shocked to see the state I had left you in. Your panties, bra, stockings and little dress, scattered all over the hallway. Your body was covered in bright red love bites, on your breasts, your tummy and the top of your thighs. All the places you wanted my lips to stimulate you. The carpet was wet where my juices had run out of you. You gathered your clothes up, your pussy and tummy aching and throbbing from the excesses that I had inflicted upon you before, and you felt sharp pains in your tummy, used, where he had pushed and throbbed incessantly, hurting you hour after hour, but still feeling sexy and aroused by the thought of me. You found your coat in a heap by the front door, put it on and then tried to find your way home, feeling abused, slightly ashamed, but happy in the fact that you had again escaped and lost yourself in passion and orgasmic fulfillment. You wished it could last forever, but I'm afraid the truth is, that any heaven would become hell if it lasted too long. Your heart was still pounding at the thought and you could hear it. You felt so incredibly tired and drained. Finally you got home and without even undressing, you collapsed on the bed. You felt a slight shuddering spasm and realised that your knickers were filling once again with more of the white, milky excesses of last night. You were too tired, too exhausted to do anything though, and as you lost consciousness, you thought to yourself, there is nothing more painful or more horrible than to be me. John X

From: Natasha <natasha_nw3@yahoo.co.uk>
Date: 14 April 17:49:03 BDT
To: john smith <appledogstime@yahoo.co.uk>
Subject: Angel

Dearest Boy

I do hope you have a nice time in Church. You're the horny angel and I the little devil. Oh dear... should not have said that, should I? I am seeing Billy this Easter, also getting hot and naughty reading your e-mails. And the next week, I don't know what will happen... 4 months without sex! God bless you and your family this Easter.

Natasha your special angel xxx

From: Natasha <natasha_nw3@yahoo.co.uk>
Date: 14 April 18:06:48 BDT
To: john smith <appledogstime@yahoo.co.uk>
Subject: You

Dear John

Miss you lots and lots already, enjoy your time at home.
Love Natasha x

April

From: john smith <appledogstime@yahoo.co.uk>
Date: 16 April 14:20:43 BDT
To: Natasha <natasha_nw3@yahoo.co.uk>
Subject: Then you must be doing something wrong

Just got back from church with the family asked fran to look at her computer as I wanted to see if there was something from you and there was. If you have time, miss me as well. Write me a two page letter of all your hopes, dreams and sexual desires in bed and your fantasy of our fourth meeting together. In the meantime have you had a row with one of your friends? Spent time in bed? Go out, write an erotic letter for me, feel good, wank and feel good again. I went to church on Good Friday. Easter Sunday lunch now. I'm back at church at four thirty and then I'm going out tonight for a nice meal with the family. Anyway have a nice Easter. I have been thinking a lot of you. Love you and miss you but not the pride and arrogance. Will write again if my sister is nice to me, otherwise I get in touch on Friday. Love and hope x John

From: john smith <appledogstime@yahoo.co.uk>
Date: 18 April 09:36:34 BDT
To: Natasha <natasha_nw3@yahoo.co.uk>
Subject: Liverpool madness

Just woke up thinking that you're driving me mad even on holiday. Can't wait to hold you, kiss you and get him all the way up in you with my hot pounding balls rubbing you all wet. I'm in pain thinking of you. My family and me are having long walks together, afternoon teas and getting to know each other. They are looking forward to meeting you soon in sep/oct. Wow! Wow! How time will fly. You will need to shag him twice a week to do it all in time. Anyway what other news do I have for you?? I have a slight cold. Ruth phones every two days, desperate for my body, yours and Billy's. Life goes on, needed the rest from everything accept you. I have almost finished the next story to you xxx Love, very much the one you are with, and yourself Wish you were here now young lady x John

April

From: Natasha <natasha_nw3@yahoo.co.uk>
Date: 21 April 11:24:49 BDT
To: john smith <appledogstime@yahoo.co.uk>
Subject: I am all for it

Dear John
I am very pleased that you have decided to spend extra time with your family. It is important to get priorities in life right and our families should be on a top of the list and you do need the rest. Little bit of mum's love and cooking will do you good. My mum keeps asking when will I be coming home. She is planning a two week walking holiday for her, me and my grandmother. Two other members of mum's family and me will have our big birthday in July and a big birthday party is being planned. I did tell my mum about you, she never asks too many questions so I don't have to tell fibs. No one else knows yet. Billy and me are getting on well. Have been to the cinema twice, we go for walks and talk a lot. Well he does the talking and I listen most of the time, he could talk for England. I feel more and more tired everyday, hopefully it will go away soon. Nevertheless I don't stay in bed all day and don't spend my days sleeping and I don't fight with my friends or Billy. Maybe you should use the state of the art camera you borrowed to take pictures of your hometown and your family and forward those on to me. One of my best friends was from Liverpool but I've never been there. He was born in Wales but grew up in your town. Hope you recover soon from your cold.
Love and kisses Natasha xx

From: Natasha <natasha_nw3@yahoo.co.uk>
Date: 21 April 15:44:50 BDT
To: john smith <appledogstime@yahoo.co.uk>
Subject: Liverpool - what an old fashioned city

Yes John,
The sites of Liverpool are not exactly impressive I have to say. Maybe that is why I have never been myself. Will I ever go? Who knows? The head of the town hall would definitely be bare if it wore a peace of my underwear and I dare say half

of it's tower too. But will you ever get your grubby fingers on them? Who knows? Will I ever go? I'm glad you have some of Ruth's underwear with you to get you excited. Though, I am glad that you are use to the larger sizes as I poses them too, but only Ruth will tell you the advantages of warm, comfy 'smalls'..And yes I do still want a picture of the family with you in the middle. If you can get all of you in the
picture I know that your talents know no bounds. Love Natasha x

From: Natasha <natasha_nw3@yahoo.co.uk>
Date: 21 April 18:12:05 BDT
To: john smith <appledogstime@yahoo.co.uk>
Subject: Tonight's the night

My Dear John,
Well I do hope you talked me into an ok and safe thing. Tonight I will try it out... I have your lovely silk blindfold you sent me and I will keep you, my pet psychiatrist informed. You work so hard John, why do you bother with my little problems? I can't think. Hope your holiday's going well. Think of me tonight. Stay ok
Natasha xxx

Poem from Natasha

Billy you don't know what's coming to you
Tonight you'll get sex you can only dream about
When I lay there helpless and submissive
My heart beating faster
My pulses racing
My lips so red
Your eyes so blue
In the dark
That is all of you
Your dreams come true
I'll really make your dreams come true

April

THE BLINDFOLD
Friday 21st April

I pulled my Jaguar up outside the house. I was not sure what I was in for. I had to wait for the call on my mobile. She had informed me, like a military operation, that she would open her front doors and her door to the bedroom at 8 O'clock. It was now 8:35 and she had still not rung. I was practically a nervous wreck and becoming more so by the minute.

I was expected to enter her house, then her bedroom and give an Oscar winning performance in a completely blacked out room, with no talking, and just some quiet music playing. With her wearing a mask, this was like some strange Venetian rhapsody. A masked charade ball. Could I do it? I did not know. The minutes ticked by and my legs were shaking in anticipation. I had been sitting in the car nearly an hour and it had been a long time since I had been anywhere near her completely physically. We had played but that was all. Suddenly the phone rang twice. The signal. I felt a feeling of shock and horror which I could not explain. The whole thing seemed so bizarre. I was wearing just jeans and a t-shirt. No pants underneath, to make things easier for her. I remember as I walked to her door, making a quiet silent prayer that she would not get my cock stuck in my zip.

I passed through all the doors, climbed the stairs, and as promised, the bedroom door was on the latch. I pushed it open and all was dark inside except for one tiny candle on the table. She was standing, and I could just make her out, and the music was playing low. She had on just a tiny silky white pair of knickers, and some black hold up stockings, a white matching tank top and a silk blindfold over her eyes. She held out her hands in the dark to try to find me, and then her hand caressed my jeans. Her other hand went up to my neck and she started to kiss me hard. As she pulled down the zip and reached inside she gasped at the size, and gave away just the tiniest giggle. I had taken a Viagra tablet in case the nerves and the strange situation would blunt my libido.

She wanted to say to me, 'You're not wearing pants.' I felt it. But the exercise called for no talking.

She led me to the bed in the candle glow, and the idea got

me more and more excited, as she could see nothing. For her, everything was just touch and smell and feel and warmth. Skin to skin. She pushed me down on to the bed and pulled my jeans off from the ankles in one swift movement. My cock was ramrod hard with excitement and Viagra. Then she straddled me from the waist down.

My eyes closed, opened, then opened wide again, and I watched her pert little titties bounce up and down as my Viagra increased hard on slid straight into her. She let her long blonde hair cross and re-cross my chest and nipples, teasing me with it. She bent and kissed me passionately, and I said to myself as quietly as I could, 'God, you are fucking gorgeous… unbelievable.'

Her finger went over my mouth to stop me talking. She was vivacious and stunning in her silk blindfold. The chemistry was mind-blowing, even though we were both nervous. She had a ticking time-bomb between her legs. The hunger, the skin-touching-skin, the hot fire, her body on my body, her knickers still on, and for the first time, just pulled to one side, the way I love it. The silk of them rubbing on her bum as I held it. My cock was rubbing against her clitoris now, and in the sensuous absolute quiet, everything centered on a few inches of red hot gasoline nerve endings. A four inch area of fire and flesh, her body burning with need and desire. We had both forgotten over the long months, it could be this good.

She was now soaking wet, and I was deep inside her. She moved up and down my shaft and was in control. Squeezing, tightening her pussy, like a mouth and hand all rolled into one. I was thick and hard and filling her up with me, and hitting her cervix over and over again. We both felt so fucking good.

We had done everything in our sex life together, tried every perversion that you could think of. Even two men fucking her at the same time. We had done the woods, the car, everything. But this was different. This was so different. No talking, and just the sounds, this was such an incredible turn on. Just a cock and a wet pussy slurping, skin bouncing and banging against skin. Lips sucking on nipples. The shape of her body in silhouettes against the candle glow, onto her window blinds.

I started to fuck her hard now, and she, holding onto my bum, mirrored my movements so that it was like we were carrying out some strange ritual African dance. I was hitting her G-Spot over and over, taking her roughly now, and she loved it. Holding onto her hips and her arse, for a good fifteen minutes, I was punishing her and pounding her with her on top all the time, still in control. Then suddenly she pushed herself off me, and fell on her back with her legs spread wide. She grabbed me with both hands by the hair and pushed my head down between her legs. She reached for a pillow in the dark and pulled it quickly under her bottom. She then pushed and forced her clit into my mouth. I could not remember a time when she needed it so strongly before. I could hardly breath. My whole mouth and nose was full of her pussy. I worked my tongue up and down carefully so as not to catch her or hurt her in my eagerness with my teeth. Then sucking her clit in and out of my mouth whilst flicking it with my tongue and keeping it wet and sweet with my saliva. Two of my fingers pushed in and out of her with a nice rhythm. Roughly the same rhythm as my heart was beating. Breathing out my hot breath onto her pussy lips, she moaned and was starting to breath more deeply now, more and more. Giving out tiny cries, like a seagull, small little moans, as my tongue flicked harder and harder. Then a sigh, then a louder one. Even in the dark I could see her face was flushed hot and red. Her little sighs were coming faster and faster now. She was on fire. Her hands pressed tightly on the top of her pubic bone, parting her own pussy lips. I pushed my mouth right in, and flicked four or five times hard on her already blood gorged, swollen clitoris. Expelling it from my lips and then re-swallowing it inside my mouth once more. I gave her ten more quick rapid flicks like music, and suddenly, she really started to moan loudly. She opened her legs wider, pushed her bottom off the bed as my fingers thrust into her faster and faster and faster. She was into it then… shouting and moaning as she came with a massive orgasm. My fingers covered by her thick juices, she was still coming, and still coming, and I gently licked her clitoris, very slowly. Shock-waves engulfed her body as I strummed her pussy and clit for another few seconds, like an electric guitar. Then she grabbed me by the hair again and pulled me up to her, her legs wide open and crossed over my bum.

I pushed into her deep and hard into her… it had been a long time. She bit my nipples for the first time in her excitement. She held my head and kissed me deeply. I was losing my mind. I knew that I could not last much longer. I drove my cock deeper and deeper and deeper into her. Her throat made guttural noises, low down like an animal as I hit her cervix over and over again. Then I ejaculated into her slamming against her body hard. One, two, three, four, five… in quick succession, and I collapsed onto her body. Her arms wrapped around me, and both of us were shaking. Shaking for the moment. Shaking for the surreal ness of it all. Our sex life had started again.

I held her tight and rolled onto my back, taking her with me, so that her head lay on my chest. All we could feel was the beating of our hearts and our hot breathing. Through her window, the only one she had not pulled the blind down, I saw a cloud of shooting stars fly across the sky, similar to tiny fireflies. We stayed motionless, thoughtful, just hugging and holding, for a full twenty minutes. Then as instructed, I got up, put on my jeans, felt around the floor in the dark for my black t-shirt, slid it on, bent over, kissed her sweetly, my tongue just running along her bottom lip gently, and left her lying there with her thoughts, her blindfold still in place.

I sat in my car for a full twenty minutes looking up at her window. The lights suddenly came on in the bedroom and the exercise was over.

As I turned to drive home I noticed a man standing at a window opposite Natasha's flat. About 40 feet across the road, he was holding a pair of binoculars up to his eyes, and peering straight into the one window we has left the blind left up on.

Fuck! I swore to myself. She still had her blindfold on! But the agreement was that I was not allowed to talk to, or even call her. I stopped the car and got out leaving my lights still on. He saw me and pulled his curtains across straight away.

She would not be the first woman to have a peeping tom.

I've been so lonely without her
The last time she took my hand
The last time we held each other
So very, very close
Was it a hundred years ago?
A month?
Or just now
Was it a promised land?

April

An uncertain place
A new beginning?
My heart alone
Hearing hers
Has she been with someone
Who only hears his own
I knew she lied
But I forgave
And given time
We both changed our minds
We were meant to be
I tried to believe
I'm getting used to playing the pain
The game
A roulette wheel
I'd rather lose my money
Than my heart
You bet my shirt
That's why we've been apart
We had reasons
That we went our separate ways
But our souls have met again
Nothing will be left behind
As she was so very hard to find
The flowers were dying
And now the Spring is here again
My hands held hers
And our rhythms are one
And only her and I can hear them

April

From: john smith <appledogstime@yahoo.co.uk>
Date: 23 April 02:07:47 BDT
To: Natasha <natasha_nw3@yahoo.co.uk>
Subject: Such words out of the mouth of a pretty girl who sent me her pussy, wet and dry

O Ho! Someone must be helping you and reading my mail to you? A mature girlfriend or something? You reply was too cool. If I have been reading you correct. Who is helping you baby to draft your replies? If no one then I really do love you more and more. You are very intelligent, not just bright. So you never rose to the bait, no angry words..clever girl who's growing up fast. My mum, dad and sister hate their pictures being taken but here is my dads office with me sitting alone in it and one of me thinking of you lucky girl. Baby to think this is all yours and yours alone soon. Do as you wish, your own plaything. You will be the last girl to enjoy it. I will never go with another after you. Yours for life X Kiss my darling xxx love only for you xx John P.S. They are all in bed as you are with Billy. Or have been i hope..?? Kiss X JOHN

From: Natasha <natasha_nw3@yahoo.co.uk>
Date: 24 April 17:32:09 BDT
To: john smith <appledogstime@yahoo.co.uk>
Subject: The middle of our universe

Dearest John
When I said I wanted you in the middle of the picture I didn't mean you, yourself and the middle of your universe. Though that is a magnificent specimen, finally you are getting the hang of the photography business. John your charm knows no bounds and you could master a picture of the family. I know he does not talk back like people would but such a sweet and lovely boy. How can anybody resist you asking? Did you watch the Liverpool game or are you not in to football? I suspect you are not. Hope you are continuing to have a nice holiday. Billy's coming over later to take me to a surprise film.
Love and kisses Natasha xx

April

ON THE BEACH

Mondays were usually bad days, but not this one. This was a good news day. We were off to the South Bank together to see one of the last of Ava Gardner's films called 'On The Beach', which was set after a great war which had left the earth in disaster, with a huge cosmic cloud slowly circling the globe, wiping out each all life on each continent as it circumnavigates. The film follows the escapades of the last remaining members of the world's population.

We set off to the Italian restaurant we had visited before, and after the obligatory walk, we had a quick look at the book stalls.

She told me her internet lover John was in Liverpool with his family, and had sent her another picture of his gargantuan sexual organs to get her excited. I went a bit further this time, and asked her where she thought it would all end. She just said he was in love with her, and that he was very selfish, and had a high opinion of himself, and would stay at this stage, as an internet friend.

'I don't really like him, I don't like him at all. He is manipulative, self-centred, and thinks he is sex on legs.' That was all she would say of the matter. As usual with Natasha, she only told half the story, and I knew that she was becoming more and more fascinated by him, and his exceptional body every day,

The film was brilliant, and gave us a lot to think about. What would we do if we were told, we had just two months to live? Gregory Peck and Ava Gardner, after two months of an incredibly deep and beautiful love affair, they say their goodbyes. He takes his nuclear submarine with his crew out to sea and sails her all the way down the coast of Australia to reach the bottom. At the same time, Ava Gardner takes her little sports car and drives the sea road, keeping him in sight, and he her, permanently, till they could both go no further, then he blows her a kiss for the last time, opens the water-tight doors off his submarine, and goes down with his vessel. She sits in her car crying and maybe, the last person left alive on the planet. She takes out two small blue pills which the government have issued to everybody, so that they do not suffer from radioactive toxins and pain. The pill puts you to sleep, and within half an hour you are dead.

As the sun sets for the last time on the sea, she smiles to

herself, dries her tears and says, 'I'm gonna' beat ya' this time Mr. Radioactive.' She pops the two pills and the credits roll.

'God, you certainly leave this film with a lot of thoughts in your head! After a film like that, what would we want to do? I expect the majority of people would want to be with their loved one, and make love for the last time. Or perhaps, if you were a mountain climber, climb one last mountain and die on the top, or like one gentleman in the film, die with his beloved racing car after having taken it at a 180 mph drive for the last time. The film had touched her and me, as you realised the finality of death, and how quickly and unexpectedly it may creep up on a person.

We got to her place and she asked me up. She said she was very tired.

'Let's do it quickly' she said, not meaning full sex. She went straight onto the bed, took her knickers off, and I went down on her. She must have been as horny as hell. She came in two minutes, the fastest ever. She then started to give me the most beautiful wank, bringing me off with her mouth for the last 20 seconds. I ejaculated and she swallowed, and then held her arms up for a cuddle. She said she was sorry it was not a big hot fuck, but she was just too tired after the work, the film, and the glass of red wine she had had in the Italian restaurant. We cuddled for a short while and she said she reminded me she had an early start at work tomorrow.

I drove home thinking it was getting better and better with Mr. John Smith's help. It was making her happy, randy and nice, so I thought we were all pressing the right buttons.

April

From: john smith <appledogstime@yahoo.co.uk>
Date: 25 April 09:03:01 BDT
To: Natasha <natasha_nw3@yahoo.co.uk>
Subject: More interesting is the middle of you. Where the magnificent specimen…

should be till the day we both leave this planet. Your bit and my bit to give us both ultimate pleasure and fun
till death do us part. Any way my dad hates having his picture taken (as much as I hate football) my mother goes all silly in front of the camera and shy and my sister ha ha ha she just runs as fast as she can. So we wont put them through that torture on this trip. When you come to meet them yes they may condescend to please you. Have to hurry as sis coming back soon. Left early, they've all gone to market today that's in a little village outside Liverpool. All home grown and homemade etc home spun products. I'm here thinking of you again. I hope it works out with us as the final break with Ruth will be very bad. I know it. She wants me so much but I have to move on to you. I do get very depressed, down and suicidal thinking of it but I want you so much. You must be starting to feel it now that you are starting to sex him again. The first one is sometimes real bad as you have to face your hatreds. That's how it should be. You have to face them and destroy them to become a better person. Next one will be better and then it will get very good when you and him are shagging really good for the ten. You will notice things changing around the fifth shag and you start to feel that this is nice and ask yourself "Why? Why did I not get this close before" He can be on top if you wish but you are in total control. Then comes the final three where you are his complete slave, he can do with you as he wishes. Make you do what he wants. That's when he sets you free, you will feel like a brand new person and so so good. Lots of women started to cry quiet a lot after it was all over. They felt so good to be free of everything. After a week or two away from each other you meet together with the lights on, sound, talking as normal and you will think he is the most wonderful man on the earth. Always remember though..you did it, not him. You should try to be up to once a

week or twice if possible before I'm back next week Monday. Idid not say it would be easy... it will be hard but that's it. You are DETOXING your brain and soul. IT WILL HURT. Then hopefully you come to me a new woman and I to you a new man. Don't worry, I have a lot of stuff to go through with Ruth. You can see with the panties she's still crazy for me but her family hate me now. I wasted their little girls life, they had to put the blame somewhere for their hard stance. We two did not think it through, to busy being in love and shagging all the time. That's why I want it as near perfect for us. Love you my darling Natasha. Stay as nice as you are my sweet kind girl. Love you so much x Take care and love yourself John xxx

From: Natasha <natasha_nw3@yahoo.co.uk>
Date: 26 April 22:47:31 BDT
To: john smith <appledogstime@yahoo.co.uk>
Subject: Re: Have not heard from you since I told you that I loved you, wanted you and adored you

Dearest darling,

As I told you, you love, want and adore a fantasy created by your over active creative mind. I am not trying to belittle your feelings but honestly speaking you don't know the first thing about me and the same goes for me. I will love you the first time I set my eyes on you but will this all go according to the John Smith big plan just days splitting up from his girlfriend of long standing? I know that Billy phoned his friend at the flower shop to ask for Ruth's number but I don't think he called Ruth. I understand that it would make things easier for you if they met now, but I am not ready for that just now and if anything, it would complicate everything for me. I am not sharing him with Ruth right now. Please don't tell me off as you are just about to do now. This is probably selfish of me but that is how it is for now. I am not having Billy going to bed with Ruth and me at the same time. I just don't feel very sharing this evening.
By the way the exercise is harder as I though it would be. I am not giving up, just saying. Hope you understand.

Love from your dearest sweetest Natasha x

From: john smith <appledogstime@yahoo.co.uk>
Date: 27 April 08:42:14 BDT
To: Natasha <natasha_nw3@yahoo.co.uk>
Subject: Double standards! If you don't tell how can anybody know???

Well, well, well. So total mix up of the brain cells. You are 30 almost and you still drift along in a haze of dreams and black hate and so called injustices (many of your own making). May the First is upon us. May day, time to grab yourself firmly and say, grow up Natasha! before it's to late. Grow up, be positive, make lists, set timescales. Do something. Set mountains to climb and climb them. Don't talk, don't think, just do. If he starts to see Ruth now, it won't be so bad for him. Do you really love people and want the best for them or just say WORDS? You have to mean them. Really mean them. I know and have been told by more than one person that Billy really, really loves you and would do anything for you and always puts you first. Is it not the time to do the same for him in return in everything?? Especially before you run off in to the sunset with me as you know you will. You know it will work with us so stop running Natasha. Total body, love, kisses, soul, hot deep kisses. We will love being together and will love making babies. Billy will be your best friend for life. Back Monday night John x

From: Natasha <natasha_nw3@yahoo.co.uk>
Date: 30 April 12:06:10 BDT
To: john smith <appledogstime@yahoo.co.uk>
Subject: Not true, love you to bits and appreciate all you write to me

I do love myself. Why would you rather somebody who hated them selves? How can I expect anybody loving me if I do not love myself? I watch and learn..from the masters.

Love Natasha xx

Natasha's Prayer

I love me
Who else is there?
I'm the only one who knows me.
It's not selfish to be true.
I'm never unfaithful to me like I am to you
And I can please myself
So much better- it's true.
I know what turns me on
And what turns me off
Every pain, every ache
Every sneeze, every cough.
And when I take my panties
Off, that as well.
No-one can kiss me as I kiss
Myself.
No-one can miss me like I
And if I sigh or cry or laugh,
Or joke or sleep or die,
There's no-one in the very end
Who has to face the truth, but I.

May

From: john smith <appledogstime@yahoo.co.uk>
Date: 1 May 08:44:07 BDT
To: Natasha <natasha_nw3@yahoo.co.uk>
Subject: You do need help.

As the rest will sort themselves out in the end. The sex life of a young girl, boy, young man or woman is very important to their well being in general. If you can get
that sorted out, the rest nearly always comes out ok. So listen to me please. I'm back in London tonight at eight, straight in to work at six tomorrow so no Ruth or sex tonight. Love you. Will write soon xxxxx John x love yourself x

From: Natasha <natasha_nw3@yahoo.co.uk>
Date: 1 May 10:00:43 BDT
To: john smith <appledogstime@yahoo.co.uk>
Subject: Re: You do need help.

John I have never doubted that you are trying to help me. It is just the patronising tone you take with me. I don't disregard your help or your suggestions. I am almost thirty but you talk to me as if I was five. I know what Billy is, how old he is, what he does for a living and what he is doing for me. I don't need reminding all the time unless this is a part of your therapy. I try to do my best by him there is no doubt about that, you know just little bits of our life from what I told you and from what you have heard from his friends. I do need help, but I don't need to feel like damaged goods every day? And that is exactly how I do feel after reading some of your E-mails. Maybe the E-mail coupled with luck of time, it's not the best medium of communication to try to sort somebody's problems. I should stop obsessing about my problems and myself and get out there and get on with it. Whatever life consists of. Maybe you know more than me but ultimately I have to live with myself and with my problems and with my job and with my boss - have work to go to for the first time on Saturday and it needs to feel OK because the only person I don't want to run away from anymore is me.
Kisses Nxx

People can be frustrating sometimes. Especially when they don't want to do what we want them to and they can't see what is good for them. Or they take too long over it.

From: Natasha <natasha_nw3@yahoo.co.uk>
Date: 1 May 12:23:05 BDT
To: john smith <appledogstime@yahoo.co.uk>
Subject: Still too proud to be proud
John, I did not say that I refuse to carry through what you suggested, I did say that it is not easy. Not impossible. Believe me I have to trust you to have started all this. And it was you yourself who said that the first few times are difficult and being on the receiving end of it I agree. Don't give me a hard time I blindly trust you, a person who I have never met and as you said may never meet. I do get on my high horse when I get pushed too much. Also when I am constantly reminded of all the particulars of Billy such as his age, work, experience and his love for me. Maybe you should tell me what is the reason for you reminding me constantly? I am out of the few, who knows the most about him. We are getting closer everyday on your suggestion and it feels really good most of the time. So am I following what was prescribed to the last letter or do I not dear John. If you were here I would put my arms around you. Love Nxx

From: john smith <appledogstime@yahoo.co.uk>
Date: 1 May 17:32:12 BDT
To: Natasha <natasha_nw3@yahoo.co.uk>
Subject: So what you are saying (even if you don't want to face it in your self)..

Is that you find it difficult to really shag a man who you shagged thousands of times? (your words). A man you love very much and is your best friend? Meaning that out of thousands of fucks you had with him, half the time you were not trying and the rest of them you just went a long with it. Most of the time you were fucking your dad over as you made him a dad person. When to him you were his girlfriend. How could you say he was and is a good lover and the closest person to you? You have used him and abused him for your own way and security whilst giving him half hearted sex in return. Now at last after all the years you are making your mind up to give him the real thing at last. You could have been having orgasms and good times years ago but you wasted his time and your own. All this time. You better start putting things right ASAP dooting the eyes. I love you and want you still but you really are or have been up to now a hardhearted self-centered girl who used a man. Can you ever repay him for what he has given you and the way he has taken it all from you and is still there. You chose him x john

From: Natasha <natasha_nw3@yahoo.co.uk>
Date: 1 May 19:00:53 BDT
To: john smith <appledogstime@yahoo.co.uk>
Subject: Re: So what you are saying (even if you don't want to face it in your self)..

Dear John,

I have been facing it all for a while. Sometimes I feel that it would be easier to be ignorant to it all but I am very aware of most of the facts listed below. He was there for me as well as I was there for him in a good way. I worshipped Billy for years but there is no excuse for what I have been doing. I feel guilty every time I think about it and you are right. Living with me was Hell most of the time. And still is I suppose. I have wasted lots of time, his and mine and I wouldn't want to waist yours as well. Why oh why would you want to be with somebody you call shit I don't know. I don't want to think what you would call me in few years time. I did tell you to do your analysis well. I am not going to apologise anymore I wish I could tell you all of it but I am pretty sure you have worked most of it out already and if you have not you will. I feel sick of feeling guilty and miserable all the time and I am not doing it anymore it makes me very ill. If I have become hard it is only because I had to. I do wish we had met five years ago, I was a nicer person in a way then. Nxx

From: john smith <appledogstime@yahoo.co.uk>
Date: 1 May 19:57:54 BDT
To: Natasha <natasha_nw3@yahoo.co.uk>
Subject: Blame

It's called cause and effect. What did you do? Fall in love with a client as well as everything else while he stood by to help you? God you have so much hate in you. I can do no more for you. God helps people who help themselves but as you are hell bent on destroying yourself and living with the guilt for the rest of your life. What can anybody do???? Three months... are you ill still? Yes! Have you written a letter telling me what you like in bed? No! What is your big chip? Everyone gets a bad hand of cards sometimes. You give up before you look at them. In fact you just do nothing. It's much easier to blame Bill and while you're at it blame me as well and Ruth. Blame us for your misfortunes, your boss, your best friend, your dad, mum? Could it be you that has to change??? But when do you start tomorrow??? Next year or the year after? No the year after that! Nat in gods name make a start and do something xxxxx John

From: Natasha <natasha_nw3@yahoo.co.uk>
Date: 1 May 23:17:37 BDT
To: john smith <appledogstime@yahoo.co.uk>
Subject: Re: Blame

I don't blame anybody apart from myself and nobody can help me unless I do it myself. Whatever the time scale, how ever frustrating you find it. I am not giving up, far from it so stop jumping up and down my friend. As much as I don't want you to, maybe you should resume a search for the miss right because I am definitely not her judging by the last letter. Nx

May

From: john smith <appledogstime@yahoo.co.uk>
Date: 2 May 23:55:10 BDT
To: Natasha <natasha_nw3@yahoo.co.uk>
Subject: 17 hours of work, on my way home to bed..yes on my own
Well what can I say.. I made you a real good offer, a life of happiness and prosperity for as long as we both last. Best I can do. I tried to help you solve your problems, I did my best. You can take a horse to water but you can't make it think. But if I can't help you no one can, I did my best with the highest degree from my university in thirty years but some horses will never drink or want to? If someone chooses not to help themselves you can't make them. God helps those who help themselves. God bless and good luck love you x John X

From: john smith <appledogstime@yahoo.co.uk>
Date: 3 May 08:15:47 BDT
To: Natasha <natasha_nw3@yahoo.co.uk>
Subject: Been working for one and a half hours already. Another 16-hour day.

Hope you are still dreaming. Good sex, then wellness and feeling good everyday. It's got to be worth it has it not??? Have a nice day x John x love you and you love yourself x

From: Natasha <natasha_nw3@yahoo.co.uk>
Date: 4 May 22:04:08 BDT
To: john smith <appledogstime@yahoo.co.uk>
Subject: Re: Been working for one and a half hours already. Another 16-hour day.

I am sure that it will be worth it, all of it. Hope you are not working too hard. N

May

From: john smith <appledogstime@yahoo.co.uk>
Date: 7 May 10:19:29 BDT
To: Natasha <natasha_nw3@yahoo.co.uk>
Subject: back home after a night of silly sex

Hi. You write to me you bitch. Well yes I did spend the night with Ruth but you were on my mind all the time, even when I was on the job so to speak. Two hot solid hours of it, she came twice and I made my excuses and left so I did not have to do it another three times. Anyway thinking of you all the time helps but makes it difficult as well but to be truthful it is exciting with you there in front of me, as her body becomes yours as I fuck her. But what can I do? We can't help who we fall in love with and I had finished with her when I met and found you. Anyway I had good sex with your help. Wish it had been you. Roll on September. I told her that I had to leave early as I wanted to test drive the new car up to 120mph on a quiet bit of the motorway. She begged me to let her come but I put my foot down and said no as I wanted the experience alone. I treated myself this week. I got myself a new car with my own plate. In Jan, Feb and March I made £55,000 so I bought a new Porcshe. It's black with john 1 as the plate. It sounds a lot but I sold the old one for £18,000 so not much more then your average car at £37,000. A new jag would cost that and I get the plate as well. Can you send me some more sexy pictures of you to keep me happy till September? It's a long time still and I'm wanking myself silly over you. You make me so horny but need some new images and if I give you my address what about some panties? I will send you some replacements. Love you and want you lots. What did the doc at st johns wood say? Having fun? I bet you never realised you could feel such things. Anyway I'm home alone with all your pictures laid out in front of me. I need some new stock please. Get Bill to take some. You know the kind of pictures us men like. Real slut stuff! You know legs open wide and slut knickers on or just showing it as they fall to the side. Dog shot with your bum in the air. Some dirty pics to keep me on boil for the next four months. Well my little sweet girl kiss thousands of them xxJohn love yourself lots.

May

From: Natasha <natasha_nw3@yahoo.co.uk>
Date: 7 May 12:31:54 BDT
To: john smith <appledogstime@yahoo.co.uk>
Subject: Why do you have silly sex?

Hi John,

Billy told me he had seen your car outside where you said Ruth lives. I suspected that the car was yours anyway. JS1... John Smith 1 couldn't belong to anybody else. Personalised number plates are a bit silly but I am sure it will give you lots of enjoyment. I believe we should enjoy what we have and if that makes you happy then why not, though I must say it is extravagant to say the least. Make sure that you don't upset anybody, as they will know what car to go for straight away. Actually I just wanted to say - nice car Mr.Smith enjoy it. I was depressed all evening feeling sorry for myself. It was a stupid day at work, I don't get as stressed as I used to before I got ill. The boss is getting better as I told him that if he doesn't I will walk. I will go anyway but not yet. Such a pretty boy, innocent face and he wants me to send him dirty pictures of me? Unheard of. I don't want to have anything to do with you, first you call me 'worse than a shit' and now you ask me for new pictures.. how cheeky can you get. No chance. The pictures I have are all from the time when I was 'working' and I am not going to send you those, they
are hidden and bring out all the wrong kind of memories and feelings. Sometimes I get them out. I would have to have some done and I might just for you but I am not promising. Anyway why would you want to drive your car at 120 MPH in here? Aren't you risking a speeding fine? The only country you can do 120mph is Germany isn't it? What ever you do don't smash yourself, it would be a shame. I am going to Hendon to a talk on colitis, it seemed a good idea when I agreed to go but I don't fancy it anymore. Can't not go as it would be rude not to.

Love Nxx
What are you doing later?

May

ILLNESS

She called to ask me if I would go with her to listen to a talk on Colitis and its alternative forms of treatment at an old church hall in North Finchley. I agreed and was happy that she was finally considering other remedies other than the hard and toxic drugs she was currently taking. The talk was apparently an extensive look into foods, vitamins and specialised diets that can be followed to alleviate symptoms.

When we arrived, the hall was filled with men and women of all ages and different backgrounds. It shocked me how very young some of the people were. Some scampered around with their arms full of books and leaflets on the condition, which were readily available on the many stalls all over the hall. Others were sat down waiting for the lecture to begin. It really did surprise me just how many people actually suffered from this illness.

I had a feeling that, although she had made the effort to get herself down to this talk, she was not all that prepared to put in any more to change her life for the better. She was always so tired all the time, and big changes meant a lot of effort, which tired her out even more. But I was still pleased that she was here in the hall with me, and at the very least, we would walk away much more wiser on the subject, though we were not any closer to a solution for all her deep-rooted problems.

We did walk away much more informed, and it saddened me to think it how it could not be much fun to be a poorly, sexy thing like Natasha, being constantly ill and having to work every day regardless.

Back at her flat we cuddled for half and hour on the bed, and I left her to sleep, gently pulling the duvet over her. I quietly prayed for better times for my little angel.

Tears, Looking For True Love, Eternally

My poetry starts to tell how I feel;
It's tinged with sadness, my tears are real.
I was born without my name,
Raised along with the wind and rain,
So I can give all my love-
Eternally.

All I ask is to love a girl,
Who I know will want to stay.
All I ask is to love a girl,
For much more than just one day,
And that this love will last,
On its own-
Eternally.

Perfect soul mates, meant to be;
Welcome dreams and broken schemes.
The wave washes over, breaking me,
Like a pebble by the beach and sea.
I get so wet and cold, I'm growing very old,
Looking for my true love quest-
Eternally.

From: john smith <appledogstime@yahoo.co.uk>
Date: 9 May 2006 20:34:10 BDT
To: Natasha <natasha_nw3@yahoo.co.uk>
Subject: Still nothing from you. You agreed a truthful start to you and us

Can't take it, just silence. Nothing. No more emails. Nothing. Just silence. What do you want? We may be forty years together to start by not telling you the truth, letting you get away with whatever you want to say. Even if I know it's wrong and not the truth, well I don't know anymore. O.k. I will wait for you, if I don't hear from you in ten days I will presume you don't want us and that will be the end of us. Nothing more I can say or do I tried to get to know you and help you and love you. May be some people can never be helped. Kiss x John x love you and all them that love you will give you till the 20th then call it dead in the ground and walk away. Pity it could have been real good xxxxxxxxxx

From: Natasha <natasha_nw3@yahoo.co.uk>
Date: 9 May 20:40:55 BDT
To: john smith <appledogstime@yahoo.co.uk>
Subject: Re: Why do you have silly sex?

Dear John
What a beautiful day it was today. I love this weather before it gets too hot. Can't stand all the heat of the sun in the summer. There are only two men who want me nobody else, and I am not complaining. More than I can cope with wouldn't be able to cope with one more telling me off, actually there is one more but he tells me off for different reasons (just in case you take it the wrong way he is my boss). Wouldn't want you to get the wrong end of the stick. I am having a very positive and enjoyable day. I have been on a high all day for some reason. I can't post you anything I don't have your address. Can you imagine us meeting in the waiting room at the doctors for the first time? How bizarre would that be and what a romantic place. Would you hold my hand while I described to the doctor all my symptoms? The doc would think that I am

having a heart attack if he took my pressures and my heart beat. God save me if he did an internal examination, I would need a spare pair of panties. It is very nice to offer though - and I mean that without being sarcastic. Anyway this is all bizarre and mad and funny and silly no not silly I got myself into trouble using that word last time so not silly. And if silly than silly ha ha. Hope you are doing well let me know my dearest man who thinks he knows everything. When will you be ruling the world? If you are nice to me I will come and help you. No silly me you don't need any help.
Love and kisses
Natasha xxx

From: Natasha <natasha_nw3@yahoo.co.uk>
Date: 9 May 20:49:32 BDT
To: john smith <appledogstime@yahoo.co.uk>
Subject: Re: Still nothing from you. You agreed a truthful start to you and us

Ultimatum? not nice at all. Give people a chance my love. World wasn't built in a day.

How happy are you today? Nxxx

From: Natasha <natasha_nw3@yahoo.co.uk>
Date: 10 May 08:07:45 BDT
To: john smith <appledogstime@yahoo.co.uk>
Subject: This evening

Hi john

Hope you are having better day today. I will write to you this evening as I am working all day and it might be impossible to do so during the day.

Love Natasha x

From: Natasha <natasha_nw3@yahoo.co.uk>
Date: 10 May 22:41:37 BDT
To: john smith <appledogstime@yahoo.co.uk>
Subject: What went wrong yesterday?

John

I don't know where this came from. It was only the second day yesterday that I hadn't written to you. I just reread your E-mail and somewhere you are suggesting I am not telling you the truth. Let me tell you that I have been totally honest with you right from the word go. I am not sure what else you expect from me but I am not guilty of not telling the truth. You should tell me what wasn't true. I don't really know what prompted you to write all
this stuff. What is happening in your life apart from me not writing to you for two days? It can't be just me. Ten-day ultimatum is not good and I don't want to live through another one of these. John if I didn't want to have anything to do with you I would tell you, maybe you should tell me what is the matter and what upset you so much to give me ultimatum of this kind. I was upset when you decided to call me names and when you gave me long speeches on horses and water and on free sex. I don't always need explanations I am not silly. I get upset when you talk down to me and patronise me (because that is how it feels sometimes). I am almost thirty years old but you make me feel as If I was five and needed my bum spanked for not doing as I am told. And this is the truth and exactly what I feel. I did have a really good day yesterday though I feel very, very tired all the time. I am shattered most of the time. Now that I go to work I don't need and want stress. I like you very much my lovely but I don't need blackmail and ultimatums. Please let me know what upset you so much to feel the need to write what you did. What is happening in your life? What are you doing? Are you still working the killer hours? What do you do when you don't work?
Hope you are Ok
Love me xx

From: john smith <appledogstime@yahoo.co.uk>
Date: 11 May 07:56:10 BDT
To: Natasha <natasha_nw3@yahoo.co.uk>
Subject: Re: This evening

What is upsetting me? It's easy anyone can work it out! It's the frustration of not being with the woman I love. Having to wait so long is driving me crazy! I can't hold or kiss the woman I want to be with. What do I do when I am on my own? Sit, think of you and wank to you. Only the pictures are old now my life is. You work and sometimes Ruth in that order so don't ask me why I get angry. It's also getting you to do anything like now, like this min, everything takes ages which can be so frustrating for someone who likes to get things done. My Mum and Dad are action people, if something needed doing it was done end of story. So that's why I don't understand someone who can put things off for days, weeks or even months. All most like a different planet. So my little darling that is what makes me angry, so make me happy. Cure it all for me kiss x John

From: Natasha <natasha_nw3@yahoo.co.uk>
Date: 11 May 08:49:31 BDT
To: john smith <appledogstime@yahoo.co.uk>
Subject: This morning

John

but this is me, the woman you say you love. I am working on it but you must understand that this has been an integral part of my life for many years. I am not trying to excuse it or apologise for it. I am just saying that I am working on it and if you met me years ago you would have found me impossible. Paralysed with fears of all sorts. I am going well at this moment. You can't just love one part of me, so please do not get angry or frustrated. I am not trying to please you or fit a mould. All this must feel ok for me. I had a lifetime of letting people make decisions for me. Now I would be glad if I could be allowed to make some of them myself. I understand how

frustrating and alien this all is for you but only you must know whether this is worth fighting for, I think it is, but you must let me know what you think and not get frustrated and nasty my dearest darling John.
I am on it.
love and kisses only for you Nxxx
Don't work too hard today. What time do you finish?

From: john smith <appledogstime@yahoo.co.uk>
Date: 11 May 10:24:07 BDT
To: Natasha <natasha_nw3@yahoo.co.uk>
Subject: I'm sure you are my sweet little pink knickers lady. All I'm asking is you to try harder

A little harder. Otherwise we both may be collecting our old age money from the post office and you may still not have sorted our and your life out. 85 years old nat asking what have I done with my life? Well I thought about sorting my problems out. When will you do it tomorrow? But tomorrow never comes. That's right that's why I can't do anything or sort them out. Any way I'm running out of people to blame. But your 85 now and you still have the same problems? I know but at 85 is it worth it? Well it's your life? I know and it's nearly over.. and what did you do with it? Was it a good one did you have fun and enjoy it? Well for one thing I had a lot of problems. Did you sort them out and get on with living? Well, no... Is that going to be you?? So ask your self the question...yes or no? And do something. The other thing is that I'm a man with needs I can't change that. Love you lots be good xxx

From: john smith <appledogstime@yahoo.co.uk>
Date: 12 May 00:12:04 BDT
To: Natasha <natasha_nw3@yahoo.co.uk>
Subject: Strange day, three hours working as a carpenter

Won't go in to the details but the little girl was crying down the phone so big cave man was wanted. Go urgently in case somebody brakes in and rapes me in the night (she should be

so lucky). Window broken and half open. Sash has broken window open, madam was so hot in the night that she had to take her knickers off. To cool off she opened the window wide. The poor thing this morning was leaving for work, the window would not close so ring daddy urgent "quote" but I will loose £3000 coming to fix your window. She says you have to come I will get robed, things taken, raped in the night.. little green men from mars etc etc. So I left work to fix it and it took me three hours. I drove by your house on my way home gazed longingly hoping I might see you but no... I'm told later that a freelance carpenter would have fixed it for £120. Oh well so now I'm the most expensive carpenter on this
earth! Will my talents never stop?? So that was my day. Speak soon love xxJohn love yourself and them that loves you...wanking off in old knickers pretending they belong to you. I'm on my back, your pictures have a most deserving place now..on my ceiling stuck there with great pride. So when I open my eyes in the morning I see you looking down on me kiss xxxxx j

From: john smith <appledogstime@yahoo.co.uk>
Date: 12 May 09:18:06 BDT
To: Natasha <natasha_nw3@yahoo.co.uk>
Subject: Hot weekend. Wish we could have spent it together

If we got together the weekend could get even hotter. Hope your starting to get the big Orgasms. See you soon, get ready for the big one in September. September 27th you and I will fly to New York and if it's wonderful as I know it will be we will get your ring at tiffany's. Kiss x Have a nice one. I will think of you shagging Billy this weekend and hope your starting to let go of everything in your past and are at last giving yourself to a man. Total and complete even if you are calling the shots kiss x Love, the one you're with and love yourselfX John X

From: Natasha <natasha_nw3@yahoo.co.uk>
Date: 12 May 18:18:26 BDT
To: john smith <appledogstime@yahoo.co.uk>
Subject: Re: Hot weekend. Wish we could have spent it together

Wish we were spending the weekend together too but I am working all Saturday. Why New York?
Will write later.

Nxx

From: john smith <appledogstime@yahoo.co.uk>
Date: 12 May 23:31:20 BDT
To: Natasha <natasha_nw3@yahoo.co.uk>
Subject: Why New York? Because it's there!

You have never been there, and I have to pop into the New York office for four hours one day and it has the best Tffany's in the world. You deserve the best in the world on your finger… kiss John x love all who love you and yourself x

From: Natasha <natasha_nw3@yahoo.co.uk>
Date: 12 May 23:34:35 BDT
To: john smith <appledogstime@yahoo.co.uk>
Subject: Re: Hot weekend. Wish we could of spent it together

Dear John

It was so hot and what a wonderful evening. Yes I am looking after the man and he loves every minute of it. When are you taking your holiday with Ruth? And how soon after that do you propose us going away? Just let me tell you that I didn't say I am going yet. I have to go to bed I am so tired again.

Will write later love Nxx

May

THE WOODS
Friday 12th May

Things were getting better and better. In truth, they were th best times we had ever had together. We never fought at all, I never needed to ask for sex; in fact she would want it more than me on some occasions.

The job in the opticians was putting a huge amount of unnecessary stress on her. In hindsight, it really was not such a good idea for her to be working at all. Her boss seemed to delight in finding various ways to wind her up, which she did not deserve in the slightest.

However, she had a day off from it all today, and so we went off to the woods with a picnic hamper to have a nice refreshing lunch. She looked stunning in her pretty little dress, and God knows what exciting delights lay hidden beneath it. She was happy and relaxed to be free from work, knowing that there were be no stresses chasing her for the day. She knew the woods off by heart, and it calmed her to be here in her place of comfort.

We had all her favourite songs on the CD player in the new top-of-the-range BMW I had bought, which was almost as wonderful as she was.

It was another hot, warm day, with all the colours of the rainbow falling upon us through the trees above the parked car.

There was a stillness over everything,

It was now 12:30. The 12th of May. My mother was born on the 15th, and I had given Natasha my mother's ring as a present. She wore it all the time.

It was one of those special days. She was so happy. She held my hand, laughing, playing, flirting. She was making me 20 years old again and ten feet tall. This is what it should have been like for the last 8 years, but other people, and so-called friends got in the way.

We found a fallen tree in the sunshine and we were eating pate sandwiches, cheese and tomato, and cold chicken. All the misery and pain in her face started to go.

She lay across the old tree trunk, and the sun was coming through the trees in long shafts of dappled light, with the dust of the forest rising through it. Birds were singing, and she had her long full gypsy skirt pulled up higher than her knees.

When she shifted her body to get more comfortable from time to time, she tantalisingly, knowingly gave me a brief glimpse of her tiny red panties. She had one of the most beautiful bottoms I have ever known in the world. Almost like a black woman's bottom. Wonderfully firm, round and shapely. I felt like we were both in the middle of a Constable painting. A lad and his lass. Birds were chirping, tiny flying insects buzzed, the heat in the 80s hanging, a stillness over everything, and not a single person in sight.

A spider was spinning her web between two twigs at the bottom of the tree trunk hoping for a prey to land. A fox ran across the little path through the woods near where we sat, stopped, looked at us for a few moments, and then passed on her way, her tail flying out behind her. A squirrel dropped some nuts, clambered down the tree to retrieve them and went back up again. A long way away in the distance, you could hear the running water of a stream over rocks, almost making the sound of tinkling music.

She wore a light blue top with bare arms, bare legs and no tights. The curve of her breasts under her skimpy top was exciting. Constable would have certainly liked to have painted her! She was angelic with the sunlight framing her head and face, catching her blonde hair from behind. The hush and yet still sounds of the deep forest had an incredible stillness. Perfect.

I turned to her smiling face, and I said to her, 'Why don't you take your clothes off and let me take some pictures of you? These woods are so beautiful. Let's remember this forever.'

She didn't refuse. Instead her reluctance almost showed eagerness.

'Not here by the path.' She said with a cheeky grin, 'But I will. Why not?'

'Yes, let's.' Like an eager young school boy, I followed her deep, deep into the woods. Somewhere nobody knows. To find and enjoy forbidden delights, given willingly.

We came across a small clearing. She took all her clothes off, and then she put them on a tiny tree stump. She put her arms around a large tree and stuck her bottom out at me provocatively. She knew, as all women do instinctively, what she was doing to me. I began to take lost of pictures, as she jumped around and made different poses. Sometimes half in shadow, sometimes posing in a sunbeam, sometimes just visible in the darkness of the forest. Long shadows and sunlight mixing and breaking up through the leaves, as she ran around laughing.

'Come on!' she said, 'Take your trousers off! And your pants.' She said laughing. 'Relieve the pressure on him! Let me do pictures of you as well!'

These were some of the nicest pictures of me standing with my cock hard by a large oak tree. Today, everything about her was beautiful. She ran around snapping away with the camera, and laughing. Her wonderful body, alabaster, like a statuette. Her legs sometimes spread wide and bent as she peered through her camera. I came up to her and put my arms around her in the middle of taking the photos. Nature and these woods must have seen this moment many times. This is how life should be.

She kissed me, turned her back, put her hands on the tree and slightly spread he legs. She left the camera laying on the ground. In this soecial moment, her bottom was slightly pushed up for me, and her knees slightly bent. I slid him into her in one smooth thrust, deep, deep. She let out one tiny cry and gasp. She said, 'Oh god… he's so big today.' I started to fuck her with long strokes, the sunlight on my shoulders and in her hair. All of nature went suddenly quiet. Even the birds stopped singing. The only noise in the forest, was the noise our bodies were making, and the slurping of water in the ground. As my hard cock went deeper and deeper inside her wet wet pussy, I could not control myself anymore. I came deep into her after 20 minutes, and the cry I let out rang through the forest like the sound of a male lion. Neither of us had any condoms, and as she pulled her panties up, she laughed and looked at me.

'You'll have to pay if I get pregnant!' She wiped herself with a small bit of tissue, and with that beautiful bottom upturned, inviting even more pleasure from me. The forest waited and held its breath in anticipation.

'I hope it's a little girl, darling!' I said. 'We can call her Sunlight, or Forest Glay, or something silly and beautiful like that, and tell her she was made here in the forest.' There were still no people except us two. It was as if it were our forest. We owned the world at this moment. It was ours and nobody could ever take it away from us. Corny, it's true, but we felt like Adam and Eve with forbidden fruits. Time flies when you are having so much fun. We had been here 5 hours and had done all the nice things that a boy and girl should do.

She took my arm and we walked back down the long path. I fretted whether we could find the car or not, as always. She laughed at me and chirped, 'Yes yes! I know where we are. I come here all the time!'

It had been a wonderful day and we had pictures to prove it. No stress for her. This is what this girl needed; a stress free life. I loved her at that moment more than I had ever done, and maybe she herself did not realise it, but one day she would treasure these pictures forever.

I saw and felt the call of nature, and we both heard it at the same time. It was 5:30, and we had gotten there at 11 in the morning. Then we realised, it was not the call of nature, it was not a bird or an animal, it was the sound of a saxophone being played. We found a man who lived in flats 3 miles away. His neighbours complained when he practiced at home, so he came to his woods to play. It was the only place he could go and not disturb anyone. So we had a free concert. I took some pictures of him, with the sunlight falling on him and his instrument. We left him in his world and I was sure that all the squirrels, the stoats, all the little animals came to listen, as we started the long drive home through the rush hour.

It was so nice to not work today. We had both found enchantment. She was clinging onto my arm, and kept squeezing it from time to time. The music on the wireless was playing the song 'Angel' and my mind went back over the day's events. Why couldn't it always be like this? Other people would always get in the way. Other people would always try to ruin couples. Well-meaning friends always wanted to put their 20p of unwelcome advice in to a relationship. Problems and hang-ups are there in plenty anyway, without interfering friends or relatives.

I looked out the window as we drove down the long road to the north circular, endless forest on each side. I saw a large beautiful oak had been felled at the side of the road. A magnificent oak. It must have been at least 400 years old. To think that it was standing when Shakespeare was still standing on this earth. Why had they felled such a beautiful tree? They are so very special. A little bit of the England that we all love. Where is life leading, tell me friend? In what far shore will it end?

We saw a charming old Inn and restaurant at a little roundabout in the woods.

'Come on, you don't need to cook anything when you get home after such a lovely day, let's have dinner here.'

We were slightly shocked when we got inside though, because this old inn had been turned into a Thai restaurant inside. Still, why not have Thai food?

We talked of the stress of her new job, her future life, what she wanted to do, but no mention of her internet friend. He was forgotten on this day. This day was ours, and ours alone.

She put her hand on my knee and squeezed it gently. We looked at each other and we knew that we would always feel something. Whatever happened, there would always be something there. What storms, what disappointments, what bitter blows? The more you are loved, the more you feel love, and the more love you give out, the more you get back. I always tried to be her rock.

When we got back to her house, she and I went straight up to her room. She took off all her clothes straight away, and lay face up on the bed. It was years since I remembered her doing that. She spread her legs, and I took her in my arms.

'My turn now you lovely man! You had your fun in the woods today!'

Soon I was next to her naked and she opened her legs even wider, and held her pussy herself, just above her pubic mound. I slid two of my fingers up inside her and slowly started to push them in and out, feeling for her g-spot. I then started to lick and suck her clitoris into my mouth at the same time, breathing hot air from my lungs into it, flicking it with my tongue. She was already so sexed up and so horny. Thick cream started to flow into my fingers and into the palm of my hand. It was the fastest she had ever come. After 5 minutes her breathing started to get heavy and deeper and deeper. She gave a little tiny moan and a little cry, like a cat when you accidentally stand on her paw. Then she was screaming, and she really came, her body shaking more and more, thick juice pouring out of her fast. Then she closed her eyes and lay very still. It was already 10:30, and she gave me a hug. We both thought of the beautiful 400 year old oak, that someone had cruelly cut down, no doubt for some stupid counsel reason.

She hugged me tighter and tighter, and kissed me strong and for real. Her tongue, like a serpent tongue, flicking back and forward inside my mouth. Then she said she was off to have a bath. We had spent 12 beautiful hours together. She looked at me with a great deal of love in her eyes, and I went home to feed the cats.

'A perfect day, Billy' she said. I loved her to bits. Why is it not always like this? Why did we need someone, an outsider on the internet, to bring this about? Maybe everything dies in the end, like the beautiful tree. I made up my mind at that moment. To enjoy her and everything about her for as long as it lasted.

May

I Used To Be A Tree

I used to be a tree
Lovers hearts were
Scratched on me.
Now I am a note pad,
Basildon Bond.

Boys and girls
Sending dreams
Through the post
Love, hope, happiness
It makes me miss the
Wind, snow and rain
Of when I was a tree.

Now there are so many parts of me.
Some makes the news,
Others envelopes tined blue
Rose pink, various tints and hues
Perhaps you wrote upon me too.
Some things never change
I used to be a tree.

People read messages from my bark
When they walked about in the park.
Now they read me everywhere.
Paper, paper.
Get the news
So much of me now is front page news.
I feel quite faint
That's progress for you.
I used to be a tree.

I hated to be cut down
With my branches tall,
Up to the sky, several stories high.
But now I bring so much
Pleasure: 10,000 pads they

May

Made of me.

Boys and girls
Send love to each other
Lovers still sit on my stump
That's all that's left of me
A young girl cried
Her poor heart sad
For the love that was
Not meant to be.

Her tears fell,
Old seeds long blown free
The sun, air, earth worked its
Magic spell, and grew another me.
Something's never change,
I'm a tree.

From: Natasha <natasha_nw3@yahoo.co.uk>
Date: 12 May 23:40:49 BDT
To: john smith <appledogstime@yahoo.co.uk>
Subject: Re: Hot weekend. Wish we could of spent it together
Because it is there - what an explanation. Almost original. I have not been to lots of places and lots of those places I would not want to ever go so that is not a valid reason. Your office is there well that might be a good reason and that Tiffany's is there, that is very sweet and that might be a reason too I suppose. I don't really like big cities. That is a good reason for not going. Love me

From: john smith <appledogstime@yahoo.co.uk>
Date: 13 May 15:38:35 BDT
To: Natasha <natasha_nw3@yahoo.co.uk>
Subject: Don't forget if you do fall in love with Billy again
Or should they? Or condemn you. Age or any other reason is not a reason, it should not be. After all look at my mum and dad, real love defies all barriers and it's not for your friends, your family or for anyone else in this world to have a right to tell you what you should and shouldn't do. It should not be. For in the end it's better to spend ten more years with a man who truly loves you, wants you and cares for you then to spend 30 years with a man who does not know you at all and who could leave you at any time. Who can know how deep his love is? What ever you my say, think or hate about Billy I have to say that his loyalty is with out question there always. I ask anyone to say it's not. A man who sticks by a woman through thick and thin bad and good is worth a great deal. I'm saying all of this because one it's true and two you talk now as if you don't think we can work it out and who is to say you might not be right. You might not have such a bad life with Billy and as my dad says better the devil you know then the one you don't. Anyway early days, lets see how things shape up as the deep blue sea is very deep and who knows what you might find out about you in this time of inward looking and change. This is grow up time Natasha as you're a woman now with all those initials. As you give more and more to a man who loves you and get back more and more in return you

will start to get rare and surprise gifts from people. Karma is strange and we do not understand it fully. Your parents, family, even a sister or brother (if you have one) will start to be nice to you. Give you gifts, try to get closer to you. Will want to tell you things, will want you to be closer to them. The mysteries thread that runs through the universe lets the force be with you etc etc. The Buddhists call it deep karma. By being kind and loving towards a cat or dog you open up new windows in yourself, you never knew that feeling existed.So yes lets see how the next four months pan out and what new windows will open up in this new world we both enter. I still want to fuck your brains out as you do me and if it worked I would want to spend my life with you but lets love the ones we are with now with everything we have. Give our until our time comes?? Then lets see what happens. Love him and yourself lots xxxJohn

From: john smith <appledogstime@yahoo.co.uk>
Date: 13 May 16:04:39 BDT
To: Natasha <natasha_nw3@yahoo.co.uk>
Subject: As I sit at home in my office with my little maid running around cleaning everything…

With her feather duster even me?? I look at the pictures of you, the one which I have had blown up big now so you sleep next to me in bed...Ruth does not come here anymore, the dog and her.. It's to upsetting. Too many sweet and sour memories. I think to my self. What will be will be. The only thing we can change is ourselves. XxxJohn

May

JOB LOSS

I received a call from her asking for me to pick her up from work, which I thought was a little odd, as she had never asked me to do this before. The moment I saw her walk towards me in the car, I knew a disaster had occurred.

'What's wrong?' I enquired as she stepped into my car. Huge tears welled up in her eyes and rolled down her cheeks. She was shaking a little.

'He sacked me.' She said, bluntly. 'My services are no longer required…'

I paused for a moment.

'I'm so sorry darling. But you were fed up with the job anyway, weren't you?'

'I know! But I still didn't want to be dismissed!'

I took her for a meal at the Chinese restaurant opposite the Post Office on Finchley Road. She was so upset that there was no way she was going to go home and cook for herself. She was in quite a state, and was only just managing to keep herself together. During the meal she ranted on about what a mean, horrible bastard her ex-boss was.

'So what will you do now?' I asked.

'I have some baby-sitting jobs, and a few more cleaning clients… what else can I do?'

When we arrived back at her flat, she threw herself on the bed, howling and weeping and so very messed up. She just kept crying. Nothing could console her. Nothing could make her come round.

'I'm useless at everything! So utterly useless!' she kept saying over and over again into her pillow. After about an hour she was beginning to exhaust herself with her own grief. She had calmed herself down enough so that she could talk, and started to tell me about how her father had been right all this time. She had grown up with him telling her how useless and hopeless she was all her life. I did my best to cheer her up, and wrapped her up in a blanket, pulled the blinds down, turned the little kitchen light and small lamp over the cooker on, and switched the main lights off. I looked at her sleepy face, so tired and unhappy after the day's events, and left her to drift off as I laid her down to rest.

May

I walked out of the building and looked up at the sky for a brief moment, when I noticed the light switched on at the flat opposite hers. I looked towards it, and saw him, staring straight across at Natasha's closed blinds. Standing, just standing, staring at her window. If I caught him again, I thought it might be a good idea to call the police in future. It all seemed a little too bizarre for my liking.

The Light Across The Street
So you're a young man
The light across the street
Your body burns for her
And envies me
This warm and painted night
With shining sky
Take three pebbles from a brook
And the brook no longer sings
Who are you mystery man?
What licentious thoughts
Are in your head
Nobody knows your name
You just stop and stare
From your window up there

May

From: Natasha <natasha_nw3@yahoo.co.uk>
Date: 13 May 18:56:20 BDT
To: john smith <appledogstime@yahoo.co.uk>
Subject: Re: As I sit at home in my office with my little maid running around cleaning everything

Hi John

I believe that I am in need of some gigantic changes in my life. You write about karma, if all that is true I must not have been very nice or good person. I have been politely told today that my services will no longer be required at work and that we have not gelled as much as he expected (my boss that is). And lots more and more and more. Bottom line is I will have to look for a another job very, very soon. With my experience and my education it is always a fun thing to do. How depressing can it
get. The job hunting is probably less scary then turning up to work on Monday. As you say what will be will be and I will just have to get on with it. I just feel a bit pissed off and alone today.

love me

let me know what you are up to.

From: john smith <appledogstime@yahoo.co.uk>
Date: 14 May 00:12:35 BDT
To: Natasha <natasha_nw3@yahoo.co.uk>
Subject: Karma and all that jazz. You knew it was coming just like everything in life you know it,

You knew it. We all do. Some people try to forget the signs, others take heed and remember everything you think is possible. It will happen if you let it, people worn you but you worn yourself. Take no notice at your own peril, in future if you think something act on it don't put it to one side. Still I'm very sorry very sorry but you knew it even I knew it. You told me you did not get on over and over..your mistake if you made one at all..was to let him know that...KARMA. Be nice. If you had been really nice to him he would have not been or could not have found a reason to let you go. So until you do go bend over backwards to be nice to him and he will find it impossible to let you go. It's all still karma. You can then leave when you feel like it. Play him at his own game. In the mean time be cool don't panic or go crazy. Go on holiday with Billy take it easy, look after babies, do something non-stressful, no harm in that or no shame. If the wife of the future king of England could do it so can you. Diana was a kindergarten helper. You will have time to think doing that. What do you want to do with my life besides have kids etc get married etc make a man happy etc? Take your time, believe me you have it. There are men who I work with who were full time students till they were forty so be cool, take your time this year you have been through a lot. Don't rush, rest, make a little here a little there, be kind, give out good feelings and things will come to you wait and see. Get your sex, health and your own feelings of self worth sorted first as the rest will come of it's own accord. Kiss X Be happy everything is meant in life, you knew it was coming. Learn next time, don't show your feelings to people who employ you. I never do. I hate my bosses but never let them know. I just smile and say ok. Those ok's mean consider it done. Big smile on my face but underneath I think...Fuck you. Take care xxx john

From: john smith <appledogstime@yahoo.co.uk>
Date: 14 May 08:17:19 BDT
To: Natasha <natasha_nw3@yahoo.co.uk>
Subject: Go and have fun today with someone who loves you forget it for a few days. Who knows

Who you might meet, job and opportunities will open up for you from nowhere. I had ten jobs before this one. I'm working today all day and one place I threw a chair across the room smashing my bosses desk. In another I got him by the throat (different boss) and wanted to kill him. Not too much but when I do I have a wicked Irish temper, when it explodes you better run and hide until I calm down. My dad gave me a good talking to about four years ago, since then I have been a good boy. When they get me angry and upset now I just look at them and say yes sir no sir three bags full sir but inside I think you fuck! Shit face! Get the fuck out of my life...anyway have fun as they are not worth it, especially if they won't meet you half way. Go out! Have fun! x kiss John

From: Natasha <natasha_nw3@yahoo.co.uk>
Date: 14 May 08:34:05 BDT
To: john smith <appledogstime@yahoo.co.uk>
Subject: Re: Karma and all that jazz. You knew it was coming just like everything in life you know it,

Thank you for your kind words my dear John. I couldn't have been nice to that man. But as you say I will be nicer than nice until I leave. There is no time limit on when I have to do it so he said. I appreciate very much all you said you are a clever man but I never doubted that.

Love and kisses
Me xx

From: Natasha <natasha_nw3@yahoo.co.uk>
Date: 14 May 08:42:30 BDT
To: john smith <appledogstime@yahoo.co.uk>
Subject: Re: Go and have fun today with someone who loves you forget it for a few days. Who knows

John

That is quite a temper you have there! I was invited out today but I cancelled it maybe I should un-cancel it and will go later on. Thinking of you. See you very soon

Nx

May

From: Natasha <natasha_nw3@yahoo.co.uk>
Date: 14 May 22:14:33 BDT
To: john smith <appledogstime@yahoo.co.uk>
Subject: Re: Go and have fun today

Hope you are not working too hard my dear john.
Nxx

From: john smith <appledogstime@yahoo.co.uk>
Date: 15 May 17:30:21 BDT
To: Natasha <natasha_nw3@yahoo.co.uk>
Subject: It's not the money you have, rich or poor it's the quality of life that's important

So don't worry that's just ego that's used to saying we do this or that. We can work as a window cleaner (man or women) we may have a very small flat, a cat or a dog, a man or woman who truly loves us, we have only have six dresses in the cupboard, ten tops, two pairs of shoes and we take two small cheap holidays a year. We have ok helth but we have everything we need to live. We cook cheap but simple food, good love and sex twice a week. We have a cheep car but go to the country once a week, the cinema once a month. That's all you need, that is real happiness to love and be loved. A roof, a cat or dog, a countryside not to far away and a seaside to visit twice a year. You need no more then that. So if you find a little job with no stress and you feel happy and you look forward to seeing your man when he can see you and when you do spend time together. Make each other happy, what more do you need in life?? Nothing. We have two-dozen men working with me that are worth over six million. Are they happy, no their lives are so fucked up. You got to believe it. They are so fucked up, all of them. We have a young girl (25 years old) that cleans our office, she earns £15000 after deductions about £300 a week she has a boyfriend 21 years older then her, a little dog, and a tiny one bed flat in Wapping and that girl is so happy and content. So the men try to pull her but no she does not want to know. She says no thanks and yet they could change her life. They may even fall in love

with her as she is sexy and very pretty. I spoke to her the other night when I was in the office on my own late working and she was cleaning. I said don't you ever want to leave your man for one of these rich boys here? and she said no my man works in a photo lab he earns £300 and lives with is old mum, we help each other as we are together. No life is perfect look how unhappy these men are, do you think I want to be with one of them and be unhappy with them? No thank you I'm happy with what little I have. You know something Natasha darling if I lost everything I had and could be with a girl I love in a nice tiny place, what more can any of us want? In the end it comes down to quality. Money does not get you happiness..it brings you more problems and how to be very unhappy in comfort which is not comfortable because you don't know if the person loves you for you or for the prestige and money. If you have nothing they must love you for you. There is nothing else She was so right. Kiss don't worry about the job you get as long as your stress free John kiss xxxx love all
that love you and yourself x

From: Natasha <natasha_nw3@yahoo.co.uk>
Date: 15 May 23:34:25 BDT
To: john smith <appledogstime@yahoo.co.uk>
Subject: Re: It's not the money you have, rich or poor it's the quality of life that's important

Dearest John

I was getting so sad when I read that, you will not write to me until Wednesday and here you are a few hours later-a letter. This is all so true what you have written. It is not the money, it is how you feel in yourself which is important. The little cleaning girl is right. I have a friend - well somebody I know, he is worth more than all your work colleagues combined and he is the most miserable person I have ever met. Never sure whether people want to know him because of him or because of what he owns. But lets be realistic, certain level of income is necessary as we do have to pay the bills and the Jewish landlord. If I forget my rent, which hardly ever happens (it must be in cash as he is on the fiddle, I am sure of it, he will drive me to the bank and wait outside for his money). We don't need much to be happy. And being happy is a feeling inside of you, nice little moments here and there, it is not directly linked to your bank account. I believe that simple pleasures don't need a lot of money spent on them. I just miss having the cat or the dog, I am not allowed to have one, not even a gold fish. I had a little white dog I loved at home but it died few years ago and so did my cats. This job I lost is not the only work I do as you well know (I know that you have your spies on me) so I am not totally without work. I have been working for my self since I came to England. I work for some very nice people who appreciate my work, I got rid of the horrid ones. But this was a real blow to my confidence, I was in bits yesterday. I am more positive today. Thinking of you a lot. Sending you some pictures which Billy took of me on Friday we went out to the country. I don't particularly like them and they are not what you wanted but anyway let me know what you think, I am sure you will. Love Me xxx

From: Natasha <natasha_nw3@yahoo.co.uk>
Date: 18 May 21:25:46 BDT
To: john smith <appledogstime@yahoo.co.uk>
Subject: Don't over do the working

How is New York? I was walking down West End Lane today, and I had something to tell you for a split second. I thought I must call you, it felt so normal and natural. After I realised that I can't - no number. The brain is a funny thing. Anyway will write to you later my dear John.
I am working all day tomorrow and Saturday. Love you lots. Nxxx

From: john smith <appledogstime@yahoo.co.uk>
Date: 18 May 23:15:18 BDT
To: Natasha <natasha_nw3@yahoo.co.uk>
Subject: The implant and how good it is

Here I sit with my laptop on my lap waiting for my flight to be called should be in new York at nine thirty tomorrow. We had a professor come in to invest some money and he said the implant was so good that every women in the world should be treated with it, even if they are well and ok and nothing is wrong with them. It gives you pain free use of pads and nothing changes, same time every month. It makes you feel really good and sexy so there's one for you. Will write when I can xJohn
P.S You must be up to the 6th or 7th hot shag by now and having real fun with billy xxxxxxx

From: john smith <appledogstime@yahoo.co.uk>
Date: 20 May 14:29:42 BDT
To: Natasha <natasha_nw3@yahoo.co.uk>
Subject: In my hotel room thinking of you.

Where are my new pictures to helpd my raging hard on? Suffering, need to come. Thinking of you. Pictures please. If anything ever happens to me, if I ever had an accident or anything, (as I'm a bit crazy at times) marry Billy. Well here I am for a month working hard. They also want me back here for three weeks on October 10th so that is the final date now when I am taking you with me and after three weeks you and I will be mad in love. If you change your mind I will give you the tickets to do as you wish with. Have a holiday in New York City. So your ticket is booked, a return flight from Heathrow 12 noon on the tenth of October, first class. Kiss X Missing you already, feels good to know that you are just up the road. Will write soon? You must be having fun, you will be real nice and hot for me
Take care xJohn

May

From: Natasha <natasha_nw3@yahoo.co.uk>
Date: 20 May 2006 19:29:57 BDT
To: john smith <appledogstime@yahoo.co.uk>
Subject: Here are some pictures from last week country walk

John you are a naughty man. I did say that when I split up with Billy that I didn't want to go looking for anybody else and that marriage, children and all that was the last thing on my mind. I am not a nice person to be with now though, I do try very heard. Billy is very disheartened by the whole situation of you and me. I am very down because of my job and because it was partly my fault that I lost the job. I am not just up the road you are very far away and I am here. Here are the pictures Billy took of me last week, I don't like them but he thinks they are lovely. Let me know what you think. love Nxx

From: Natasha <natasha_nw3@yahoo.co.uk>
Date: 20 May 19:42:30 BDT
To: john smith <appledogstime@yahoo.co.uk>
Subject: Re: In my hotel room thinking of you.

John maybe we should meet first before we go away for any length of time and then decide whether we want to go away together. I can be an incredibly miserable person and I know for sure that that would not be fun for any of us.
I am sorry to be so pessimistic all the time.
Nxx

From: john smith <appledogstime@yahoo.co.uk>
Date: 21 May 00:18:34 BDT
To: Natasha <natasha_nw3@yahoo.co.uk>
Subject: The photographs of you are so beautiful

The photographs are wonderful so sensitive and yet sexy. I got an instant big hard on when you come with me it will be great... God you are so sexy, really sexy. I love the pictures, this will be short as working all day tomorrow. You said he won't be down, you said it. The words came from you. The best lover, best friend, closest person to you in the world. So why would you not consider marriage to him if I weren't around crazy lady? Speak soon xx John

From: john smith <appledogstime@yahoo.co.uk>
Date: 21 May 2006 08:39:31 BDT
To: Natasha <natasha_nw3@yahoo.co.uk>
Subject: You bloody, fucking beautiful gorgeous little tramp

My god that arse is fucking great!!! Hard on all night! You might be a crazy, mad, depressed stupid mixed up kid in a woman's body but have you got a great arse! God I can't wait to bend you over the bloody bed here in New York pull your panties to one side holding you by the neck face down on the bed giving you the greatest fuck you ever had. My god almighty we are not making babies first, we having some fun when we do it. Yes, yes, yes that arse of yours will get such a seeing to. Your pussy lips will be shouting stop! Stop! While your body shouts no more No more! You will be sore for a few days each time but so, so happy. My little Natasha Nemcova fucks are what you need, you need it now as well. Why are you so down pissed off etc. If you don't get it at 30 you don't get it. I told you, your body is made for sex you need sex real bad. Good hot hard sex. That's why when you are not getting it you are like you are I bet you have not even started on the body course. Put it all off again? No wonder you are down. Your body is brighter then you. Why don't you listen to it? You need a damn good seeing to! A real hot fuck! Get drunk, rip the skin off his back. Fuck me shag for god sake Natasha. Get down to it! Get on with it start living your life. I can't wait to get my hands on you. With in a week you will have a smile on your face everyday you just wait and see. I had a smile on my face after three hard, hard wanks to your pictures last night. Get down to some good hard shagging and love, love, love it. I cant wait to get my hands on you love you, sex you, kiss you, love you, cuddle you and then shag you some more. Our life will be work hard and play hard together. Work, shag, cuddle, dream, shag, work and then create loads of excitement. Babies, babies and more work. Take care of them and each other. Stop giving me the hard sell all the time. You

know you want me. Got your pictures out again now on the bed yyyyyyyyar yar hoooooooooooooooyar o god o god o fucc o god yyyyyyyyyaaaaaaaaaaaaaaaare god fucking hard what an arse what an arse goddddddddddd arse what what a fuckingloveleyyyyyyyyyyyyyyyyyy fucking arseeeeeeeeeeeeee o god o my god heaven heaven come here you pussy come here you dirty beautiful little tramp let me get my hands on them love handles now your really going to feel it there and there and again deep deep in you fucking deep in you you beautifull fucking woman and
again fuck fuck fuck
oooooooooooooooooooooooooooooooooooooooooooooo
ooogoooooooooooooooooddddddddfuckgodiwantyounatash
aaaaaaaaaaaaaaaaaaaaaaaaaaaaaaaaaaaaaaaaaa
aa

From: Natasha <natasha_nw3@yahoo.co.uk>
Date: 21 May 11:40:43 BDT
To: john smith <appledogstime@yahoo.co.uk>
Subject: Re: You are one very hot sexy babe, one very horny woman with a great arse

This is telepathic and not the first time. I am checking my e-mails and at the same time I get a letter from you. I am glad that you like the pictures, and thank you for your kind words. Billy is coming over in half an hour and I intend to please him no end. Hope you are fine and enjoying your work time in the Big Apple. Thinking of you most of the time.

Speak soon
Natasha xx

May

21st May

Blimey. My life with Natasha had certainly turned around. I hate talking about sex all the time. We have had and still had so many beautiful times together. She made me feel so young. What could I do? She was a changed girl. She always was the girl of my dreams. Someone I always wanted in my life, but this now was the full feast. It was no longer a famine. It was a Sunday English breakfast. This was baked beans on toast. This was a beautiful woman with the sunlight in her golden hair. This was a beautiful woman on a starlit night. This was bliss. This was May blossoms falling in cascades of trees. The sun was shining and whatever she may have been thinking in her head, whatever she may have been fantasizing about, for me at this moment she was a dream come true. Whatever she was on, whatever was making her adrenalin run, all I could say was, that I wished all women were on it! Four months ago, I did not think I stood a ghost of a chance, but now night and day, she did something to me. Out of nowhere she came.

Well, it had been a warm Sunday morning, and I had read all the Sunday papers as I always did on Sunday. I always tried to read at least three papers to get a balanced picture of what was happening in the world. The Times, The Mail and then the News Of The World, just to find out if other people are pretending to have a better sex life than me. But I did not think that was at all possible at that moment.

I got to her place at 1 o clock, and she looked fabulous, beautiful, an angel. It was warm, very warm, and she was in a cotton dress with a large flowery print on it. I was in the mood for everything. I could not sleep a wink last night, thinking of today. I guess I'd had the best dreams ever, and now we were here.

We drove to the Spaniards at Hampstead and sat in the sun. They had a big aviary with thousands of tiny birds in a big cage. All through the meal, they would chatter and sing, serenading us while we were eating. As do the babble of voices merging into one low hum. The mothers, the dadas, the kids, the young girls chattering away together about the men they didn't pull on the Saturday night, the lovers staring into each others' eyes over bangers and mash. Why do people always look so much better when the sun is shining? If England was like this all the time, no one could ever want to leave it. We talked of her sister, her mum, her dad, her disappointments, the other people in the pub, and the birds, the ones in the cage that is.

We went for a walk in Kenwood and all the way round across Hampstead Heath. We walked and walked and talked and talked till we got to Jack Straw's castle at the top of Hampstead Heath, and then walked all the way back to the Spaniards to pick up the car.

Everyone was in a spring mood. She received many admiring glances from boys, and a few girls. Rain was expected tomorrow, so I was glad we had such a wonderful time today. London could be so much fun at this time of year.

We started to drive back to the flat after the long walk. Then I saw a little patisserie at the bottom of Hampstead Hill. She ordered a nice cake with strawberries and cream and a Darjeeling tea, and I had a hot chocolate. The girl serving us looked like she was Polish or Czech, but she looked bloody familiar. As she served the tea and cakes, I asked her, 'Have you been here long?' to which she replied, 'I haven't been here for years, but I'm sure you were here then, ages ago.' Yes she said, I've been here nine years and I've worked here 9 years!

'Has fate caught us up again?' We came here on our first date, and here we were again many years on with the same waitress. She was still pretty as a picture, and I must admit, I upset Natasha a little by having a tiny flirt. Natasha looked at me and said, 'Let's go to my place now. Can we please?' The way she looked, I started to feel rising excitement. She looked radiant, beautiful, desirable.

The minute the door closed to her little room she put her arms around my neck and pushed herself up against me really hard and kissed me. 'Come into my bed you silly man' she said. I said to her 'Be careful with my heart.' Her hand brushed the hard-on in my trousers. Her eyes opened large and she said, 'Do you want some "tea"?'

'Yes please darling, I never say no to a cuppa! I thought you'd never ask!' I don't know why, but I wanted to picture her as she was today for the rest of my life and I knew she felt the same.

She wanted to make me happy, which I was anyway, just to be with her. So instead of flopping onto her bed like a lazy fat walrus, I lay on her floor flat out after the walk, as I had a little ache in the base of my spine. But what she did next, soon made me forget this!

She walked back from her little kitchen, put the tea on her bedside chest of drawers and stood right over me. Her legs were wide apart, one foot either side of my shoulders. I was looking right up her pretty dress. My brain shut down. The very thought of it, besides the sight of it, you'll never know. A tiny triangle or v-shaped silk… a tiny g-string just covering a little pulse started to beat hard inside my head, and a rather bigger pulse inside my pants.

I sat up, my head under her pretty summer dress, my hands holding her buttocks lightly. Tenderly I pulled her to me, and buried my face in the triangle of silk. She just stood there without moving. I smelt and licked her panties from the outside as they started to change colour and become wet. I licked the outside of her panties with my tongue. I was completely covered by her dress, I couldn't see her face, but the change in her breathing told me she was getting excited. I could feel her heart beating even through her pussy lips on the other side of her knickers.

I slid my hand up her legs to free her pussy from its silken prison. She was open and wet, her pretty clitoris already glistening and full. That old feeling… I just closed my eyes and took her clitoris into my mouth, flicking it from side to side over and over. She was still standing over me as I held her cute little bottom in my hands, pulling her body and pussy into my mouth as hard as I could. Her breathing was getting ever heavier. She was fizzing with excitement. I peeled down her knickers, and she stepped out of them. She pulled her own dress over the top of her head. She was so horny now it was unbelievable. She fell on the bed, her feet still on the floor, with her legs dangling over the edge and wide apart. I was still licking and sucking her like mad. It was the first time I had eaten a whole pot of honey for sweets after lunch. She giggled just for a moment, and then she was into it again. Her hands holding her own pussy lips apart as I sucked her clitoris in and out. My mouth was full of beautiful honey. Her little pussy started to fart with excitement and she stared to moan. I knew it was going to happen any second. She started to shout, her voice rising to a high pitched squeal. Her hands were playing with her own nipples, and she came with a fantastic orgasm.

'Fuck me now Billy! Fuck me while I'm still coming! Put

it in now! For God's sake man!' she screamed.

'What about a condom?'

'Don't worry about that, I'm on my period tomorrow! Shag me now for god's sake! I want you to come with me! Hurry man, hurry! Get inside me now!'

Every bit of me was cock, all of me was cock. I was losing myself in her body. I felt her wetness everywhere, even in my toes. I lost everything for a few moments, my mind. No woman had ever come close to what she was doing to me at this moment. I was not conscious of anything else.

'NATASHAAAAAA….' I screamed at the top of my voice. I bit into her nipples, hurting her but she was loving it. She held my arse in her hands, pulling me in tighter and tighter, wanting the fuck of her life, and you know what? We were both on form. We were flying to the moon. This was what life was about.

She was reawakened. She was a new woman. She was so groovy, she had changed completely. I could not believe who I was with now. The smell of her body, her tits, her pussy, the taste of her would stay with me till I died. Her legs were curled around my waist, and my cock drove into her hard hard deep deep, hitting her cervix. I altered the angle so I hit her g-spot, and this caused her to moan like mad. She was not acting, this was the real thing. She was having fun and loving it. She smelt of hot sex. Peppermint tea. I left tiny love bites on her tits, but she did not complain. It was 20 minutes or more, and I had been shagging her hard, but at a time like this, who looks at the clock?

Her legs loosened slightly on my waist, and she let out tiny sighs on the back of her throat. Her teeth were biting her own lips with the pain and pleasure mixed. Her nails dug deep into the cheeks of my arse. Her body started to jerk and shag me back hard. She was so fucking clever. She could make it happen for a man, just when she wanted it to. I was crazy, I was mad, I was insane. I wanted to eat her. I came, and screamed at the top of my voice. The room smelt of sweet honey sex. My cock was red and hot and her pussy lips were swollen.

'That was nice!' she said as she swung to face me on the bed. She hopped off and walked naked towards the window. She was so bewitching… such a naughty witch. She pulled the blinds down as it was dark outside now.

'God, how long have we been at it?' I said to myself.
'I have some soup in the fridge,' she said, 'Shall we have some?'
She dropped a damp Kleenex in a box in the kitchen and put a pot on a ring to heat it on the stove.
We sat at the table and had the soup with a special rye bread. She put her silken house coat on, that hides nothing. She moved about the room and the house coat kept flicking open, giving me memories of what we had just shared.

'Shall we have a sweet?' I said.

'I will.' She said, 'And you will too.'

'What will that be?'

'My pussy again…' she whispered seductrively.

She lay there again on the bed, her legs spread very wide this time. A wave of heat raged over her and her face was red. She had one glass of wine with the soup. I could not take my eyes off that tiny hard sweet little clitoris. Her brown eyes with a tinge of hazel were looking at me. She was drinking me in. She had only left the tiny light of the oven on. My mouth was full of sulphur and mint and smoky sweet honey. The pain of the past and all the other hurts were gone. Her whole being, her mind, her head, every part of her was concentrated on those 6 milimeters of lust between her legs. It pulsed through her body and her fingers twirled through my hair. She pushed her pussy onto my lips as hard as she could. I teased her and drover her crazy with my tongue, as only two people who had been together for 10 years could do. My tongue followed the edge of her pussy. Her body was on fire with her needs. Her scent, her eroticism, her sex. It was always where everything started, and it was always where everything ended. Her body was in my brain. It was the reason why my heart beat so fast. It was the reason I was alive. I knew I would never stop loving her.

Natasha, naked is mind boggling for any man. She was the sunny side of the street, she is I-Don't-Know-Why, she is 'I Am In The Mood For Love', she is between the devil and the deep blue sea, she is moments away, gasping and losing her breath. She told me with her breathing and tiny moans. She even said, 'Don't stop. Don't stop Billy.' Then she came. A second orgasm. I slid a finger into her and started to fuck her with it, and with each thrust of my finger she screamed more and more. 'Oh god!' she shouted, her legs closing on me and opening. Her bottom moved up and down. This was the best we both could do. I was next to her now. Could I shag her again. She read my thoughts.

'Sex is an important part of this relationship. It almost defines it. If the bedroom went pear-shaped, so would we. But she was a master. She was too good.

She pushed me back on the pillows and took me in her mouth. She sucked and teased, pulled and played with my balls, as only she knew how. My bum came off the bed as I moved with her, into that red round sideways pussy of a mouth. She knew how to use her tongue on the top of my cock.

'I love your cock.' she said, 'I really can't deal with circumcised ones.' She sucked me deep down deep into her throat. My balls were against her lips, I could feel her hot breath on me. She was moaning with excitement as well. Difficult with a mouth full of cock. I could feel her magic starting to work. My balls were begging me. We were both so excited as my hand came up to her head. I was going to mouth fuck her. I pumped her red lips, thrusting into them, and then I came shouting her name. Madness as I filled her mouth and throat with my cum. She gulped it down swallowing like mad, like a tequila sunrise, as if she hadn't had a drink for a week.

She bent over me to kiss me and it was long. Her tongue flicked across my lips, and I tasted myself on her lips and she tasted herself on mine. It was 11:30, and I had to get home to feed my other pussies. She kissed me again and told her I loved her.

'I love you too.' She said.

As I looked into her eyes which said, 'Stick with me baby, I'm the sort of girl you could live with.' And I thought to myself, 'You are such a naughty baby.' But I had a feeling the best was yet to come. However, it did not matter what she said anymore. I was floating. It had been the best Sunday for months, and I thought about the poor Polish girl still working at the tea and bun patisserie after 9 years. How different all our lives were.

May

The Tea and Bun Patisserie

We had tea, a bun or two
Feelings, sad-so, so blue.
You will soon go away
The sun won't shine, rainy day,
Earl Grey, Grey, Grey.

The girl who served the tea
She looked at you and me
A muffin and a bun
Darjeeling or Earl Grey,
She chirped in her cockney way.
Placed the cake beside my cup,
The pain inside I can't
Conceal the tears- She looked away.
Pretty and sweet
She worked seven days a week
She saw love's tragedy
Played out upon the cake shop floor,
She doesn't want to ride love's carousel no more,
Works from nine to nine
This patisserie- a university,
A degree, sociology.

Because I love you so,
How much you'll never know,
The sun it won't now shine
Until I know you're mine.
The girl who served the tea
The bread and toast and me,
She knows our love will never be,
Cleared the crockery away
This table next will be free.

The girl who served the tea,
Hair white as snow
Shuffles, shakes and sways,
Now all bent and bowed.

May

Cakes, buns and me
Now at last the tea.
Takes a little longer,
Has time killed the pain?
Could we ever be the same?
The buns I hope are not to blame,
Twenty years on?
Tea remains the same,
Must be Brooke Bond Dividend.
Collect your money on the way out.

From: john smith <appledogstime@yahoo.co.uk>
Date: 22 May 2006 07:26:12 BDT
To: Natasha <natasha_nw3@yahoo.co.uk>
Subject: Three o clock in the morning in Manhattan New York City

Can't sleep. Why should I sleep, I'm thinking of you and all the dreams I have for you and me. Anyway don't know what you are up to today? Are you getting ready for work now? Let me check it must be seven thirty in the morning London time. You staying in bed all day without me? Poor me with no you again. Only a few pictures. Poor Ruth off to her beauty parlour to do nails all day. Lucky Billy making pictures of some beautiful creature I expect. This is life it moves on and we are frozen in time for a short while xxxxxJohn

From: Natasha <natasha_nw3@yahoo.co.uk>
Date: 22 May 07:50:32 BDT
To: john smith <appledogstime@yahoo.co.uk>
Subject: Re: Three o clock in the morning in Manhattan New York City

You should be asleep my friend. I would be if I could. I am getting ready to go to work. You will feel tired like me if you don't sleep. Have to go or I will be late. Will write later. Sleep, sleep, sleep......

Love Nxx

From: Natasha <natasha_nw3@yahoo.co.uk>
Date: 22 May 07:51:44 BDT
To: john smith <appledogstime@yahoo.co.uk>
Subject: Re: Three o clock in the morning in Manhattan New York City

What are your plans for you and me?

Nxx

From: john smith <appledogstime@yahoo.co.uk>
Date: 22 May 11:35:09 BDT
To: Natasha <natasha_nw3@yahoo.co.uk>
Subject Marriage, babies, life long happiness, till death do us part

-in one word, that's all we need… MARRIAGE xJohn

From: Natasha <natasha_nw3@yahoo.co.uk>
Date: 22 May 19:26:07 BDT
To: john smith <appledogstime@yahoo.co.uk>
Subject: Re: Marriage, babies, life long happiness, till death do us part
Why so much emphasis on getting married my dear John? Apart from the religious aspect which will be important to your family and mine? Is there any other reason?
Natasha x

From: Natasha <natasha_nw3@yahoo.co.uk>
Date: 22 May 19:36:58 BDT
To: john smith <appledogstime@yahoo.co.uk>
Subject: Re: Marriage, babies, life long happiness, till death do us part

London is drenched in water. It has been raining since the morning and there will be more this evening through out the night. I have just come back from work. What a horrid day that was. Never mind I am home now in my lovely little flat, turn the heating on, cook some dinner (though it would be nicer if I was cooking for somebody else). Looking forward to tomorrow as I am going to see my pregnant friend. She is due to give birth on the 5th of June. Last visit before the baby is born, I am sure that she will have another little boy, what a horrid prospect two little monsters if the first one is anything to go by. Well he is not a monster he is actually very sweet most of the time. Have to go and cook or I will collapse. Speak soon my dear John.Nx

May

From: john smith <appledogstime@yahoo.co.uk>
Date: 23 May 21:29:22 BDT
To: Natasha <natasha_nw3@yahoo.co.uk>
Subject: Where are you tonight my hot potato?
Getting ready for my thick white creamy salad cream with hot butter. Can't wait for you and your hot cream to cover him all over as he slides in and out of you driving you wild and crazy till your shouting for more. Sore but happy x john X

From: Natasha <natasha_nw3@yahoo.co.uk>
Date: 23 May 23:22:32 BDT
To: john smith <appledogstime@yahoo.co.uk>
Subject: Re: Where are you tonight my hot potato?
Hot potato? Who you calling a potato? You sausage. I did tell you that I was going to see my pregnant friend today. Do you read my E-mails or do you just look at them. There is a Punk Rock Girl playing on the radio I love the song not sure who is it by but she started from her bedroom broadcasting via her web cam. I have a really bad and painful stomach today probably not enough food in it. My friend is nice and rounded but the more I look at my godson the more I go off little boys. Were you a nice little boy or a little horror? Sweet one day and insufferable the other I suspect. Have to go to sleep I am finito today again. There are not enough hours in the day. How is the hard work going you sex pot?
kisses Nat xxx

Ps: There is nothing nice about being sore I know I have been there ... number of times with Billy ... take care of yourself and don't do anything silly.

From: john smith <appledogstime@yahoo.co.uk>
Date: 24 May 00:22:46 BDT
To: Natasha <natasha_nw3@yahoo.co.uk>
Subject: New York. 7.30 at night, home early. Off out to get some eats
Well you must be in bed as I'm off out to town. Time zones and all that jazz. English time 12.30 night. Wow feels strange like we are behind, which is what we are. Did you know that I

was always a good boy?..Why? Because I was brought up in a fairly strict R.C. family and I was afraid of what terrible things god might do to me if I was bad. I had this fear installed in to me. I don't blame them, they had it installed in to them as well but sometimes they wouldn't act on it to much but sometimes I think what will god do to me? I'm wanking to sexy Natasha tonight and poor Ruth who I once loved is all alone and I'm not thinking of her. God forgive me. Then I look at your face and sexy Garden of Eden body and think fuck it! I love her and want her so fuck it! If I can go to hell for wanting a woman I love and desire forget heaven. Yes I know it's not good to be sour but sometimes if you are sour you really remember the good time you had getting there and the horny feelings you felt so I've been told.
Anyway I can't wait to love hold and fuck you. I'm alone and want you here with me. My belly is empty so time to fill it. Think of me and the future xxxJohn

From: Natasha <natasha_nw3@yahoo.co.uk>
Date: 24 May 22:37:06 BDT
To: john smith <appledogstime@yahoo.co.uk>
Subject: You won't go to hell if you behave

I don't think that you can go to hell for wanting a woman - as long as it is me (only). I was born into a RC family too but my parents didn't go to church at all. It was my grandma who installed the fear of God into me. At least one sole saved as she says. I love her to bits, I spent a lot of time being ill when I was little and she and granddad would look after me. Both my parents come from very strict families and that was the reason why they didn't carry on with all the church thing. We were all christened (my sister and brother) but I am the only one who is confirmed. Must go to bed, look after your little self in that big city my lovely man. Kisses all over Natasha xx

May

NIGHT

She phoned at 5 O clock to say she'd just finished work. She seemed more cheerful and happy than ever. How long could this thing last? I thought. Who was stoking her fire?

'Are you free tonight?' she said.

'I can arrange it… why?' I replied.

'I want you to come over.'

'Not another crazy internet exercise,' I said.

'No no… just you and me. Let's see what happens.'

There was an instant twitch. She always managed to do that to me.

When I arrived, there was only a low table lamp on. She had just come out of the shower, and she smelt of soapy, creamy shampoo and oil of olay, and she had her silky house coat on with a tiny pair of white silky knickers she must have slipped on when the doorbell rang.

I joked with her, 'You all ready for me then?' She laughed. 'You might just be lucky tonight! I've just finished my period. I came on last time you fucked me, but it's been a very short one this month, so there's practically nothing there.' Her dark brown eyes penetrated me more deeply with one million question marks over her head. 'I just want you to trust me at the end of the day.' She said. 'I know I made a few silly mistakes, but if you could always hold me at the end of the day, tell me you always love me, and you're always there for me, and that I'm doing things okay… it could always be like this.'

My hand moved to her gorgeous arse, and she grabbed it and moved it up to her waist.

'You're a bad boy Billy,' she whispered as she snuggled her face up to mine. I could smell the talc, soap and her shampoo in my nostrils.

'But you're what bad boy needs.' I said, 'And you're a very very naughty girl when you want to be.'

'Well I want to be tonight,' she said as she ran her finger down my black t-shirt and put two fingers into the waistband of my blue jeans. She tugged them away from my tummy, unclipped my belt, and undid the tiny buttons, one by one, ever so slowly.

Natasha had a degree, an MA in driving a man mad. I

gathered the hem of her silk cover and turned her back to me, pulling it up above her waist so that I could enjoy the perfect view. I loved her bottom so much. Her body shivered in anticipation. My jeans had fallen to my ankles and the raging hard-on that pressed in to the crack of her arse told her she was working her magic. She was such a clever minx.

I kissed the back of her neck, and she dragged me to the bed. My mouth was lost in her neck, her ears, her long blonde hair. I flipped her over on to her back and let her hair spread out, a massive gold on the pillows. She started to flip my nipple with her tongue. She pushed me onto my back and climbed on top of me, letting her long hair brush up and down my chest, and then up and down again, driving me insane as she pulled my pants off.

He stood stiff, hard and proud. Like all the cucumbers you see in the supermarket. She ripped her own knickers off and threw them to the side of the bed, and sat on me lowering herself slowly onto me, savouring every moment as he pushed his way up deep, deep inside her. She rubbed her pert little tits over mine, her small breasts pointing upwards. Then she came down on me hard, gripping tight with her pussy, pushing herself off me, leaving just the tip inside me, before pushing down hard again. She let out tiny moans from her painted lips. They were parted slightly. She was splitting the red spectrum. She was so fucking good.

One of her hands caressed my hot swollen balls as she started to pound me, and my back arched to fuck her back. I could feel the heat. It was like I was in a silk oven. All over him, pure lust took over, as I fucked her and she me. We danced together, and her sense of timing was perfect. We had a song and we were singing it together. In the back of my head as lust took over, I could hear the unchained melody as the dance of sex goes on.

Oh my love, my darling, I hunger for your touch

She was in rapture. She had me in her complete control and we were now both breathless. My overheated balls were brushing over and over and over again, against her swollen pussy lips. I turned her over on her back once again, pushed her knees apart. She moaned, half in disappointment, half in anticipation, as I buried my head into her pussy. My fingers carried on fucking her, just like my cock was doing a few seconds before. I plunged my face, nose and mouth into her pussy, my tongue lingering, accelerating, and I let my sense guide me as I gently licked. I tasted a slightly acidic, tiny green lemon on my lips as I sucked her infinite sweetness, slowly in my mouth. And it was silky.

I had one finger on her anus, and I just slipped a tiny part of it inside so as not to hurt her. Her pelvis strained upwards. I felt like her whole body was opening up to me. I was sucking and licking her, moving in and out, my fingers continuing. Her mucus poured out as she stretched and offered herself to me, but my tongue was determined and resolute. I could feel the moisture and rising excitement. I played with her nipple with my free hand as she became breathless. It was coming in quick gasps. She started to scream, her moan getting lower and drawn out as her orgasm overwhelmed and set me on fire.

My fingers fucked her like mad. The tempo of our song had gone from a tango to a jive. This was rock and roll time, and I could feel her whole body at once. I imaged all the things she was thinking. Maybe Mr. Smith's massive cock she showed me a picture of. She filled my hand with her love juices.

It went on… the moaning, the screaming… then she pulled my hand away as it all became too much. I climbed on top of her while her body was still shaking. I was so fucking horny for her, that it went in all the way in one hard quick stroke. I fucked her hard. Bang, bang, bang, bang, bang, bang! There was no pillow under her bottom this time. She arched her back and moved with me. I could only manage 20 hard deep thrusts. I played her like a violin, and the music was fantastic. I was randy, mad and screaming. Her concerto had reached fever pitch. She was killing me with her song, her music. Her face was hot and her breath was fanning my face with fire. Her mouth was open and was still on the last seconds of her orgasm as I came with her. Her perfume filled my nostrils, her pleasure all over me. Her legs were still spread wide open. Then she pushed me off her as she crouched on the bed where handfuls of man sized tissues covering her pussy. She pushed me out. All my juices.

'Why are you so jealous, you silly man.' She said, 'You're still the best ever.'

Will I ever find such perfect rapture and sex again. She will, but my chances were low at my age. These were the days of wine and roses. These were my swan songs. My final grand love

and tease.
The song had almost finished, but the magic was still with us. Her orgasms were getting bigger and bigger, every time we did it.

'I'm getting so close.' She said.

'So close?' I asked.

'So close to the Big O on penetration.'

'You shouldn't get so jealous.' She said again. 'You are the best.'

'But others are new and exciting and different. That's why I get so bloody jealous. And if I did not love you, I would not get jealous.'

'Do you want to take a bath with me before you go and feed your cats?'

'It's so good now between us. Let's have five minutes more. Let's have five minutes more in your arms.' But I declined her offer of a bath. If I had a bath with her, I knew I would end up fucking her again, and I'd want to stay all night, which was okay as my wife was away on one of her endless business trips, but my little cats would be hungry and starving.

Anyway, it was perfect as it was now. She wrapped herself around me like a python. She hugged me so tight, she did not want to let me go, and I could hardly breathe. As I went down the stairs, I shouted up,

'Marry me!'

She shouted back.

'Get divorced, then maybe baby!'

May 24th Swiss Cottage

A lonely girl sits crying
In a health food shop café
The tears that run down her cheeks
Are the same as the rain
That runs down the window frame
She loves her boyfriend
But she does not know how to live with one
She cannot control the emotions she feels
Is it all make believe?
Is anything real?

May

She seeks to experiment

Life
Date other men
Can she dare to break up?
Lose what she has?
Can it be all make believe?
If she believes in me?

The rain falls
Her tears fall
A blossom, a leaf
Falls off a tree
The same as the love
She gives to me
It's washed down the gutter
And out to sea

People who love sometimes
Don't last
Who said it?
It has to be
The blossoms in spring
Nestle on the lips
She turns to me
Are they lips that lied?
Or deceived?
Just to set herself free

I laugh, I cry
I need a life belt
Was I not wise or foolish?
To take a chance
On a girl who grew up
Maybe too late
In Swiss Cottage
On May the 24th

May

From: john smith <appledogstime@yahoo.co.uk>
Date: 26 May 00:55:38 BDT
To: Natasha <natasha_nw3@yahoo.co.uk>
Subject: How are you?

Sorry my mind was on your body and I was thinking of the fun! So how are you x John

From: Natasha <natasha_nw3@yahoo.co.uk>
Date: 26 May 08:32:13 BDT
To: john smith <appledogstime@yahoo.co.uk>
Subject: Is it getting good between you?

I am fine, very tired but fine and yes I was entertaining Billy last night and it was very good. Will write later, work all day today and tomorrow.

love Nxx

From: john smith <appledogstime@yahoo.co.uk>
Date: 28 May 09:18:41 BDT
To: Natasha <natasha_nw3@yahoo.co.uk>
Subject: Well not much from you, in fact nothing so you can't expect much from me

New York City is hot! It's party time all the time and the swinging summer is here. You see people strolling in the streets smiling with the sun radiating through their smiles, people lounging and enjoying the city heat and atmosphere. People sitting outside and enjoying the restaurants all fresco watching the girls go by in pretty summer dresses, taking nice summer breezy walks in the colourful parks. Everything captures the word fun here. Healthy free fun. When the sunsets and the radiating beam of darkness and light hits the sky it's party time. This city can party the night away. People get on with their lives here and tomorrows just another day in paradise. A girl picked me up last night, she was really something else. We came back to my room, we had two bottles of bubbly. I told her no sex as I have two wonderful women waiting back in England for me, whom I will gaze at in one way or the other in 13 days time. Anyway I couldn't throw her out so we talked, had a cuddle and kissed for 15 mins. Nothing else. She left five mins ago. 4am New York Time, must be about nine thirty London time. It seems that you are the only one having fun at this time. Smile. A night on a comfy bed having hot, steamy sex. Ruth and I have no one and no sex so why's the lucky girl talking about luck? How is the job-hunting going? Is it fun? A nice up market kindergarten like sweet princess Diana is what you should be.. she took it for this reason.. No stress, just fun and games and a lot of fun with the little kids. My sister knew Princess Diana, she met her four to five times. She told my sister that she did it to get away from stress as her mother and father had broken up when she was 13 years old. We all found out later she was throwing up all the time so that was why she took a stress free job. Hope your being a good girl and saving yourself for me. It's what infidelity brings. Don't want you getting ill again no way. Those days are over forever for you I hope. This is why I am so truthful with you regards to the girl from last night. We snogged for 15 mins, only to keep her happy and not let her down or hurt her too much. Come on girly updates from London please. What of your hopes, desires and future? How is the sex? Great? Getting better every time? Lucky girl big OOOOO soon I'm sure. Come on speak..what do you really like in bed? Tell, tell, tell as I am on the bed now after a hot snog thinking of you and only you. I'm having a glorious wank to your pictures. Fuck me I have to try and come! It's five in the morning. Come on girly tell all, keep me up to date. Read my mail carefully xxxxx john

Love the one who loves you

From: Natasha <natasha_nw3@yahoo.co.uk>
Date: 28 May 10:10:36 BDT
To: john smith <appledogstime@yahoo.co.uk>
Subject: Re: Well, not much from you

Dear john

I am glad that you are having so much fun in the big city. I was meaning to ask you John what constitutes infidelity in your book? How far can you go for it to be ok? Where does fidelity end and infidelity start? I struggle with this concept as everybody has different opinions on it and different sense of value. But I do appreciate and acknowledge that it is me you are thinking of....
Love Nx

From: <appledogstime@yahoo.co.uk>
Date: 28 May 10:41:33 BDT
To: Natasha <natasha_nw3@yahoo.co.uk>
Subject: Re: Well not much from you
Real infidelity can and always will be when the hand or cock enters the females knickers, pussy or the females mouth. When you are thinking of her or him and pleasing them instead of thinking about your partner. In other words you are mentally and physically giving yourself to someone of the opposite sex. The fact will always stand that you will always know in your head and in your heart when you have been unfaithful. Last night madam I was not unfaithful to you or to Ruth in any way. I did not think of the girl. I merely acknowledged that she was beautiful and intelligent. There was no breast feeling or hands in or on knickers or hers on my cock. It was a straight snog when standing at bedroom door before she left, giving her all as she wanted to see me again with me holding back and letting her down lightly as I'm sure men have done with you when they have had some one else? Anyway minx another sore bum for you! Can't wait! Your bum will be so sore! If there was anything more I would have told you but you snide attack me without answering any of the questions I asked you! Time to answer all the questions

like a good girl. Stop running please. I want the truth about everything please. xxxxx kiss love you x Read my mail, don't just jump to the thing that upsets you xxxJohn

From: Natasha <natasha_nw3@yahoo.co.uk>
Date: 28 May 11:13:19 BDT
To: john smith <appledogstime@yahoo.co.uk>
Subject: Upset? Me? No?! I don't know how that is done.

The thing which upsets me? I am not upset, can't you see that? I just pick the most relevant and interesting bits. I wasn't having a go I just wanted to know an answer to a question which bugged me for some time. There are lots of different explanations as to what constitutes infidelity. You seem to have it all worked out and I wanted to know where you stood on this. Not having a go. As to getting upset - well un-understandable even by your standards. The mind boggles and imagination runs wild, didn't you say something about a cuddle? What would you say if I came up with a similar story, how far would you trust ... or wanted to trust me?. All this is opened to many different explanations and we will have to discuss it in depth when we meet. As nothing is black and white though I wish it was, it would be simpler but who wants it simple anyway.. I am not surprised that she wanted to see you again ... you are an almost perfect specimen of a man.

Have fun my friend I will answer your questions later.
Love Nx

From: john smith <appledogstime@yahoo.co.uk>
Date: 28 May 12:57:14 BDT
To: Natasha <natasha_nw3@yahoo.co.uk>
Subject: Up now. Can't sleep. Off out for a walk in central park

If that's allowed have a look at all the pretty girls parading themselves. God don't say that to her john she'll hire a professional assassin to come and shoot you. John you can't look at anybody else either. Natasha has low feelings and everyone is better than her yet she turns men on all the time and has two very desirable men who both want her live all the time. Love you. Positive thinking my love..men do want you and you can hold and keep a man. You know that so shut up you silly wench xxxxxx JOHN

From: Natasha <natasha_nw3@yahoo.co.uk>
Date: 28 May 13:19:29 BDT
To: john smith <appledogstime@yahoo.co.uk>
Subject: Re: Up now. Can't sleep. Off out for a walk in central park

Don't know what you are on about my dear friend. So you are desirable now - are you? Well I will have to think about that for a while. And as far as my low feelings go, one day they are low and another day they are high. I am not perfect like you and the other desirable men in my
life. But I have my moments.

Love Nxx

From: Natasha <natasha_nw3@yahoo.co.uk>
Date: 28 May 20:17:14 BDT
To: john smith <appledogstime@yahoo.co.uk>
Subject: The update.

Hi John,

How hot was it in Central Park? And how were the pretty girls? I believe that most things in my life are meant to be and Billy was one of them. And you are another one. The job I lost too was meant to be as well I guess. I also said that I consider myself to be a lucky and positive person, spite of my lows, depression and ill health. Things always come right in the end.

The exercise is going well we are doing lots of extra caring and loving apart from the blindfold ones. The first one was the worse as I made the mistake of wearing the clothes I used to wear for my clients. Though Billy appreciated all the stockings and high heels it didn't feel right, even he said in the end that it was very strained, as we didn't know what to really expect of it and instead of fire works at that time we had a lot to talk about the day after. He knows the exercise was your idea. The atmosphere is much more relaxed now though, I find it strange not to be able to talk at all, I have not had the big O yet but I believe that I am not too far off it now. I now come twice, which is pretty good as normally it's just the once as it would be enough. Well it is enough, but I don't mind Billy trying to make me come the second time, as it makes him really happy. We are so much closer now. We are much more tolerant of each other. I had the dreaded implant done, didn't like the doctor at all and was in two minds about it. But couldn't afford to think about it for too long as I wouldn't have had it done at all.

So I went for the first appointment one week, and made an appointment for the next to have it done. I don't know what you have heard about him, but he seemed to be a bit shaky. He could talk for England but all his answers to my questions were very vague. Billy said that he must have fancied me, which I strongly doubt, in Billy's books everybody fancies me. I got a long lecture on safe sex and on responsible way to have babies and to find a responsible man to have them with. I was told to take the stitch out my self, never heard that form a doctor. I did as I was told, hoped for the best, paid my dues and went. I believe that it is working, as I am impossible to be with. Irritable and cranky all the time which means most of the time I need little bit of loving and tender care well not quiet - mostly I just need a hot and hard shag.
How can I talk like this, nice girl like me I never talk like this. Goody goody too shoes. We went for a walk to the Hill Garden it is next to Hampstead heath and I love it there. Never seen so many people, so we just went to the park, which is on the way to Golders Green. Punk rock girl on the radio again, love that song, have you heard it? Got my self a Saturday job babysitting in the road where Ruth lives. Three children. Otherwise not much luck from the adverts I

answered and put up yet but I feel positive about it all. Job hunting is stressful and I hate it but it has to be done, stating the obvious. I am meeting my friend tomorrow, I will emerge from my hermit hide hole and go out (only to her place though). Not doing anything too wild, if it rains we will go to my place and then swimming to the new sports centre around the corner. Might even tell her about you, haven't done it yet, the only people who know are Billy, my mother and a friend who comes to stay with me every month though we don't speak about you. It is so lovely outside this evening, nice enough for a walk. Might go later. Let me know what is new, how is the lovely Ruth keeping? How many of the pretty looking girls chatted you up.. Love me Nx

For Billy

Our paths will surely sever
He will go his way
But I'll remember him
Until my last, last day
Days go by so fast
But the memories
Of the love we shared
Will last
The nasty parts will fade
The good will last forever
He has set me free
Every step of the way
I was his love
His heart
I'll hold the dream
And he will too
Rays of sunlight, morning dew
Days will go by, for him and me
New loves will come our way
As new loves always do
Remember

May

HILL GARDEN WALK

She had lost a lot of her indecision as the years went by. She was now happy with her naked body, happy to look at it and happy to walk around the room in it. Happy to ask for tampons when she went in to the drugstore. She had lost her self consciousness and was happy to talk of serious matters, like anal sex, and whether she liked it or not. Why men always seem to want it. We actually managed it on three occasions together, and the last time she did enjoy it as far as I was aware.

She never had an orgasm by penetration, though having said one, she may have had a small one, because she was always too aware of what she was doing and her surroundings, and could not lose herself completely during sex, unless she'd had one or two glasses or wine, and then too far gone to concentrate on anything. She nearly always came 99% of the time with my fingers or tongue, but she could never really relax long enough to get the Big O. But sex was always pretty good, especially after lots of foreplay.

When I arrived today to go for a nice walk over Hampstead, which was what she had invited me for, she surprised me completely and said, 'Get those bloody black pants off you low life, and go give him a good wash!'

'But I thought we were going for a walk over Hampstead Heath?'

'We are' she said giving me a sexy smile, 'But there's the soap and towel. Go to the bathroom and give him a really good wash, and make him really nice for me.'

When I returned, she was lying on the bed, and she started to rub her nipples over my cock and get really hot.

Her finger slid over my skin. Such a surprise. She pulled me closer, pressed her breasts together so that my cock was trapped between them, and she started to wank me with her breasts and tease me with her hands and tongue. She kept smiling at me. Her tongue teasing my mouth.

'That feels like a married kiss!'

'How would you know, you've never been married!' I said to her.

'I know. It feels like we have though. For years and years…'

I stopped talking as I saw that look in her eyes. She was getting serious. Hot and damp, her pussy was catching the light as it glistened as she got more and more wet. She started to flick the head of my cock with her sexy tongue. The excitement, the nearness, her touch. She could feel my cock now expanding, twitching in her mouth.

Her teeth just glazed the top as she took him down her throat. I started to fuck her beautiful mouth, deeper and deeper. She was wonderful. There were no complaints in this department. She was one of the few girls who could really take it and really deep throat it all the way down and then some. I came so hard, screaming, so much of my cream spilling out over her lips. The lipstick that she had put on for the walk mixed together.

She wiped her lips with tissue and smiled.

'Why?' I said.

'Oh don't worry,' she said, 'You are taking me for a walk, and we are going now. But I knew you would want to shag me afterwards, and I have a very bad tummy pain, and have had it for the last two days, so I really didn't want that today, and I could not have taken it. Anyway, sometimes I love to do it. I really enjoy it, especially when he is clean and nice and nice-smelling. I really love it, and enjoy sucking him so much. I love to feel the power of my lips over him, teasing him, making him come exactly when I want him to. Come on low life! Let's go to Hampstead.'

Hampstead is one of the finest and one of my most favourite parts of London. Picturesque streets, bushes, flowerbeds, tall trees with large stretches of wild grass, ponds, swans, and some very interesting people and houses. Many artists, actors, musicians, publishers and the like lived here.

She loved to go for walks and collect things. Mushrooms, which she'd dry out, bottle and preserve. Autumn leaves, which she'd press between book pages. Country girl sort of stuff.

We finally reached Hampstead Heath in the car, and after passing Jack Straw's castle, we arrived at the nearest parking bay to the Hill Gardens.

The Hill Gardens are unique as they are a Victorian folly. Hidden away on the heath, they can be reached via a small dirt track. They were built by a multi-millionaire philanthropist and have Roman columns with neat little flower beds, tiny ponds and

Japanese cherry blossom trees that he had imported. He had spent a fortune importing exotic plants from every part of the world. We walked through the gardens with the strong smell of the spring blossom in our nostrils. There were little groups of Jewish families, with their scull caps screwed on to their heads, with one or two kids in tow. Fish were swimming in the ponds, koi carps. Girls wore summer dresses with pretty bands in their hair and many of them wore minis with nipped in waists, which looked in some ways, very old fashioned. But it was incredible what a bit of spring and a touch of sun could do. It was nice to know that girls still dressed up in pretty things to attract the male of the species when the sun comes up. Everywhere the smell, the feel, the air, there were changes visible, and that the new season was here. A thrush pulling straw out of a bush to make a nest, a teenage couple laying on the grass, snogging and making love, oblivious to everyone around them. An old couple in their 80s both with grey hair, still holding hands and walking together and grateful to be alive. A young girl of around 17 was asleep on a park bench, with empty cans of lager around her. Her skirt was pulled up high enough to see her thong and the crack in her bum. Yes, spring was certainly here.

We sat on a bench and watched the world go by. I had not seen her so relaxed and happy for months. We walked again through the woods and ended up in Golders Green park, which can be reached from the Hill Gardens. She had a soft drink, and I had my usual cup of tea at the tiny café surrounded by mothers with children and much of the life and population of Golders Green. People walked their dogs and I could see an artist painting a picture with his canvas on an aisle. Bees sniffed flowers, butterflies chased each other and when you looked into the distance, a haze of heat hung. It seemed incredible that at 4 o' clock in England, it could be like this on an April day. The climate change was obviously starting to take effect. A black man passed us, 6 foot 3 inches tall, with his little girl sitting on his shoulders.

We finished our tea and icecream and took a slow walk back to the car. I dropped her home after another wonderful day. I was getting sick to death of having so much fun! How long could the good times last?

From: Natasha <natasha_nw3@yahoo.co.uk>
Date: 29 May 12:24:39 BDT
To: john smith <appledogstime@yahoo.co.uk>
Subject: Bank Holiday

Dear John
I am sure that you know it is Bank Holiday here in England, I am expecting my friend this afternoon. Good job it is not as hot here as it is where you are. I wasn't feeling very well last night was still awake at four in the morning.
Write soon Nxx

From: Natasha <natasha_nw3@yahoo.co.uk>
Date: 30 May 08:57:14 BDT
To: john smith <appledogstime@yahoo.co.uk>
Subject: Re: sorry

Dear John it should be illegal to have to work so hard, you poor little man. You must be absolutely tired.

Thinking of you everyday
Natasha x x

From: john smith <appledogstime@yahoo.co.uk>
Date: 30 May 15:30:01 BDT
To: Natasha <natasha_nw3@yahoo.co.uk>
Subject: 10am tea break. Must be about three thirty in London
Off to the rest room to have a hot steamy wank over you and your latest pictures. Come on girl, only four months to go. Where is my story like the three I sent you? The story can tell me what you like to have done to you at the same time, nipples pulled, rough, spanked etc. So you write the fourth date and tell me what I do to you, where it is, how I do it and for how long. With detail please. What do I have to do to drive you crazy? I need it bad to keep me on the boil... come on girly tell me a story that will blow my mind xxxxxJohn

May/June

From: Natasha <natasha_nw3@yahoo.co.uk>
Date: 30 May 22:32:09 BDT
To: john smith <appledogstime@yahoo.co.uk>
Subject: Just don't over do it!

I don't feel sorry for you my dear I just worry about you, that you might be overdoing it. You won't be good to anybody if you are ill. One thing I do agree with.. if you think too much about me during office hours you will definitely be in trouble. Speak soon, must go to bed. Not well again today and I'm working tomorrow until Saturday.

Love Nx

From: Natasha <natasha_nw3@yahoo.co.uk>
Date: 1 June 22:09:57 BDT
To: john smith <appledogstime@yahoo.co.uk>
Subject: What a day.

How are you keeping sexy boy, was going to write sex mad but apparently you are not. Any more parties to go to or are you too busy working? I have been invited to one this evening but am not going. Billy is greatly disappointed. He gets very stroppy if I don't go with him, though I go almost every time. I haven't been feeling well since yesterday. I have a temperature, a splitting headache but I should have gone. He was going to check my temperature in case I was lying about it. No I wasn't lying. I have
been telling him since yesterday that I wasn't well enough to go. Oh well can't please everybody all the time. Hope you are well, I am of to bed, got the little
Saturday job. Keep well lovely boy I have been looking at your pictures lately, not all of them just the one. Don't
wank to it though ... like you do. Wish you were in London - though it doesn't make a blind bit of difference where you are as I only write to you.....
Love Me xx

June

From: Natasha <natasha_nw3@yahoo.co.uk>
Date: 2 June 08:05:32 BDT
To: john smith <appledogstime@yahoo.co.uk>
Subject: 8am in the morning

Dear John,
No email from you, you are either very busy or all the pretty ladies of New York are keeping you well occupied.
Oh well off to work speak soon.
Nx

From: john smith <appledogstime@yahoo.co.uk>
Date: 2 June 16:49:03 BDT
To: Natasha <natasha_nw3@yahoo.co.uk>
Subject: No I am working all the time. But yes, a lot of the other lads are fucking...
...girls every night. The American chicks jump on you. Knickers off in 30 mins of meeting them. Not for me, I like the thrill of the chase. Anyway we are edging the sixth month, where is my story?! You know the one that tells me what you like in bed and what you like having done to you. I have been good waiting. First it was you'll get one next week, then you wrote it all and lost it and then you were going to redo it and send it again. Nearly six months now and still nothing. Start as if you are telling a story (your sexual fantasy) and then incorporate in to it everything you love to have done to you that people may not know. Tell all darling, come on. I'm being faithful as I cling to your pictures and I hope the story can release me from the pressure I feel of pure sexual frustration. How much longer will you keep me hanging on! Kiss thinking of you xJohn love and shag silly them that love you x

June

From: john smith <appledogstime@yahoo.co.uk>
Date: 4 June 08:36:43 BDT
To: Natasha <natasha_nw3@yahoo.co.uk>
Subject: Are you dead?..

Or are you having so much fun in the sun that you thought forget him till October when he will be all mine? Until then you've decided that you will go out and have fun in the sun... and why not?? I just hoped for a nice sexy letter to keep my old man up and hard till I see you xJohn

From: Natasha <natasha_nw3@yahoo.co.uk>
Date: 4 June 10:23:56 BDT
To: john smith <appledogstime@yahoo.co.uk>
Subject: Re: Are you dead?..

Dear John,

I don't think anything of that sort! I am not forgetting you, how can I? But I am in a great danger of becoming the woman who moans the most on this earth if I am not careful. I feel like I complain all the time. My stomach is getting really bad again, I have a continuous headache. I don't feel well at all... I am no good to anybody at the moment.
So I am sorry, I have been ignoring you, can't forget
you though - you are simply unforgettable ...
Speak soon my dear friend Natasha xxx

From: john smith <appledogstime@yahoo.co.uk>
Date: 4 June 17:15:26 BDT
To: Natasha <natasha_nw3@yahoo.co.uk>
Subject: Come on girl think positive.

You are letting things get on top of you. You would not be so down and negative and ill if you let go and had some fun. The sun is shining and it's tiny knickers and pretty see-through summer dress time. It feels good. Love the sun and yourself. Sex, good food, fun and games, those are what you need to put all your negative thoughts away. You need to also (if you are) to stop thinking about bad times and terrible things that might happen. Think positive as good times are on the way and they will be. Things will get good trust me xx John xxxxxxxxx

From: Natasha <natasha_nw3@yahoo.co.uk>
Date: 5 June 21:21:37 BDT
To: john smith <appledogstime@yahoo.co.uk>
Subject: Re: Come on girl think positive.

Think positive, think positive, think positive, thinking positive, is it doing the trick - think positive, think positive, maybe later... yes, yes yes!

Got told off by Billy for tending to your plant, I was only spraying the moss around it. He said that it looks like your private parts - red, tall, erect, proud and exactly the same size and that I should stop watering your balls and come to bed. Obscene plant that, it doesn't do much though, doesn't grow much at all either.

Anyway off to do some more positive thinking if you think it will help... Are you still coming home on the 10th or are they keeping you there longer? I wouldn't blame them as you are a bit of a treasure... on occasions.

Thinking of you
Nx

June

BEDTIME AND FLOWERS

It was June and the relationship was wonderful, or at least seemed to be on the surface. Regardless of what may have been hiding underneath, we were having some of the best times of our lives. We were going out together a lot, spending days in the country, visiting the seaside, restaurant hopping, going to the cinema and much more.

The sex was phenomenal. And there was more of it. More and more and better than ever. It was all going so well. Her illness was not affecting her as much as it had been, and she was hot for me all the time, which made me feel bloody good about myself as well. Since she had the implant, our sex life continued improving incredibly.

This was quite the perfect ménage-a-trois. The beautiful Natasha, a certain Mr. Smith who never touches her but gives her a reason to live, survive and hope for her dreams and her future in his messages, and then me, who gives her physical support, sex and entertainment.

She wanted sex all the time now, and at times I did not even have to instigate it. Today after she had fucked me on and on for more than two hours like a crazy bitch on heat, this had turned her on even more and she became a fucking machine. She got off the bed, bent down on her knees and started to wank his silly, giant plant. She just loved a big, hot cock, standing proud with a big red head on it, ready for action.

Her hands stroked and caressed my balls as well, and it was all getting so erotic that I was surprised she did not give me a blow job because her lips certainly looked like they wanted to. He must be one of the most loved and talked to penises in the whole of London, I thought to myself. The plant that looks like a cock that is.

Something about him drove her mad today, and she quickly returned to bed and started to shag me silly again. Every new day was bringing great new surprises.

June

Life is Crazy

Sex, sex, sex, sex, sex, sex, sex
Coffee in bars
Disco playing
Sex, sex, sex
Man in a hat
Watching you
Car door slams
People straining
Thinking about sex
So are you
No knickers tonight
Some girls love for a pound or two
I've left you a minute
The strangers lips
What are they saying?
Funny how violent love can be
We go play hide and seek
The lift door closes

June

From: john smith <appledogstime@yahoo.co.uk>
Date: 5 June 23:20:14 BDT
To: Natasha <natasha_nw3@yahoo.co.uk>
Subject: Glad you're still getting me hard and making me grow

That's some sense of humour. Stop watering my balls. Smile. Until it's with your pussy juice I won't be happy. I hope they will be soaking wet for three hours after a hot shagging you'll get. Your little bottom will be worn out from moving, pushing and receiving a spanking from me. You are quite right you bright little animal, I'm back on the 7th of July.
kiss x john X 10 hour day xxx

From: Natasha <natasha_nw3@yahoo.co.uk>
Date: 6 June 22:25:03 BDT
To: john smith <appledogstime@yahoo.co.uk>
Subject: This month next month eventually

My dearest John,

I read what I wanted to read, thought that you were coming home this month on the tenth not next. It is the three hours of hard shagging I am worried about - you and your impressive equipment. I am sure that you will be gentle with me - on certain days...well most days.
Kisses Nxx

From: john smith <appledogstime@yahoo.co.uk>
Date: 8 June 08:11:07 BDT
To: Natasha <natasha_nw3@yahoo.co.uk>
Subject: Be a good girl from now on

Sounds like you might be on your way to a good time. From now on your life will give you good times. They are coming. The hot wonderful summer is upon us, hot summer nights, summer days. Life will be good so cheer up and enjoy x john

June

From: Natasha <natasha_nw3@yahoo.co.uk>
Date: 9 June 07:57:57 BDT
To: john smith <appledogstime@yahoo.co.uk>
Subject: Working

Poor little Johnny working like a mad person and the weather is so amazing! We should be walking in the country, no people, no office, no work just you, me, the green grass, woods, lakes and the sea. Little forgotten place to stay and who knows what might happen....

Will write later have to run
Love and kisses Nxxx

From: john smith <appledogstime@yahoo.co.uk>
Date: 9 June 08:25:23 BDT
To: Natasha <natasha_nw3@yahoo.co.uk>
Subject: Natashaaaaaaaaa!!

Yes! Yes! Yes! My holiday is on the 10th of October! I'm back to work on the 24th and then we meet up on Saturday the 28th of Oct. We fly to New York City and stay there for one week, get to know each other and then I will take you anywhere in the world, you choose and it shall be done. Wherever you want for three weeks, any spot, just name it. I don't mind any forgotten place as long as it's with you. We then return on the 28th of November to London, madly in love and you may well be pregnant. We can spend Christmas at my mum and dads house, wedding in early January. Wedding if we are both sorted and are ready to start a good life together for the both of us. Great sex, heart beating love, kids, a home and lots and lots of fun. Meanwhile I sit here still waiting for my stories?? Spit it out x KISS xxxxxx love you take care of all who love you John x

June

From: john smith <appledogstime@yahoo.co.uk>
Date: 12 June 08:51:13 BDT
To: Natasha <natasha_nw3@yahoo.co.uk>
Subject: Billy fucked you for 3 hours and you died with the hots!
No news, no stories, no emails, no lines, (not even railway lines) no juicy hot stories, silence. So Billy made it in the end, he came through and shagged you to death and you died of love. Ok when he gives you the kiss of life and you come back write to me x love John x

From: Natasha <natasha_nw3@yahoo.co.uk>
Date: 12 June 16:02:20 BDT
To: john smith <appledogstime@yahoo.co.uk>
Subject: I am back form the dead now
Dearest darling and hard, hard workingman. Billy did fuck me and he did give me the kiss of life so I am back now. What a lovely sense of humour or sarcasm or however it can be described as that you have. I am not dying of the excesses of sexual exertions but of the hot weather in here. Actually I am all over the place again but don't want to complain again and again, I don't seem to be doing anything else but complain to you. I am sure that you think... well no I don't know what you think, better no go there you will have to tell me what you think... I worked all Saturday, came home at three thirty in the morning and had a bit of a bust up with Billy. I had to do a lot of making up and being good (I do that very well). Especially the guilt trip and Billy knows just the right way to let me stew. I have a nasty temper on me and I did have a glass of wine, well two, over several hours though and that is enough for somebody who doesn't really drink. No drink at all for four months. I did have to admit that I was wrong because I was. That is the reason why their were no lines and not even the railway ones coming your way my sweet man. How was your weekend and what did you do? You are not very forth coming with the weekend news since I objected to you kissing strange girls. Are you still carrying on with the self imposed celibacy? Suspect so.... Big kiss just for you from Me xx Natasha

June

From: Natasha <natasha_nw3@yahoo.co.uk>
Date: 12 June 20:35:57 BDT
To: john smith <appledogstime@yahoo.co.uk>
Subject: Now it's wedding bells you are thinking of, who knows.

Please do stop thinking of the wedding and me in the same sentence and concentrate on work you sausage. I am sure you lost lots of company money thinking of the pussies you are forgoing and weather. You are doing the right thing, after all there are lots of beautiful, intelligent and educated women in this world. That is the real reason. Yes I did hear of Mr Lawson and his money problems. Concentrate man Love Nx

I can't get you from my head
When everything is said
I try most every day
I want a Cadillac instead
I want white wall tires
But that won't help me make it in my bed
You said you had a Ferrari
Or a Lamborghini
But all I got in my bed
When you shared it
Was an old Ford truck

June

CANDLELIGHT

I answered my phone on the second ring. I somehow knew it would be her calling me.

'Yes, love?' I said.

'Billy, my electricity has gone out. Would you mind coming over to fix it?' She sounded a little bit distressed.

'What did you do – did you blow a fuse?'

'I don't know...'

'Okay, I'll come over. Don't you worry.'

I rushed to her flat as quickly as I could and rang her doorbell. I heard her hurry down the three flights of stairs to come down to let me in, and when she opened the door and the tearful Natasha, looking so fragile, standing there barefoot, wearing a clinging red-stained wet t-shirt stood there in front of me.

She fell into my arms.

'Hello you gorgeous girl. What have you done to yourself?' Natasha sobbed and clung onto me. I could feel her erect, wet nipples through my shirt.

'Oh Billy, I tried to make a special recipe from home, and then the power cut out, and I dropped my glass, and the wine…' I shushed her and tried to calm her down as small tears of frustration trickled down her cheeks, and mingled with the red wine on her top.

On the short walk up the stairs to her room she managed to tell me how while she was listening to a mix CD that her previous Czech boyfriend had made her, she decided to do some baking and make a dessert for herself. Her Moravian grandmother had given her the recipe for it, and the taste reminded her of happy memories and a more innocent time. It was a true comfort food for her.

She had done the preparations, put her masterpiece in the oven and left it to bake while she sang along to her CD, drinking some of the red wine I had given her the other day, when the power in her flat went dead. This had never happened to her before, so she panicked and as she groped her way around her room in the dark she accidentally knocked her wine glass over.

As I walked through her door I smelt the faint smell of her unfinished Czech delicacy in the air, and glanced at it through the oven window as best I could in the candlelight.

She hurried towards the kitchen and crouched down,

picking up a towel, where I could make out millions of tiny pieces of glittering glass that had just been shattered on the floor. I had obviously arrived just as the incident had happened.

I picked her up and carried her to the bed, singing a little song.

'Don't!' She almost sounded angry. 'I have to clean this mess up!' She was sniffled a little and looked at me with wide eyes that glistened in the candlelight.

I gently kissed her on her forehead.

'Later.' I said.

I laid her down and started to get her out of her wet clothes as one does a child. I pulled off her top and her breasts were damp and stained a little red. I could not help but to lean down and lick one of them.

'Umm, the Pinot Noir from the local shop?'

Her nipples got harder upon feeling my tongue on her body. In the semi-darkness, I reached down to pull off her silk white shorts, but they didn't seem to have any wine on them.

'So these can stay on,' I murmured. I loved to feel her from inside her underwear, and of course my hand was irresistibly drawn to the exotic, awesome territory that was her upper thighs and pussy. The shorts were loose around her legs and my hand glided up easily inside them. I continued to lick her nipples while stroking her outer lips with my left hand. Her tears were drying now from her cheeks and she closed her eyes and groaned.

'Stop it Billy…' she pleaded, although it was said in a submissive way that indicated she meant the opposite of her words. 'I have no time for this lark.'

I moved my mouth up to lick and kiss her neck, and caressed her hair with my right hand, keeping my left one softly flicking her clit underneath the silky shorts.

'I want you, beautiful, I want you.' I whispered in her ear. She lay passively, but jutted out her chin in a kind of invitation. In the candlelight she looked so young, so soft, so vulnerable. I proceeded to lie on top of her. My cock was already rock-hard and found its way easily up her shorts to her wet sex. On first contact with it, she quivered and drew a sharp intake of breath.

'I think that…'

'Shhh darling.' She obediently stopped talking and licked

her lips in preparation for being kissed.

I decided to fuck her gently and deeply, yet keeping our bodies as still as possible so it could be a very calming experience for her. With the moonlight shining down onto her flaxen hair and pale skin through the window, Natasha closed her eyes, moaned with pleasure and swayed her head from side to side on the pillow. In the perfect fit of my powerful, restrained member with her exquisitely soft and juicy pussy, I reached a mind-blowing orgasm that lasted ages and ages and ages, but it seemed that she was not in the mood to have one.

Then, suddenly she picked herself up in a slightly huffy mood.

'Come on man, for God's sake!' She had a strange expression on her face, which showed both satisfaction and a slight impatience. 'Help me get this mess cleaned up and go down to the hall to fix the fuse or whatever it is!'

'What about the love we just had?' I asked her, a little hurt.

'Very nice.' She replied. 'But I can't love properly with this mess not dealt with. Sorry Billy. Be practical sometimes.'

I fixed what she wanted me to fix, and left sulking slightly two hours later.

I scatter your dress my love
Wild delight
I'm a little bit lonely
When I leave you tonight
The roses are all stripped and bare
Yes, the petals falling through the air
Will you ever whisper what I like to hear

From: john smith <appledogstime@yahoo.co.uk>
Date: 13 June 06:23:34 BDT
To: Natasha <natasha_nw3@yahoo.co.uk>
Subject: Yes you're right..

But there is only one of you x John

From: Natasha <natasha_nw3@yahoo.co.uk>
Date: 13 June 09:21:04 BDT
To: john smith <appledogstime@yahoo.co.uk>
Subject: Re: Yes you're right..

But there is only one of everybody, to state the obvious. I think you are just very, very overworked and the rest.

N xx

From: john smith <appledogstime@yahoo.co.uk>
Date: 14 June 08:55:47 BDT
To: Natasha <natasha_nw3@yahoo.co.uk>
Subject: Agreed

But you are very special. Yes there are millions of one offs but who would want them? The drags of the earth. People, who live off the state, live off everybody else, use and abuse people. The one offs you can keep and consign to the waste paper basket of history but a goddess is a rare and beautiful woman who was put on this earth to make the world a better place. To also please herself and the men in her life while she lives in her life and lives it to the full with no regrets. That has to be what you strive for everyday. You are a goddess, stay one. Never dig the dirt again or mix with low lives. Keep your self above that. Kiss x love them that loves you and yourself x John from busy, busy, busy New York city x

From: Natasha <natasha_nw3@yahoo.co.uk>
Date: 14 June 22:23:41 BDT
To: john smith <appledogstime@yahoo.co.uk>
Subject: You must look after yourself

You need some good hot loving and I am sure that darling Ruth will give all she has to you. But most of all you need rest or you will be no good to anybody my dearest darling John. It does sound funny but I am looking forward to you being home too. Though I don't see you and for all I know you might be anywhere on another planet for all the difference it makes. It will be good to have you just around the corner again. Thought about you a lot
today and all the worries I have about our relationship, the things which didn't matter at all in the past are turning into major problems, but they are my problems for now and nothing for you to worry about. I am going to help my friend with the children tomorrow. She had another boy as I thought she would have. I am sort of looking forward to it. Look after your self my lovely over worked sausage man, thinking about you every day and counting the days .....
Kisses Nx

From: john smith <appledogstime@yahoo.co.uk>
Date: 16 June 00:30:38 BDT
To: Natasha <natasha_nw3@yahoo.co.uk>
Subject: Seven thirty New York City

Good night little Natasha hope you are thinking of me as your hand slides between your legs in bed tonight, just before you fall asleep x john

From: Natasha <natasha_nw3@yahoo.co.uk>
Date: 16 June 21:59:22 BDT
To: john smith <appledogstime@yahoo.co.uk>
Subject: Re: London

Dear John,

I am counting the days and have been for a while only it keeps changing and it makes the mathematics difficult. Tell them to stop messing my sums up. I am doing my best in being good to everybody in site, Billy and my friends included. I acknowledge every kind word spoken in my direction, even the not so kind words. It is proving a challenge though, you must know more about me than I do and it pains me to admit it. I used to be such a good girl, where did it all go wrong?? But I am sure that I will reform again with your kind help.

Hurry up home man I am waiting for you,

Love and all my kisses Nxx

From: john smith <appledogstime@yahoo.co.uk>
Date: 17 June 19:48:36 BDT
To: Natasha <natasha_nw3@yahoo.co.uk>
Subject: My story..

Where is my story of what you like? Where is your fantasy? Nearly half a year since you promised. You must be Spanish as tomorrow never comes. Everything is demarni, demarni sara. When??
Have you got the Big O yet from penetration? x kiss X John

From: Natasha <natasha_nw3@yahoo.co.uk>
Date: 17 June 20:37:16 BDT
To: john smith <appledogstime@yahoo.co.uk>
Subject: Re: My story..

All right, all right, I feel very guilty for it I do remember that I still owe you what I promised. I remember every day when I wake up and again when I go to sleep. It's been a long time since the promise was made, I remember that as well. I am finding it difficult especially after reading your highly sophisticated stories, you can say I do feel intimidated by them. Nevertheless I am sure that you are not expecting anything ...well just my fantasies. To be honest my sexual fantasies are normally very crude not much story to them, and I refine them according to how they work. They are the fantasies of the perfect man in my life and there is not many of those. I am babysitting my lovely two children tonight so it will not be today, but I will do it. They keep looking over my shoulder so will write later. It is bedtime in few minutes anyway. What time do you finish today and are you working again tomorrow? I will write later can't concentrate as we are watching the football. It's Italy 1-USA 1. For now. Love Nx
From: Natasha <natasha_nw3@yahoo.co.uk>
Date: 17 June 21:50:12 BDT
To: john smith <appledogstime@yahoo.co.uk>
Subject: Match over

Had to tell you. All right, all right... you made me really randy thinking of you returning, metting and taking me for the first time... I had three wanks for the first time today.
I woke up thinking about you, had a shower and brought myself off with the shower head. Very nice you are my dear John. Ten minutes ago I re-read your e-mails. Yes, for the first time in a long time, and I made myself come again. This implant is certainly doing its job.
Love Natasha xxx Hurry back xx I want you

June

From: Natasha <natasha_nw3@yahoo.co.uk>
Date: 18 June 12:56:33 BDT
To: john smith <appledogstime@yahoo.co.uk>
Subject: Re: My little baby girl you need babysitting if you want to be my baby for life

I am getting very close to it every time we do it, but I am not there yet, no doubt it will happen very soon. And if not with Billy I have somebody who is very sure of himself and is promising the earth. Have you heard of him? No we have not finished all of the exercises yet, but the in between bits are better and better. I am hundred percent sure that I will eventually get there. So I will get wet even before you touch me, it can go either way, I will either be so wet that you will have to wring my panties out or nothing at all will happen. One thing is for sure I will have jelly legs and bees in my brain preventing me form thinking and walking straight and that is even before you go anywhere near me my sex mad boy. I am working on the story, as I have been a number of times. I intend to send this one though.

Kisses all over your hot overworked body
love Nxx

From: Natasha <natasha_nw3@yahoo.co.uk>
Date: 18 June 16:35:25 BDT
To: john smith <appledogstime@yahoo.co.uk>
Subject: I have to tell you...

Billy came over this afternoon. He has just left, and we'd had lunch just after 1 O' Clock. He then shagged me hard and deep and I came the closest ever to the Big OOoooooooo. We were nearly at it for 80 minutes. In fact, I'm not sure I did not get a little bit of it... Maybe I did. I certainly did feel something 10 minutes after the shagging when his mouth was all over my pussy, eating me. God, I'm so horny John... I need to see you soon/
Natasha xx

June

From: Natasha <natasha_nw3@yahoo.co.uk>
Date: 21 June 00:27:07 BDT
To: john smith <appledogstime@yahoo.co.uk>
Subject: Here it is!

My dearest darling man, the never-ending saga of the story for your own pleasure. It is eleven o'clock on Tuesday evening and I have had three different ideas for it in my head for ages, just when it comes to actually putting it down it gets complicated. I will just have to make it simple... Fantasies ceases being fantasies once we make them possible to happen, and that is why some of them should always remain in the realms of our imagination.

I had all my windows open, the hot evening air was coming through my flat, the smell of the lime trees outside reminding me of home, making me home sick. These warm evenings would normally get me out of the house walking the streets but today was so hot I decided to enjoy the weather from here. You are still in the big city and even though we have never met I miss you like mad, and wish you were here with me. My fantasy runs wild with me and you and our life together. The door bell goes - I don't expect anybody I thought maybe it's the Jehovah Witnesses or the TV licensing people, I bend out of the window to find out. Oh dear a woman with dark hair, a little pink dress, high healed shoes what does she want? I go downstairs to find out. 'Are you missing him as much as I do?' she says in a very quiet voice. Well yes it is. The woman you have been seeing for the past five years, I have mixed feelings about this, why is she here? Has something happened to you? Is she all right? Shall I invite her up? Only the people I know are allowed in to my world and she is your ex or something along those lines. Well what can I do, she looks upset and I can't just let her stand there. We are sitting on my big bed only because I don't have armchairs anymore, chatting about our lives and you whilst drinking wine that I found in the fridge. I still don't know why she came to see me but she looks relaxed now almost happy to see me, I find that hard to believe though after all I am the one who is just about to run away with the man she still loves very deeply. Sitting so close to her I can see why you were attracted to this little lady, she looks perfect, like a fairy from the Christmas tree, not a hair out of place. All the nights you spent adoring every bit of her, never ending passion and romance and now it should all end because you are in love with a girl on a picture on the silly website she should not even be on anymore but she does not know all that and I thank my lucky star for I believe it would not go down well with this lady. Suddenly her animated hand lands casually on my thigh and I feel the electricity of her soft touch running right threw my whole body but she has no idea. It is all this thinking about you two in bed together which has done it. Can I? Shall I? Will she be angry with me? How do I go about it? Dear sweet Ruth is chatting away but her words go past me, there is just one thing on my mind for now, will I upset her? Well the hand is still on my thigh... 'Ruth can I brush your hair?' My voice is almost inaudible but she hears 'Yes' her big eyes fixed on my face, with a questioning look on her face she moves away from the wall where she was resting, she turns her head towards me. As I start brushing her soft dark hair, she closes her eyes but doesn't stop talking as if the silence frightens her. The brush makes slow gentle movements from the top of her head to the tips, I put the brush away and she finally gives up on the one sided conversation she was having with herself for the past ten minutes and I know that I will not be refused now. She will be mine and I hers tonight. Her eyes still closed she breaths faster. I run my fingers through her hair, her tiny ears, her neck, dare I touch her anywhere else? Dare I kiss her? My lips land softly on her shoulder and here arms reach for my head........ But now you have to excuse me my dear John and Ruth I have to go to bed and sleep, let me know how you find the first part of the story and I will finish it tomorrow.

Love you lots wish you were coming to bed with me tonight.

See you soon Nxx

June

From: Natasha <natasha_nw3@yahoo.co.uk>
Date: 22 June 09:19:58 BDT
To: john smith <appledogstime@yahoo.co.uk>
Subject: Re: Wanked twice already, rest please great

Dear John, how are you doing apart from wanking your self blind? You know they say. And what do you do when you don't wank and work? I am not very well again. Went to see the doctors yesterday but they are so busy there that I am lucky to get five minutes with the doc.

Have to go I or I will be late.
Love Nx

From: Natasha <natasha_nw3@yahoo.co.uk>
Date: 22 June 20:59:14 BDT
To: john smith <appledogstime@yahoo.co.uk>
Subject: Re: Wanked twice already, rest please great

He has wanked himself to death, I know it.
Nx

From: Natasha <natasha_nw3@yahoo.co.uk>
Date: 24 June 10:45:37 BDT
To: john smith <appledogstime@yahoo.co.uk>
Subject: Second part of the story.

I sincerely hope that you are just ignoring me for now and nothing has happened to you dear John. Tell the doctor that the rest of the story can be found at the bottom of this E-mail and let me know what you think, if you haven't died of over work exhaustion and frustration of the sexual kind.

Nxx

Our lips meet, we embrace each other, this is the softest kiss I have experienced in a while – soft, kind, unselfish. There is no hidden agenda behind it, as her tongue enters my mouth and gently meets mine. She tastes pleasantly sweet, our lips merged in to one hot slowly moving mass, none of us willing to brake the union for now... My arms stroke her soft face, neck, reaching the first buttons of her little dress, slowly without her noticing I start unbuttoning. I gently lay her on my bed her eyes firmly fixed on my face, her arms protesting as she reluctantly lets me go. I feel in complete control over this little girl for now... I push the bits of her skimpy dress apart, she is wearing white lacy underwear. Her little breasts standing to attention and the unmistakable fragrance of her excitement filling the room...or is it me? Suddenly her phone rings, will she leave it and let me continue? I look at her excited face for an answer and it is the wrong kind, she pushes me out of the way searches her bag retrieves the silver gadget ... 'It was John and he is on his way to me' as she hastily buttons up, shoes, bag, no goodbye, no nice to meet you, no we will have to finish it sometime... she is on her way. This evening she will be yours once again - not mine. Will she tell you, will she keep it from you???

See you both very soon.

Love and kisses for you and you only Natasha xx
From: Natasha <natasha_nw3@yahoo.co.uk>
Date: 24 June 23:39:59 BDT
To: john smith <appledogstime@yahoo.co.uk>
Subject: I'm worried

Hi John, You might tell me I'm a silly girl but when I look out my window, sometimes I think I see a man watching me from the flats opposite. Once he had what looked like binoculars. I thought it might be something of Billy's doing as he gets very jealous, but when I told him, he was just as worried as I was. I might go and talk to the caretaker who I know very well. Love, Natasha xxx

July

From: Natasha <natasha_nw3@yahoo.co.uk>
Date: 2 July 13:00:39 BDT
To: john smith <appledogstime@yahoo.co.uk>
Subject: Thank you for the card

Dear John,

Thank you so much for the card and for remembering that it is my birthday. Spending $60 on a pair of panties might be a bit extravagant so I will put it to special use. You having just a little incident as your dear sis described is the understatement of the century, you must be mashed! I am not sure if you are even able to read my e-mails. By the look of things not. I don't want to contact Ruth as she would not appreciate it I am sure. I wish I were there with you looking after you but that is impossible. I worry about you, how and why did it happen and what consequences will it have on your future life? It is so hot here today over 30 degrees and my silly birthday on the 4th. I am taking Billy and my best friend for lunch, was going to have a party but with me going home on Tuesday it was not a good idea. Anyway I am not a party person really. Might have a little get-together when I return. After lunch will make love to Billy on my birthday… then think about home. Speak soon Nxxx

July

THE GREATEST DAY OF THE YEAR

4th July

Yes, the great day had arrived. The day of the year where I had to be my most thankful. Natasha's birthday.

She both loved and hated her birthday at the same time. Nobody dislikes getting presents, and one of her girlfriends was coming over with a man to celebrate with us. Her friends and I dutifully turned up to tell her how wonderful and important she was, and we all hoped that it would be the best birthday she ever had.

We had a celebratory drink together before setting off to her favourite restaurant called 'Small and Beautiful'. It had such a wonderful, relaxed atmosphere, and the afternoon was filled with happy laughter.

Another year had gone by since the angel had been brought into this cruel world, and this was a milestone year. It was her 30th birthday today.

She had two glasses of wine which made her happy and flirty. The food was excellent and she seemed to be enjoying herself so much, it made me even happier. I did not think I had seen her this happy, this sort of happy, for months now. After a couple of glasses, I was quite merry myself, and kept breaking into song, singing Happy Birthday to her, which made her friends laugh with merriment as well.

We had arrived there at midday, and when we were ready to leave it was almost approaching 4 O' Clock, which was when it closing for a break before reopening for the evenings.

Her friends caught the bus home, and I took her back to her flat. We were quite giggly as we'd both had three glasses of wine each, and as she sat on the bed, her bare legs just slightly apart on this hot day, I looked at the expression on her face, which looked thoughtful. As if she were envisioning the big 30 in her mind. The final vestiges of herself had been washed away, the idealized romanticism that had brought her to the big city, the dreams of the girl with ambition and need to succeed and please her father. They were all of the past, and now she looked at me trying to forget the pain.

The alcohol made us both very horny, and I could tell she wanted to shag me now, and just for a couple of hours, pretend that there were no problems at all with her world, and that everything would somehow work out for the better. Perfect love and a perfect life.

The wine had transformed Natasha into the sexy little schoolgirl who had fallen in love with her head teacher, who was responding equally enthusiastically to her. The shrewdness of a potential woman, to wait and learn and see what life throws at her next.

She lay on the bed, spreading her legs just a little bit wider now. She did not actually need me anymore. She did not need this emotional crutch that I had always supplied for her, and she was now just strong enough to stand on her own. But I knew in the morning that all her insecurities would come flooding back to her after the effect of the wine wore off. She would remember again that she was 30 and a day older.

She needed me now, only for my practical value, and my expertise in any matters that needed that sort of attention. Tax etc.

She rolled on her tummy giggling, and then came up onto all fours, like an impish little dog. She gave me a sexy provocative look, and the stripped off her clothes and climbed up onto the bed again, with her legs spread wide, flat on her back and still laughing. Her face was warm, and her breasts were large and full today. It was not just the wine and her birthday that was making her randy. Her periods were nearly due. Her wonderful belly showed a deep pink line where her knickers had cut into her flesh, her tummy slightly swollen with the food, making it even more inviting and sexy. Her eyes were half closed and mesmerized by my excitement which was plain to see as I dropped my trousers and pants. I was now standing in front of her, completely nude except for my black socks.

I joined her on the bed and started to stroke the back of her neck because I knew it would please her.

'You love it today don't you? You're really switched on.' I said. I touched her breasts and nipples and let my fingers play over them. I kissed her bare shoulders down her body, and down again with my mouth over her nipples, now proud and hard. My face was buried in the flesh of her cleavage. My nostrils breathed quickly with my rising excitement, growing in short breathless intakes. The smell of her skin, the lips of her pussy already swollen in anticipation. I stroked her tummy, thighs, the top of her legs and I whispered in her ear.

'I love you. Happy Birthday.'

I touched as much of her skin as I could. My hands again, climbed up her bare thighs, and she started to arch her back. My breathing and hers was getting faster. She could feel now my pleasure mounting. What girl is not flattered when her man jumps through every hoop, climbs every barrier and every obstacle to reach her?

'God.' I wshipered, 'You're so fucking pretty and sexy today.'

Her voice was all husky with the wine.

'Make love to me now.' She murmured.

My tongue flicked and teased all her sensitive spots. I changed the pressure of the pressure of my lips on her pussy, pressing my finger on her anus hard and the other inside her wetness. I pushed it all the way into her deep, making a loop, first down, and then hard in, hitting her cervix, then up and rubbing her g spot as I circled around the entrance, as I put it in again while I pressed my tongue and lips to devour her clitoris. Her pussy reached the point of ecstasy very quickly today and she exploded into spasms. She cried out tears of emotion on her cheeks, her mouth wide open. I carried on sucking and teasing, stopping and starting, and she was screaming, totally submissive and abandoned. This was a birthday to remember.

I went on top of her, deep inside her, shagging her like mad. I felt the fluttering of her orgasm on my hard cock. I felt her pussy clinging and grasping onto it. She screamed again. It was overwhelming her and it was fantastic what a little house red wine could do. It inflamed me as well as I sucked her tongue into my mouth. I squeezed her buttocks, my nails digging into her as I fucked her hard. So hard. My cock tore her apart. With each thrust she cried out. She put her hand onto my neck pulling every bit of me into her. Her legs became tighter and tighter around my hips, and then I came over and over, yelling her name at the top of my voice.

I collapsed on top of her, and then my perverted sense of humour popped out.

'Happy Birthday.' I said in her ear.

'You silly man.' She replied, smiling.

July

From: Fay Smith <faysevencats@gmail.com>
Date: 10 July 14:30:13 BDT
To: Natasha <natasha_nw3@yahoo.co.uk>
Subject: Hi

Dear Natasha,
I am John Smith's sister Fay. He asked me to e-mail you, because he's been in a little incident with his car.
He's alright but it may take him time to recover and get in touch with you. Just letting you know, not to worry.
Best wishes,

-Fay

From: Natasha <natasha_nw3@yahoo.co.uk>
Date: 10 July 16:31:28 GMT
To: john smith <appledogstime@yahoo.co.uk>
Subject: Are you ok??
John, I got an e-mail from your sister. I hope you have recovered from the car crash and it wasn't anything too serious, do let me know.
Love N xx

From: john smith <appledogstime@yahoo.co.uk>
Date: 11 July 10:54:15 BDT
To: Natasha <natasha_nw3@yahoo.co.uk>
Subject: Back in my flat
Have round the clock nursing, flew back on a private jet with tubes stuck in me to stop infection. I have a Spanish nurse in the spare room. I'm not to good, it'll take me a month to get back in to the office. Will still marry you by Christmas if your lucky and you still want to I hope. I also hope that you have completed the exercise with Billy and finished off all 13 of them by now and you are having real good sex. Hope you are being good and while I have been out of action you have not let your heart or body go a stray again. I hope not. So anyway I do hope your love life, your job, your flat and everything else is all great and I hope you will continue being truthful with me, I have had no sex with anyone.. yes not even Ruth. I've been

a good boy, was tempted and thought of you and said to myself “do I need to fuck up my head as well as my body?” NO! Then I had the crash and could not have sex even if I wanted to. Love you lots sexy lady, be good and true and don’t get in to the old ways of telling lies and
deceiving again. Put all that behind you for good as that is self-destructive. Lots of kisses, not long now kiss xJohn

From: Natasha <natasha_nw3@yahoo.co.uk>
Date: 11 July 22:27:32 BDT
To: john smith <appledogstime@yahoo.co.uk>
Subject: Re: Back in my flat in st.johns wood
Dear John,
I am glad that you are home in one peace and am glad that you are up the road again and recovering from the accident. You shouldn’t be allowed on the road, you are a danger to yourself and others. They should take your licence away for good. I have arrived from the holiday, at home today to a mountain of problems and stuff but I will write tomorrow. If I told you now that all the tubes might fall out of you scaring the Spanish nurse. Maybe I should come and replace her but I might cause more pain then you could bare so you had better keep her for now. Love me x
From: Natasha <natasha_nw3@yahoo.co.uk>
Date: 12 July 09:05:18 BDT
To: john smith <appledogstime@yahoo.co.uk>
Subject: Do you need anything?

John

I believe you have plenty of people looking after you but if you need anything let me know. I am just up the road as you know. Anything

me

July

From: john smith <appledogstime@yahoo.co.uk>
Date: 12 July 18:40:55 BDT
To: Natasha <natasha_nw3@yahoo.co.uk>
Subject: YES

Yes I need something and you know what that is.. It's your body. Hot, steaming, naked and on fire. Your pussy hot and bubbling with excitement as I finger and lick it, getting my tongue deep in to it. The rest will have to wait as I can't fuck. I want to smell your juice all over my hand, fingers and face. I want to hear you screaming and shouting as I bring you to orgasm with my fingers and teasing tongue. I want my tongue all the way up and down you crack and in to your tiny tight little bum hole. I see your sexy bum hole in the pictures I have around my bed everywhere. I want my tongue deep in there whilst I spank your arse and finger your wet pussy. Hmmm. My mum was shocked when she came here on Sunday as she saw your pics and I said to her that at least you have met the future wife intimately. O john she says what am I to do with you. So wrap it up and send it over to me so I can use it for a few weeks. It'll help me get better kiss x John

From: Natasha <natasha_nw3@yahoo.co.uk>
Date: 12 July 21:40:48 BDT
To: john smith <appledogstime@yahoo.co.uk>
Subject: Future wife. What future wife? Some poor soul said yes to you already?

Please tell me that your mother didn't see the pictures I sent you! I am horrified!!! Dear it will take some serious work from you to get there. It might as well be sown up as far as you are concerned for now. After all you are all broke up but you can dream. That has healing powers too. You want your fingers up my hot pussy and I want to hold hands with you walking in the countryside, you want my hot body over your face and I want to hold your hand listening to how incredibly clever and sophisticated you are while watching the sunset....

Maybe I can dream on as well as the healing of dreams has

scientific basis. What did you say about the future wife to your mum?
Kind thoughts Me x

Ps: you said in your first e-mail that I am half responsible for my problems as I have probably been unpleasant to people again, well next time my council tax rises seven times to what it was for the past nine years I will try to say thank you to the officials or sing a lullaby to them. Maybe that will discourage them and they will let me off.

From: john smith <appledogstime@yahoo.co.uk>
Date: 13 July 08:31:48 BDT
To: Natasha <natasha_nw3@yahoo.co.uk>
Subject: Sweet
It's sweet that you can live in such a dream world. The rest of us have to live in the real world. Every red blooded woman knows that sitting on a mans face is one of the best ways to make your man happy. In my case getting me to a speedier recovery. Can you imagine for an active lad like me with a fertile mind how boring it is day after day to be laying here week after week not being able to do a thing! Get in the real world Natasha, do I really want to torture myself by thinking of holding your hand and walking in the woods? No. That's the last thing I want to think about. I have to be positive not negative again. My legs and arms are smashed and I can only move a few fingers so again the last thing I can think about is that. More torture? No, No. Think about what I can do. U know what will cheer me up..you sitting on my face is possible. I have to say that being a Cancer soul you are a bit insensitive. Don't let me dream when I can't move with out pain, pain and more pain. The other thing is that it's so easy for you to change the subject but lets get back to what I asked. How is it all with Billy? The lucky man taking you every night, still he deserves it after everything he has been through. Don't worry about my mum, she laughed over and over. The big pussy shot is on my wall. My mum was and still is a hot woman so she has seen it and done it all before. My dad has a high old sex drive and they both still have. Oh well

another day with my Spanish nurse and my cleaning lady on my back. I watch them walk around the room while I do nothing but just watch another hot day pass me by. I wish they would both strip off so I could get pleasure from watching them. Yes, now that would cheer me up. love xJohn

From: Natasha <natasha_nw3@yahoo.co.uk>
Date: 13 July 20:03:10 BDT
To: john smith <appledogstime@yahoo.co.uk>
Subject: My sweet little world is catching up with me

Message received loud and clear my dear. My world is probably a bit removed from the real one. I am genuinely sorry that you are in pain and all plastered up. I thought and worried about you for days when you didn't write until I heard from your sister and she wouldn't tell me anything, but the last thing I want to do is to torture or trouble anybody, least of all you my broken up John. You might as well know..the exercise is going and is on going... We got in to the practising and the in between bits too much. Billy moans there is not enough of it, I moan there is too much of it. But generally it is good or very, very good. Billy has problems with his house he is selling, I have problems with council and with the inland revenue people. And you might as well know that this clever girl hasn't been paying her dues for the past nine years with all the nanny work and the other stuff she did. The country wants to know the story of my life now. So you might have to look for another wife as there are two options, either I come clean with them or I go back to CR. I don't feel like running away as my life is here, but it is an option, I will most probably have to do what they want me to do and that is a scary prospect. I don't do very well with officials. I am sorry to tell you all this my dear John, I am sure that this is not the cheering you up but I think you should know - as you said yourself I have trillions of problems and some of them are pretty tang able for now. John by telling you this I am not expecting help or anything else from you. You have your own battle to fight. Thinking about you as always
Natasha x

From: john smith <appledogstime@yahoo.co.uk>
Date: 13 July 21:58:55 BDT
To: Natasha <natasha_nw3@yahoo.co.uk>
Subject: Re: My sweet little world is catching up with me

Will write soon as only got two fingers. Don't tell anybody this, not even me a complete stranger. You may tell it to someone and may have done so already who has shopped you to the tax people. Tell no one... I'm hopeless at this time, can't help myself but from what I have heard you have the best person in the world to help you. But my feeling is that if you want to stay you will have to pay SOMETHING. Make them an offer, everybody has to when they have no funds. My sister got in to trouble and asked them to consider £5 pounds a week. They said yes. She was £6000 in debt to them and after one or two years it was forgotten and written off. Weak now... must rest xJohn

From: Natasha <natasha_nw3@yahoo.co.uk>
Date: 14 July 20:04:55 BDT
To: john smith <appledogstime@yahoo.co.uk>
Subject: Just home

My dear friend, hope you are ok today. How are you feeling? I have just got home from work thinking about you all day but will write later. Let me know how you are? As to your last letter I have decided that you might
be a stranger but I believe that you are a trustworthy one (apart from my gut feeling I have it on a good authority). Or maybe I am wrong and you are one of these caning clever and wicked men who sweet talk little girls in to believing them. Promise them the world, the babies, the big house, the undying love forever and after they have had their wicked way with them in the woods, in the park, on top of a mountain while the moon shines, they drop them and laugh all the way home.

Anyway speak very soon love mexxx

July

From: Natasha <natasha_nw3@yahoo.co.uk>
Date: 14 July 23:10:04 BDT
To: john smith <appledogstime@yahoo.co.uk>
Subject: Nothing from you

Nothing from you still. I am not sure what to think about it? Just hope you are not getting worse my man. I know that you are very tired and that might be the reason. I was rereading your old e-mails this evening, something I don't do very often. Miss you today. Missed you for weeks. Hope the ladies are looking after you well. Get well very soon my dear. As I am not there with you here are some pictures I was going to send you just before you had the accident. So until we do see each other for real here they are stranger. All my thoughts Nxx

From: Natasha <natasha_nw3@yahoo.co.uk>
Date: 14 July 23:16:39 BDT
To: john smith <appledogstime@yahoo.co.uk>
Subject: Two more

Two more. I dare to say they are for your pleasure not for anybody else to look at. Keep them to yourself only please. Let me know what you think about them. Love Nx
From: Natasha <natasha_nw3@yahoo.co.uk>
Date: 15 July 13:05:04 BDT
To: john smith <appledogstime@yahoo.co.uk>
Subject: What happened to the two fingers?

Still nothing, they must have plastered up the two fingers, which were healthy, or maybe they fell off? Darling I don't like this at all I worry. What is going on with you? Let me know as soon as you can please or let me have a contact for you if that is possible. I will wait until you do. I Hope and pray that you are OK.

Get well quickly...
Love Natasha xxx

From: john smith <appledogstime@yahoo.co.uk>
Date: 15 July 18:57:27 BDT
To: Natasha <natasha_nw3@yahoo.co.uk>
Subject: Re: What happened to the two fingers?

The photographs are great and I got a big hard on! My Spanish nurse giggled while she treated me. She gave me a blanket bath and I had a big hard on. Why do you have such problems with people? What do you mean by I have fun with you, have good times and then drop you just like that?? I was with Ruth for five years and did not drop her SO why should I drop you? You are one very mixed up girl, why are being unfeeling again? What's happening to you? I never suggested such a thing. Are you starting to feel guilty again about something? What's your problem? Deeply shocked x John

From: Natasha <natasha_nw3@yahoo.co.uk>
Date: 15 July 20:18:37 BDT
To: john smith <appledogstime@yahoo.co.uk>
Subject: How do you look when you are shocked?

Dear John

I am so glad to hear from you! I saw you in a hospital with some complications when you didn't write and I am pleased that the two fingers are not in plaster as well. Please Don't analyse everything to the last letter. I meant nothing by it and it wasn't an attack on you on your fidelity or your person. Why do I always end up explaining my self? You should have laughed it off. I didn't mean to be insensitive, the day will come and I will get it right but for now I am not doing too well. Lighten up. I was also asking you how you were? Whether you were better or worse? I have written about my dream that involves you, now I am not sure whether I should send it because you might do your analysis on it again and tell me of. Or be deeply shocked. Or find out that I have one more problem you didn't know about yet. I presume it's due to too much pain, too much boredom and not enough sex. Maybe I should come over and sit on your face after all to cheer you up. It was supposed to be a joke my dear, I meant nothing by it. You shouldn't give me a hard time all the time but I forgive you as I am nice and caring :-) plus you're in a painful plaster so I won't make an issue of it.

How do you look when you are deeply shocked?

Love and kiss Natasha x

From: Natasha <natasha_nw3@yahoo.co.uk>
Date: 15 July 20:59:16 BDT
To: john smith <appledogstime@yahoo.co.uk>
Subject: Last night's dream

Well this is the letter I was talking about and I must come clean. I was depressed and very worried this morning as I didn't know what is happening with you, as I didn't hear anything since Thursday. No doubt you will read between the lines. These are two different stories put together. I am still in two minds whether I should let you read it as you might tell me that I am a hopeless case and I should be in therapy for the rest of my life. I had a dream about you last night, I don't dream about you ever only daydream.

I went swimming in the lido in Hampstead Heath and you were a stranger who I fantasised about for years, I knew you for years but only saw you once or twice a year. I would never allow myself to stay for the drink you would offer.. when we did meet after the few times you asked (only the once) I drank tea not wine for obvious reasons and left after the second cup. It was a beautiful warm July evening and the lido was deserted when I arrived. Only for one little person in the far end of the pool. What a beautiful strong body swimming through the warm crystal clear waters, the sun in my eyes, I watch the figure with admiration slowly falling into temptation. Fantasies springing into the overheated mind one after the other and than being pushed a side. I don't need a man in my life again I haven't recovered after the last one. I realise the contours of the body look familiar as you swim towards me, it is you but you don't belong to me any more you never really did. We ended before we ever started and you stayed with your baby girl and lived the dream, the future we never had. I can't even remember why anymore after all it was a big love affair but only on a computer screen. I get into the water and we silently swim side by side only occasionally glancing towards each other, I can't make out if you are pleased to see me, there is nothing to be said or probably too much but the moment lasts it is the most tranquil and serene of moments. The water rhythmically washes over our cold bodies, all the fantasies which weren't realised, all the dreams which weren't lived come flooding to my mind, the feelings don't hurt anymore just warmly pass in to nothingness. Why regret what never was. What are you thinking of? You are so near I can almost touch your body but I don't dare, the feeling can prove fatal. So near but so far, light years for all I care. Somebody said that I am a girl who has the best sex in her head, but sex doesn't come in to it, it is the tenderness in your look, the swelling of your muscles. I feel safe in your presence, I love swimming but hate swimming alone and you are here with me. I was truly happy for the fleeting moments while you were by my side and I thank God for these moments, they make life worth living. The evening is still warm despite the fact it is almost dark, we still haven't said anything. We just walk through the darkened pathways of the heath strangely devoid of any human presence. It is all surreal the air full of promises, you by my side....We aimlessly walk and this is not like you, at least I don't think so. But what do I know. Not a word, we reach parliament hill, I can't walk any further, too much swimming has taken its toile on my feeble body and my legs are turning into jelly. The grass smells of high summer, this is probably one of the last warm days of the year. We lay still next to each other like two dead bodies and look at the night..sky warn out, happy. My mind is playing tricks on me, I am so tired, the smell of your strong body hits my nostrils sending my mind into overdrive, my heart beats so loudly now, even you must hear it now. I close my eyes, after all I don't know whether you are free to lie on the grass with me on a summers evening and I am not just about to find out.

Though I haven't been with anybody for what feels like centuries. Is your baby girl still with you? Unimportant. Eyes still closed you touch my arm, is it by accident? I jump. Was it the electricity passing from your body in to mine or just simple fright rude awakening from me dreaming. You are so near I realise it was purposely done. Reality of it all hits, you are touching my arm very gently, my neck, my face with your strong large gentle hand, fingers caressing my soft sunburned flesh. I feel myself falling, it is not me anymore I got left somewhere at the beginning, in the water. There is some other being emerging in me, I am no more, I can't think straight and I don't try, only for a brief minute and then I let go of me, in all my silly cockiness and pride. It is hard as I am used to being in control of everything but now for the first time I am disarmed and I don't protest. My mind protests but it is far to late for that - you are gently kissing my naked body, my neck, my chest, undressing my tiny hard breasts and gently sucking them, your tenderness overwhelms and tears gently fall from my eyes. It is dark, you would not be able to see. Am I to be a prisoner of your affections YES and for once in my life I mean it. I feel your hot breath on my face, I reach for you our lips meet in an embrace of hot flesh and wet saliva with tears falling from my eyes. Tears of happiness. For eternity you are mine and I am yours..... My little white panties slowly filling with hot wetness,

I have never been so wet in my life and still you are kissing my face, my tears, our bodies pressing to each other. I feel you on top of me, the big strong hands reaching into the forbidden parts to discover all the love juices freely flowing, you are covered in me. You slowly pull them down undoing the buttons on your jeans and letting the beast out of its cage, I have seen lot on man in my life but he definitely belongs to the very top half, kneeling between my legs for a split second you take a look at my naked cold body surrendered to you like the many before. I'm begging you with my eyes to come and cover me with you. You lower your body over mine and the hardness of your cock penetrates and for the first time thrusts following intense feeling of pain and pleasure at the same time. It all gets easier as our bodies get used to each other, we move in an unhurried rhythmical way, time is irrelevant, we become one. One body, one spirit, we belong to each other. Nothing exists just us and our moving singing bodies. Your penis is so large and I took it all right up to the hairy bits, the pain is getting more and more intense but so is the pleasure, everything is governed by your increasing rhythm, pleasure, pain, heavy breathe and it is happening. I am frightened, my body taking over the whole world flashes in front of my eyes. 'Come on John fuck me Harder' I hear myself say the first words. The pain is unbearable and that is only the beginning ...... our love juices mixing inside me, happiness, pain, pleasure no boundaries.

'You fucking bitch why did you leave me?' 'To save you
leaving me my dear John to save us the heart break,
but I am here now if you are free? If you'll have
me....we can give it a go.......

From: john smith <appledogstime@yahoo.co.uk>
Date: 16 July 02:12:39 BDT
To: Natasha <natasha_nw3@yahoo.co.uk>
Subject: Re: How do you look when you are shocked?

Happy! Very happy by your last letter. That's my girl. I always thought that you are the girl of my dreams that now I defiantly know you are. I can't think to meet you till all the guilt has gone and you have worked out all your problems. I have to say goodbye to little Ruth.. I'm worn out now, the heat inside this plaster is like being in an oven. Anyway I will send you long email next Wednesday or Thursday after three big lumps of plaster comes off. I want you tell me something... What is the last big secret that you have not told me? What is it? Come on my sugar pussy, what is it? You hot little cunt of a woman, tell all!
kiss X Worn out, happy and I came on your email with out touching myself with excitement. Especially after finding out that you are my dream girl after all. Tell all now x kiss X John

July

From: john smith <appledogstime@yahoo.co.uk>
Date: 16 July 09:04:40 BDT
To: Natasha <natasha_nw3@yahoo.co.uk>
Subject: Awake all night.

Try wanking when your whole body is in plaster! Torture torture. I twisted and turned all night until I bunched up six pillows, then with two tons of plaster I fucked the pillows four times pretending they were you with a giant mammoth hard on. I am completely worn out exhausted but happy that I came five times on your pictures and story. Can't wait till December but will have to for my sanity and guilt and your sanity and guilt. Next time whenever I shag Ruth, in my head it will be you. Will try to sleep now X John

From: Natasha <natasha_nw3@yahoo.co.uk>
Date: 16 July 10:00:18 BDT
To: john smith <appledogstime@yahoo.co.uk>
Subject: Re: three o' clock in the morning can't sleep

Dear John,

I am not writing you anymore stories you messy man. Your poor nurse having to cleaning up after you (maybe she secretly enjoys it). I can't believe it, you are not telling me off! Unbelievable! I thought that I was destined to never get it right. I was driving myself mad yesterday. What are those questions? I know you don't tell me off now but now you ask me of all my secrets. Well am I a lesbian? Who knows, never had the pleasure but fantasised about another woman a lot (probably too much at times) but not so much anymore so how would I know. Anyway don't think so! Do I take strange man to my flat and secretly fuck them? No again, do I need to mess with my head? Not in the least. Not in my flat not in the park not anywhere. I am in too much trouble as it is, don't need another man to ad to it but being a clever man you will know that I do have sex with another man in my head, but only in my head. Haven't had sex with anybody since my birthday on the 3rd of July, might do this evening, I so don't

feel like it. No I do feel like it but...can I help how I feel? You and Billy in my bed at the same time fills me with horror, no thank you that is the biggest turn of, of all and again don't take it the wrong way please. Billy is the best lover but to be truthful with you, he has become a friend more then a lover, but I can't help how I feel.
Nevertheless I will carry on with the exercise as the doctor ordered, it is difficult after all what went on between me and him in and out of bed. Like you he is a very clever man. I did have and do have orgasms, I consider myself lucky on that score but never from penetration, you don't have to ask as I told you already.
I might have a bit of a commitment issue though. I can't wait to have a man to myself whether it is you or somebody else. To love and make love to, live with, sleep with in the same bed, to do all the things couples do, fight, make up, again have sex, somebody who will be there for me and I for him. I realised when you had the accident how a moment of hell is little enough to finish everything off and that there are no guaranties in life.

Love and kisses and what ever else you wish Natasha xx

From: Natasha <natasha_nw3@yahoo.co.uk>
Date: 16 July 10:08:23 BDT
To: john smith <appledogstime@yahoo.co.uk>
Subject: Re: Awake all night.

You are a dirty bastard John Smith but in the good sense of the word.
Tell me why do you feel guilty?

Love me Nxx

July

From: john smith <appledogstime@yahoo.co.uk>
Date: 16 July 11:58:00 BDT
To: Natasha <natasha_nw3@yahoo.co.uk>
Subject: Sorry but this is bad news this is the worst thing you have told me

I can't believe what you are telling me. Sorry I can't spare your feelings. You had better do something on this right away, you better start working your little panties off to put things right again. You have been telling me everyday every week that Billy was the best thing in bed ever, that he knew how to turn you on and bring you off, that he had brought you off thousands of times. Up to a month ago when I crashed my car you told me the exercise was ok and the sex was great. Like thousands of men and women are advised all over the world. You are going to have to work hard with Billy to try to fancy him rotten again and get turned on just by the sight of him. A month ago he was the best you ever had. To make the exercise work you have to work hard to fancy the mystery lover in the dark to rid yourself of all the hatred. Still making him the bad man, the dad substitute? I thought you had tried to kill that.

Yes I'm shocked by this news... What chance do we stand long term as lovers and sweethearts forever if after 6,7,8 years you suddenly decide for something else and you blame me for that? Or you don't fancy me anymore? No chance... this could threaten our future more then anything. Maybe Billy should move in with you? You should certainly go on a long holiday together and get to love and know each other. I hope you tell me you are going to work on this very hard or I can see a very bleak future for you in all the loves and lovers you take if not me and if me I'm worried. The other option is to reassure me that it was just a down day or the pills. Tell me that deep down you still do feel sexual desire for Billy. God I don't need this! One day you become the girl of my dreams forever, the next you tell me you're a fickle creature that can just switch off your desire for a man just like that. I am the same sign as him and share the same background. I can't see much future for us if you can't put things right between

you two. Do you want to end up like your parents? x john x
Worn out, now sick and fed up! Will try to sleep. Air con on full

From: Natasha <natasha_nw3@yahoo.co.uk>
Date: 16 July 12:37:47 BDT
To: john smith <appledogstime@yahoo.co.uk>
Subject: Feelings don't need sparing.

My feelings don't need sparing. I knew what was coming from you John. This is the post holiday at home blues, pills and an off day all in one. No I certainly don't want to end up like my parents and will do almost anything to avoid it, it is more then horrid what is happening at home and I end up in the middle of it. This is the direct result of it. As I said I am not giving up on the exercise and I will try hard to continue with it. I could have told you again that everything is fine and going according to plan but what purpose would that serve. I can work out what you want to hear, I am not silly, but it is pointless to say what you want to hear if it is not what is happening.

I am off to work on it once more.
Love Natasha x

From: john smith <appledogstime@yahoo.co.uk>
Date: 17 July 07:50:21 BDT
To: Natasha <natasha_nw3@yahoo.co.uk>
Subject: I have noted all your comments and I have to get well and get back to work

It's down to you now. Told you what to do and how to solve your problems. It's you and only you, no one person can help you. Read all my past letters you have, to do it you have to complete the exercise. That in it's self will get you closer to him. Again you also need a stress free job, your own hours, time, pace, no hurry just no pressure and no BOSSES over you. Go for it girly I can do no more. I will try to rest and get myself better and back to work xxx John

July

From: Natasha <natasha_nw3@yahoo.co.uk>
Date: 18 July 12:07:23 BDT
To: john smith <appledogstime@yahoo.co.uk>
Subject: Thinking about you.

Dear John,

Thinking about you. Another hot day you must be boiled alive in the plaster. Cast highly unpleasant I believe.
Keep well and positive and I hope your sausage doesn't get cooked! Otherwise I might have to send some of my eggs over…

Love Nxx

July

MORE SEX

'I want to make you dinner at my place,' she murmured down the phone line.

'Uh-huh,' I grunted. I was typing a business email as I talked with her.

'But you have to come dressed up, in a nice suit and tie.'

'Uh-huh.'

'Lovely, see you at 7 tonight!' She hung up.

'...I have to come in a what?'

A self confessed consummate romantic, I arrived with a bunch of flowers and in a sharp black suit with the red silk tie she had given me for my birthday. I wasn't sure what this was about, getting dressed up just for supper on an ordinary night in her tiny pied-a-terre, but I enjoyed making the effort, and hoped that she was dressed to the nines as well. When she answered the door, I was not disappointed. She was wearing a sexy, short black dress with tiny spaghetti straps, fishnet stockings, and stilettos. My eyes travelled up her long legs and lingered where the hem of the dress ended, before jumping up to the bodice.

'Yum! These are for you, young lady. Is there some occasion?'

'Come in Billy. Ever since we had such a lovely meal at Sofra in St. John's Wood High Street, I have wanted to try to make a Mediterranean mezze meal for us myself. It has taken me all day just to make a lot of little dishes full of finger food, but I hope you like it.'

'Well you fucking little witch, you know I love anything that has to do with finger-assisted eating...'

'Billy!' Natasha giggled and playfully swatted me with the wrapped bouquet.

As she walked away to find a vase for the flowers, I was overcome with love and care and feelings for this lady. We had known each other for so long and had experienced so much together. Yes, sometimes we didn't communicate the way other couples did, and yes, there were many issues that conspired to keep our lives on separate tracks. But in this moment, I was insanely happy to simply be in her presence, playing a courting couple or newlyweds or whatever she was up to, with her labouriously home-cooked meal and fancy outfits. 'How long can it last?' I thought to myself again. I always felt this insecurity creeping up on me, that things can never last forever.

The meal was almost over when she asked me if I had room for dessert. I responded with a wink.

'Well, it depends on how active I'll need to be later, and I get sick if I eat too much.'

'All taken care of. The mezze was not the only finger food I made for you.'

'What?' She cleared the table and brought out a tray with honey, maple syrup, whipping cream, gourmet chocolate shapes, etc.

'It's build-your-own sundae, like we have in Prague... ha ha. No ice cream though, because it would be too cold!'

She perched on the table and inched along backwards until the insides of her knees were at the table's edge.

'Interesting idea… you will be one sticky girl when I get finished with you.'

'I always am.' We both laughed. She leaned back on her elbows and I pulled off her stilettos and put them on the floor. I glided his hands over the fishnet tights all the way up the insides of her shapely legs from her feet to her hemline. As I pushed my fingers under the dress, I realized she was wearing suspenders and stockings, which I loved. I followed the front elastic of the suspenders, lifting up the dress to reveal her supple upper thighs and then her 'sundae dish'. She was wearing no underwear beneath the suspender belt.

Because of all the sauces, I didn't wear any tonight.'

'There is already some sauce here, I think – but it looks like salad cream... it is Natasha's special recipe, sweet and gooey and my personal nectar.'

She spread her legs wide for me and my eyes drank in her perfect pussy. Cleanshaven, pink and glistening. My cock was throbbing in my suit trousers, but I knew that tonight we would be love-making for hours, so there was no hurry.

I drizzled some of the various sweet potions on her pussy and ate them up with gusto, teasing her with my tongue just the way she liked. Natasha giggled and groaned while she watched. Once in a while I kissed her mouth so she could have some dessert too.

I took one of the long chocolate shapes and delicately played with it around the edges of her hole, knowing that she would be craving to feel it -- and later to feel him -- deeper.

'Mmmm,' she grunted insistently and arched her back a little, but I wouldn't rush. Her juices were flowing now, dripping down onto the tablecloth with traces of melted chocolate blended in. I then put two chocolate shapes together and slid them in and out of her in tiny increments, just to drive her crazy. She was getting hotter and the chocolate melted fast. I slurped up all the chocolate-flavoured liquid that was pouring out of her, and gently bit her outer lips and thighs. She gripped the tablecloth with her fingers and I knew she was about to come. This one was focussed solely on her pleasure, so I tolerated my throbbing rod trapped inside my pants. I gave her clitoris pressured, sideways flicks with my tongue, and put two fingers up her to press on her g-spot. It was only a moment before she came, bringing her knees together involuntarily and breathing in short little gasps of air. As her orgasm subsided and her heartbeat became normal, I wiped the dessert materials off of my face and hands and her thighs.

I snapped her suspender elastic and said, 'Right girl, get up against the window frame. Face outside.'

'But Billy, the blinds are still up, it's dark outside, and people can see in.'

'I know.' She put her stilettos back on and strode to the window. She placed her hands on the wooden frame and I ordered,

'Pull down your spaghetti straps and press your tits against the glass.' The glass was cold against her skin, which felt pleasant and unpleasant to her at the same time. Anyone who looked up from the street or the neighbouring flats would have seen exactly what this girl and her lover were doing, and the thought excited us both. I unzipped my trousers, finally releasing my manly tool which was twitching with eagerness to fuck her. I hitched up the bottom of her dress and reached round her tummy with one hand, for leverage. With the other hand, I gripped her long blond hair and jerked it back suddenly so that her head cocked back at an awkward angle. From outside, this may have looked violent, but I knew that it was just skirting the edge of her comfort zone, and therefore giving her a desired thrill. Her breathing was wild and her chest was rising up and down. She took a step back to relieve her neck muscles.

'Fucking keep your tits against the window.' I simultaneously pushed her body forward and her legs further apart with one knee, and then forcefully shoved my cock into her. She started to emit a high-pitched sound that grew higher with each thrust. Natasha was experiencing extreme pleasure, loving Billy's force and domination, not to mention the voyeurism that was perhaps taking place...

I was banging her so hard that her head was being thrown up against the glass.

'Shit, Billy, be careful!' I had complete control over myself, and I waited to explode until I felt that she would come for the second time that evening. Her pussy was dilated and blazing red hot. When she started to shudder and scream, I let loose and ejaculated my hot cum into her cavity, from where it then ran down all over her fishnet tights. I pulled back from her and walked away from the window, leaving her gripping the window lock with both hands, looking dishevelled with her hair a mess and her dress down to her waist, and panting and steaming up the glass.

'Sorry, I got a bit carried away there. You okay? I fucked you thinking of you like a hooker...'

'Don't even go there Billy or bring that up.'

I could sense her irritation.

'Okay. Let's have a cup of tea and relax together? After that why don't I take you for a walk?'

'Yes,' she said, 'I would like that Billy. Let's do it now.'

She glanced at the window quickly.

'When you were fucking me with my face on the window, I saw that man opposite again...' Her body gave a slight shudder.

'Okay, let's get out of here.' I said, taking her hand. We ran down the stairs and hurried to get the car out of the drive.

July

From: john smith <appledogstime@yahoo.co.uk>
Date: 18 July 12:20:29 BDT
To: Natasha <natasha_nw3@yahoo.co.uk>
Subject: Re: Thinking about you.

Don't worry after that story you sent I'm thinking of you and shagging you silly in the long grass. Your dress around your waist and your knickers round one ankle hanging. Most of my plaster is off and I am hobbling about with one leg in plaster. So get ready girl, get wet for me. John is coming in more ways then one x john

From: Natasha <natasha_nw3@yahoo.co.uk>
Date: 18 July 13:33:32 BDT
To: john smith <appledogstime@yahoo.co.uk>
Subject: Don't think too hard.

I am quiet brilliant, keeping two men very happy at the same time. How many women can say that? I had the shag of my life last night. I will spare you the details as you might get overheated ......

When did they take your plaster off?
Love Natasha x

From: john smith <appledogstime@yahoo.co.uk>
Date: 20 July 13:47:52 BDT
To: Natasha <natasha_nw3@yahoo.co.uk>
Subject: Think of you always

I'm in a private ward St Johns and St Elizabeth hospital. Ruth visits everyday but knows my feeling towards you so mid November or December is cut off point and goodbye to her as a lover and hello Natasha. I say goodbye she says hello. See you soon baby. Four months x john

July

From: john smith <appledogstime@yahoo.co.uk>
Date: 21 July 22:59:00 BDT
To: Natasha <natasha_nw3@yahoo.co.uk>
Subject: So no news from you..

Maybe you have fallen madly in love with Billy or are you trying to run from him? As little girl's do from daddy. Anyway you have gone a little bit cold on me again and if you knew the trouble I have to go through to get my hands on a computer to write to you you'd be shocked...it's like gold dust! I have to offer the nurses my body, especially the night nurses and the French ones. They tell me that if you want to write to your pretty girl friend you will have to shag me for 20 minutes and only then you get ten minutes of computer time. So you see, writing to you is at a price. See how much I love you? I have to sell my self just to talk to you. What a sad life! Now don't get upset...Just kidding with you to wind you up! love xxx john

From: Natasha <natasha_nw3@yahoo.co.uk>
Date: 22 July 22:50:55 BDT
To: john smith <appledogstime@yahoo.co.uk>
Subject: You little prostitute!

Put the night nurse down and learn you little whore of a man. You must enjoy every minute of the attention you get from the pretty creatures called nurses, I have known a few. Don't prostitute yourself on my account, I know how against all those practices you are. I am doing as I was told, avoiding all the stress (and you do give me a hard time) and being nice to Billy, I can concentrate on one man at a time if I don't it gets confusing. You are well looked after by the lovely Ruth - as you said she is in the hospital everyday. I have just came form that part of the world passing the hospital on my way and thought of you. But respecting your wishes didn't go in but I wanted to. Well maybe another time, when will you be out of there? How is the treatment going? Is it very painful?
Love Natasha x

July

From: john smith <appledogstime@yahoo.co.uk>
Date: 22 July 23:52:38 BDT
To: Natasha <natasha_nw3@yahoo.co.uk>
Subject: Update

I'm back home on Monday. Mum and dad are coming tomorrow to see me with my little sister. Will write next week. Very worn out kiss x john

From: Natasha <natasha_nw3@yahoo.co.uk>
Date: 23 July 00:28:01 BDT
To: john smith <appledogstime@yahoo.co.uk>
Subject: Re: Update

Keep at it my friend. You have people who love you near you, I am looking forward to the E-mail you have promised.

sleep well.
Nx

From: john smith <appledogstime@yahoo.co.uk>
Date: 24 July 08:08:23 BDT
To: Natasha <natasha_nw3@yahoo.co.uk>
Subject: Checking out now

Will do. Could have left Friday but home today, as I felt weak. I'm in some pain still. Will be in touch xJohn

From: Natasha <natasha_nw3@yahoo.co.uk>
Date: 24 July 09:33:21 BDT
To: john smith <appledogstime@yahoo.co.uk>
Subject: Please write soon...

I want to hear from you... want us to meet as soon as possible. I really think of you every night now. Nx
From: Natasha <natasha_nw3@yahoo.co.uk>
Date: 24 July 10:26:55 BDT
To: john smith <appledogstime@yahoo.co.uk>
Subject: Re: Checking out now

July

That explains it, called the hospital yesterday and they told me that you were discharged on Friday, which I thought was strange. Hope you had a good day yesterday with your family and that there is somebody responsible looking after you in your home, as I am sure that you still need it and will need it for few more days.

Look after yourself
Love Nx

From: Natasha <natasha_nw3@yahoo.co.uk>
Date: 25 July 10:50:18 BDT
To: john smith <appledogstime@yahoo.co.uk>
Subject: Work hard but keep happy

Don't get depressed my friend if you are, do what you have to do and stay positive. Does the exercise include sex or wanking? Do you have the lovely Ruth helping you out in that department? Or perhaps one of the night nurses doing overtime at your flat. I am still waiting for this long E-mail you have been promising, no hurry in your own time .....

keep well Love me x

From: Natasha <natasha_nw3@yahoo.co.uk>
Date: 31 July 22:46:27 BDT
To: john smith <appledogstime@yahoo.co.uk>
Subject: Your way or no way?

Now hold on John, would you say that we should calm down and start again? Unless you are enjoying all this which I doubt. I am happy to talk to you and joke with you, I am not getting at you or trying to be nasty to you purposely. I said it before and I am saying it again now. I don't think that we have to accuse each other all the time and make each other feel bad on daily basis. Unless that is what you want, God knows I have had enough of it. I am happy to make the first step – are you? Why don't you meet me? Natasha x

August

From: john smith <appledogstime@yahoo.co.uk>
Date: 1 August 00:06:18 BDT
To: Natasha <natasha_nw3@yahoo.co.uk>
Subject: YES! YES! YES!

But after I finish with Ruth and one last holiday. No more saying I am sleeping around, as I'm not, not even with Ruth at this time. I'm faithful in my mind and body to you so please lets be straight from now on and when it is a joke say so? Anyway I'm still under orders for complete rest and sleep with an hour of exercise as well. I'm still stiff and it's painful. That will teach me to look up girl's dresses! Never again! Cause of my accident..I was delivering the car to the port and this really sexy girl went by me on the free way. She went past but saw me as she did. She slowed down so she could drive side by side with me, she was on my right and I was on her left. She must of put the car in cruise control for this..with one hand on the wheel she kind of bent over to the best anyone could whilst driving and showed me her panties (they were small and red). She turned around looked at me and mouthed (I could not hear her obviously) three times "catch me and fuck me" and blew a kiss. Well I intended to catch her, give her a bow and say thank you but no thank you and then drive away..but then we hit a corner at 90 mph and she forced me in to a ditch and drove on with out a back word glance. Fucking cow!! Anyway I learnt my lesson, never again. Will write soon when I'm in work next Tuesday.

Still weak, in pain and not strong at all.

Kiss x John

August

From: Natasha <natasha_nw3@yahoo.co.uk>
Date: 6 August 21:16:12 BDT
To: john smith <appledogstime@yahoo.co.uk>
Subject: YES

Dear John,

Are you feeling any better? I hope so. Don't over do it at work tomorrow if you are still going.

Thinking about you
Keep well Natasha xx

From: john smith <appledogstime@yahoo.co.uk>
Date: 8 August 07:33:52 BDT
To: Natasha <natasha_nw3@yahoo.co.uk>
Subject: He fights and runs away. Will live to fight another day

Back at work today thank god! My flat become a prison. Back to my old self, well not quite but a lot wiser. Hope you are ok? Sorry about the lack of letters but kept myself to myself, I had a lot to think about like where
my life is heading? That's the third time I almost killed myself..so I better think and learn fast. Better drive only in to pussy in future and only yours at that. It's much safer driving in that part of the world. Kiss X John

From: Natasha <natasha_nw3@yahoo.co.uk>
Date: 11 August 22:44:53 BDT
To: john smith <appledogstime@yahoo.co.uk>
Subject: Have the brain cells recovered too?

Dear John,

How was your first week at work? Did you still remember how to do the sums and work the computers? (only joking of course). I have been taking stock and thinking of where I am going as well. The road of self discovery.. wonderful thing. Other than that I am working very hard, don't get paid much for it, started sowing again..the only downfall of that is that I spend a lot of time in my flat. Went to Epping Forest on Wednesday, I needed the break, picked lots of blackberries which are still in the fridge. I haven't had any time to do anything with them yet.

Let me know how is it going at your end.
love Nat xx

From: john smith <appledogstime@yahoo.co.uk>
Date: 13 August 23:46:38 BDT
To: Natasha <natasha_nw3@yahoo.co.uk>
Subject: Re: Have the brain cells recovered too?

Weak but ok. Spent the weekend fucking Ruth, it's been a long time, almost two months. Hope your ok? You seem changed as of late, can't describe it much..The only thing I can say is that you have become much harder. Maybe you always were and I did not realise? Hey what the fuck do I know anyway?! I just based myself up and nearly killed myself over a pussy that flashed by! A moment's weakness could have killed me. Anyway it was nice to fuck Ruth again, it was nice to fuck somebody to get the old feelings again. Feel the old cock throbbing hard and lusting for it. She was more of a little girl then ever before...lying there like a little girl completely submissive and passive. Not sure I like it anymore..? I needed the fuck real bad though, real bad. I could of done anything to her..anything. I felt like treating her like a real whore but in the end I just wanted to fuck her hard for 30mins and come, which I did. She blew her top and came like mad! She came at least twice and then on the end of my mouth as well. She was happy...Me?? I just felt I needed a body to use. The old feelings were not there. I kept thinking of you and that kept him good and hard. I was so weak at work but I will get stronger. I learnt a bitter lesson. Hope you are well. Anyway the dog was all over me, I really felt a lot for the dog. I missed him more than Ruth...it's been so long but it was good to be in a pussy. Still life goes on, to where I don't know. Hopefully towards your direction. I still hope for you but you seem to be changing everyday. Oh well I guess there's tomorrow, tomorrow and tomorrow and work. Kiss john x

From: Natasha <natasha_nw3@yahoo.co.uk>
Date: 14 August 00:43:17 BDT
To: john smith <appledogstime@yahoo.co.uk>
Subject: Re: Have the brain cells recovered too?

Dear John,
A lot has happened as of late. You yourself are not a bundle of joy either understandably. You could have died? My friend there are worst predicaments than death it self, you more than anybody knows that. It was stupidity to the highest degree on your part and that is all I have to say about you and your car crash for now. I was so worried about you. So very worried.

And so we go on..

Love Me x

Ps: Don't over do the work tomorrow my dear John and look after yourself.

From: john smith <appledogstime@yahoo.co.uk>
Date: 14 August 22:44:58 BDT
To: Natasha <natasha_nw3@yahoo.co.uk>
Subject: There can be no reason to break your word

I may have done a very stupid thing but I don't paint the pot black over and over again as I have heard on the grape vine you do..over and over again. I hope I have learnt by my stupid mistake, I hope you begin at long long last to learn from yours. If you say something and tell somebody you intend to do something then do it and never go back on your word. If you don't people can never trust you fully again. I gave my word to you and I intend to keep it. Don't keep repeating history. John xx P.S. My incident was a one off

August

From: john smith <appledogstime@yahoo.co.uk>
Date: 15 August 09:11:10 BDT
To: Natasha <natasha_nw3@yahoo.co.uk>
Subject: Back to normal and winter is on it's way

I'm off to Israel with Ruth. We are leaving around the last week of October for three weeks and that's it..goodbye my lover good by my friend, you have been the one etc etc and then it's all you, you, you! I have been in since seven this morning and it's killing me. After two months off I can't get back in to the swing of this no more. Still, the moneys good thank god. It's getting cold, I can feel a chill in the air already but that's just your heart. Lets not talk about the weather. Come on girly lets get warm again. I am starting on some new stories for you and me to think about. Make sure you tell all your clients that you will be away in New York from the 20th of November onwards. Anyway a big kiss my darling XXX John

From: john smith <appledogstime@yahoo.co.uk>
Date: 17 August 08:54:15 BDT
To: Natasha <natasha_nw3@yahoo.co.uk>
Subject: So, my brain cells have rotted and it's so very cold
The ice and snow of Natasha sweep over me like a gale, feeling the raft of her frozen heart from deep down in Siberia. Ruth tells me that Billy sold his house in West Hampstead? Billy asked you to have nothing to do with the studios and you agreed and promised to put the keys in an envelope and post them to the new owner. But that didn't happen did it? Billy found out and the shit hit the fan apparently but you knew it would did you not?? You can't say and promise one thing to one person and another to another. Meanwhile I sit here thinking of you, waiting for November, cock in hand, frozen solid in Siberia again and for what? In the end honesty is the best policy all round. If you don't lie and deceive you can never be put down or caught out. Just be truthful. Simple. I have another three hours till I finish this part then European market, Tokyo and then New York six hours later. I'm so worn out. Kiss x John

August

From: Natasha <natasha_nw3@yahoo.co.uk>
Date: 17 August 19:26:40 BDT
To: john smith <appledogstime@yahoo.co.uk>
Subject: It will get even colder!

John dear,

I can see that you are doing very well fishing news from all over the place. Had you asked me, I would have told you if you really wanted to know. Especially how that story came to be and all the ins and outs of it. But no, you are still going and listening to all the people around you. I wonder why? Why would you want to? Why would you not come to me and ask me before you accuse and use harsh words? People will tell you only what they want you to know, you with your ignorance and mistrust in me are ready and willing to believe all you hear.

Your choice my dear. I am grateful to you for all the lovely letters you have written to me, when I felt really down, when I was going through awful times in my relationship and when I was in the hospital. I do treasure them. You made me very happy indeed. I couldn't wait for your letters to come fast enough, you made my life worth living again at those times and I thank you for it. But I don't see how we can go on if you don't trust me. I can't and don't want to be with a man who will believe the whole world over me. You accused without Asking..my end of the story! I have no reason to lie to you or to anybody else. For me, trust is the most important thing in a relationship and if you don't trust me enough I suggest you go and find somebody who will fit the bill better then me. Somebody you will not have to spy on to satisfy your presumptions. Go and find a perfect girl as I am not her and never will be, but I deserve to be trusted, like you. As far as I am concerned

I trust you. It was a conscious decision on my part and I don't trust most people on this earth but clearly you find it difficult. But why? What prompted all this mistrust? I asked you for your address to send you a card, just like when you asked and sent me a card but no sign, no address. I will not go in to how you got my address. I asked you to give me your phone number when I was worried about you and you said no. I am sure that there was the Ruth issue, but I would never do anything to upset her or you. So there we are and life goes on.....back to the sowing and the tax man and the council tax and whatever else my life consists of at the moment ....

I hope you have a lovely holiday with the baby girl and find what you are looking for in a girl or a woman. You are not a bad bloke and I like you, but not even you know everything.

Natasha

Ps: Look after yourself and I mean that, get strong and well again.

From: Natasha <natasha_nw3@yahoo.co.uk>
Date: 17 August 23:33:20 BDT
To: john smith <appledogstime@yahoo.co.uk>
Subject: I don't treat you bad

And I thought that this was about you and me – not Billy or Ruth. Or any other ex in our lives! How silly was I?! You can rant about them till the cows come home.

N x

From: john smith <appledogstime@yahoo.co.uk>
Date: 18 August 00:27:34 BDT
To: Natasha <natasha_nw3@yahoo.co.uk>
Subject: Fantasy World!

It really seems that you want to live in a fantasy world of your own making basically meaning nobody can help you because you believe what you write and think it happened the way you see it..but deep in your heart you know the truth. You know it. You wanted your cake and wanted to eat it as well! There is no trust or mistrust in this story. This is you deceiving yourself and trying to make everyone happy. But why would you want to make a stranger happy over Billy and go in and clean his house when you know Billy did not want you to do that? Nothing to do with trust or anything else, you blind and kid yourself with that. That is just stupidity, plain and simple. I guess you have to be what you want to be, fine. I tried to help you solve all your problems and put your life right but no, nothing. You don't try, you give up on everything to easy and when things go wrong because of something you've said or done it's always the other persons fault. A simple request... "Don't go to my old property anymore" Billy says. Where is your trust and respect for Billy? What was so difficult about that request from such a good friend? So where is the trust? Blaming people for things you don't have yourself. Yet he is still there. He should grab you, put you over his lap and spank you till you can't sit down for a week. How sad John

From: Natasha <natasha_nw3@yahoo.co.uk>
Date: 18 August 09:58:59 BDT
To: john smith <appledogstime@yahoo.co.uk>
Subject: My world is too real for a fantasy

You go and fish out a few more stories. You didn't think that Billy was going to let me go to you without a fight did you? And by the look of things it is going according to plan and you are too blind to see it. Enjoy it John.

Throwing insults as freely as promises and words of love. Go and find somebody who is better and someones whose opinions you are interested in as well as what they have to say. No trust, no relationship. What do you think that does to a proud man like Billy? According to you our business needs to be run passed lots of other people. Never mind you just go on. If you never wanted to see me you should have said not launch a huge attack on me like that. It is easy. It is not important what happened and how it happened. People make mistakes (I know you don't as you are perfect). I never ever want to see the house and it's occupants again. That house is a curse and it nearly destroyed lots of people, Billy and me included and now you are going on about it. Will it never go away? I have sorted my differences with Billy over the house and you have still not an idea about what happened. Only what you have heard. I will give you good advice if you want it, so drop the subject and stop insulting me. I have lots of patience but even mine will run out very soon. Very, very soon. It is you who is acting like a spoilt child not me. Standing on your moral high ground and preaching to us mere mortals on how to behave. By the way what happened to your address and the phone number? I suppose I don't really need it do I? Not if you carry on like this any longer. I don't need any more hurt and with somebody looking at me all the time from the window opposite... I have had it with all of you.

Have a lovely day my darling John

From: john smith <appledogstime@yahoo.co.uk>
Date: 18 August 09:59:59 BDT
To: Natasha <natasha_nw3@yahoo.co.uk>
Subject: I really did fall in love with you.

If this is the end so be it, I won't write again. You have a man who loves you, another who wants to love you and be with you in the future and a chance to make a life for yourself and you throw everything away all the time. How lucky in life you are to have that person who loves you. Not just treat them as if you are doing them some big thing giving them a present, there are millions of women in this world... but there are not many. But it's your life and your choice so if that's what you want you go your way. Thank you for writing to me. I will hang on for one or two weeks and then give up on you. So I will say goodbye as you want beautiful girly and I hope things work as you want. Goodbye lady Kiss

Kiss John X X X

P.S.
As regards to my address and phone number...I always said (it came from you in the first place) that Me and Ruth have split up for good you would have it all. As you know mid November will be when I split from Ruth. We could have talked then but the girl who is to proud to be proud has made her mind up. So who am I to fight? Bye my love x John x
From: john smith <appledogstime@yahoo.co.uk>
Date: 18 August 10:11:32 BDT
To: Natasha <natasha_nw3@yahoo.co.uk>
Subject: At work

I just made 2 million pounds for the company so that's £35,000 for me. This is a good month. Pity about you... could have got you a really nice ring for that. Well you live in a fantasy world of your own making, maybe you can live safe there all your life. Everything is so different from the reality. Take care, hope you truly find happiness xxxx John

From: Natasha <natasha_nw3@yahoo.co.uk>
Date: 18 August 2006 22:02:58 BDT
To: john smith <appledogstime@yahoo.co.uk>
Subject: Re: At work

Dear john,

My work.. I cleaned two flats and looked after a little two year old. Sweetie pie of a girl. She is the loveliest kid ever. It does feel like I am on a totally different planet but only according to you. I didn't want Billy's money and surely I wasn't writing to you because of yours. I am sure you will find a good cause to spend it on even if it isn't me. Mind you I am not a cause at all. There is so much I want to talk to you about. I can't do this writing, everything gets twisted and taken out of context fuelled by gossip. Have you ever asked yourself why he might be with me for the past ten years? I am sure you did. I am insecure but not to the point that I would be unable to have an independent life John. I just don't have the faintest why would YOU still want to be with me after all you called me all the names under the sun - today a new one a schizophrenic. I know why HE wants to be with me but it is beyond me why would you, after all you have said. If we should carry on writing, this should just be about you and me. I will get on with my life and you with yours but if you think you would be better of with somebody else then I am sure you will be quite a success with all the girls.

Please tell me again why you want to be with me as if I described somebody as you did, I would not really want to be with them. Unless you fancy a screwed up girl with severe psychological problems in your life as you described me. I did love the idea of a perfect man to be with but there is no such thing is there?

Only you sounded as one, too good to be true. As they said in Some Like It Hot, nobody is perfect......

Have a lovely weekend John and look after your silly
self my lovely man

From: Natasha <natasha_nw3@yahoo.co.uk>
Date: 18 August 22:27:44 BDT
To: john smith <appledogstime@yahoo.co.uk>
Subject: What was the reason behind all of it?

Dearest darling John,

Which ever way I look at it I can't see a way out. I miss the lovely person you were when we started, the sweet man has turned in to a menace. I wish I knew why? I was worried about getting in too deep and I couldn't sleep most of last night after what you wrote to me, which means I am in too deep. I think about you every day, most of the spare time I have. All this rubbish predominates my life with the rest of the stuff I am going through. You were absolutely ghastly to me and if you can't see that then I don't know. I don't talk about you and Ruth because I don't think that it is my place to judge and comment, but that is me. What is between two people should stay between two people, the third parties involvement is not required unless invited to comment. And it wasn't your place to comment. What was the reason behind all this rubbish you came up with John? What did you want to prove? Tell me.

Natasha x

From: Natasha <natasha_nw3@yahoo.co.uk>
Date: 19 August 08:56:27 BDT
To: john smith <appledogstime@yahoo.co.uk>
Subject: The past and the future

John you don't realise one thing..no friend of Billy's will tell you that I was there for him 24/7 everyday all day when he was going through the worst part of his life. I was always there when he needed help or a shoulder to cry on and he will confirm that. I am not always the menace you are trying to portray me as (though we all know that I have one or two issues). I don't want a lap dog, far from it. A man with an opinion who knows what he is talking about straight and honest will do. Since last Christmas, I have turned a leaf in my life and started listening to people with more experience. I got my self an implant, I went and got my work sorted on the advice of my elders. I am doing a job, which was suggested, and I am trying to get my life in order. I am carrying on with your exercise as it deserves my best shot if it should help. I am not perfect but I try, maybe not hard enough at times but I do try john. You could give me credit for that in your writing. I need to change and only I know how much and I am working on it even before you came on the seen I was seriously thinking of getting professional help for my problems as there were times which were not easy for me to put it mildly. I still think that I should have gone and talked to somebody who could help, there is so much to deal with and to get over. I sometimes feel that it will be impossible to do. And I am sure that you even in your wisdom shouldn't get involved in my problems. Nevertheless I am working on it slowly but surely

but the change is so needed. Most of the stuff you have written about happened five years ago and yes I agree I was wrong to be unfaithful but first - I told you all about it- and second I have turned a new leaf which is learn from my mistakes and never do it again, but only I know that. But you still talk about it. It was the lowest of the low but I have to move away from that or I will end up killing myself with the guilt generated from it. It happened it is finished and bringing it up will not make it any better. Billy's kindness and willingness to help people. My concern was that Billy was going to be there all day long running from his flat to mine as we are just next door. And my other concern was that I would be accused, as I already have been in having something to do with the man, as he is supposed to be very popular with the ladies and I can do without that. Since Christmas there hasn't been anybody else and I will keep it that way to the point of me staying alone if I do split up from Billy and don't make it with you. After all I have been through I need somebody who will trust me. As I told you previously, if you wanted to know you should have asked me and I would have told you everything. And I mean everything. You are the first person after bill who I have openly talked about my
life to and that is something I would never do. Not in a million years. I have not lied to you and I tried to be truthful with Billy too. John I am the only person who can appreciate what the man has done for me as I said previously. I am aware of his worries for me I worry about him a great deal, but that is what people do if they share life together. We have all done stupid things in our life that includes you, him and me. But it doesn't mean that we can't change and move on from that, you after your three car crashes must appreciate that. I am sure that you didn't purposely smash yourself on any of the occasions. The same here.

Love Natasha

August

From: john smith <appledogstime@yahoo.co.uk>
Date: 19 August 11:51:55 BDT
To: Natasha <natasha_nw3@yahoo.co.uk>
Subject: I have read what you have to say.

My little maid is round singing at the top of her voice. Nice to see her happy. She has a new boyfriend he's Irish. He gave her a right hard seeing to last night for two hours she says. He is 28 years older then her. She is 26 so it's put her in a real good mood. She told me she had not had sex for a year so now she is singing like a bird. It's wonderful how women get so much from it and what it does to them. Anyway us..I will get in touch with you when Ruth has left for good and see how your life is and where you have got to with sorting it out. Hope he spanks you hard, which is what you fucking need for all your wrongs as well as a good fuck after, and at last you would of grown up. Anyway pencil 20th Nov in your diary, I will get in touch and we can go from there. After our holiday Ruth will go to live in Israel for a year so that's really good by Ruth. I hope you love animals beside me that is as I get my dog back. Hope you can handle him he is big as I am. Anyway lets first see how you get on with your life. Get lots of non-stress jobs and calm down. Maybe, yes maybe you might turn out to be a real nice girl. Until then take care of yourself, have fun, be good and god bless. God will look after you till we meet kiss x John...let me know all you have been up to around the 18th Nov. The day she flies out. My last letter for now xxxxxxxxx Kiss John X

From: john smith <appledogstime@yahoo.co.uk>
Date: 28 August 16:45:13 BDT
To: Natasha <natasha_nw3@yahoo.co.uk>
Subject: I had to tell you.

Shagging all the time like mad I am. I'm like a rabbit, she loves it and can't get enough of it. She would like it five times a day and night but me, I, myself can't stop thinking of you all the time. Even when we are both on fire I think of you, she says I have become a wonderful animal but it's you that's made me one. I fuck like mad and think of you, it's your legs that are spread wide, it's your pussy I eat kiss x John

From: john smith <appledogstime@yahoo.co.uk>
Date: 16 September 13:39:40 BDT
To: Natasha <natasha_nw3@yahoo.co.uk>
Subject: I'm counting the days till the 20th of Nov

I have not and never will forget you, I want you more then ever and I'm counting the days till Nov 20th. Don't forget, I have tickets booked for New York nine days later. Love you lots xJohn xxx
From: Natasha <natasha_nw3@yahoo.co.uk>
Date: 26 September 19:00:58 BDT
To: john smith <appledogstime@yahoo.co.uk>
Subject: New York

Dear John

I have read all your E-mails that you have sent me. I feel that I should write to you...I would not be able to go to New York with you. I just can not afford the time off. I have still over six thousand pounds of tax to pay which I haven't got, and my council tax has gone up considerably but it is not just my money problems, I will not get the time off work as I work for a new family now. They are expecting a new baby in four weeks time and I will be expected to help out by working more hours. But I also don't feel that going away after knowing you just for a few days is the right thing to do.

I am very sorry Dear John. Speak in November.
Love Natasha x

From: john smith <appledogstime@yahoo.co.uk>
Date: 27 September 14:32:43 BDT
To: Natasha <natasha_nw3@yahoo.co.uk>
Subject: Re: New York

I understand how you feel..I'm up to my eyes in tears and

have to sort her head out before she leaves for Israel. She is in a bad way. Anyway will write soon kiss X John

From: john smith <appledogstime@yahoo.co.uk>
Date: 28 September 20:34:00 BDT
To: Natasha <natasha_nw3@yahoo.co.uk>
Subject: I will marry you one day, I know it

Hi... I think of you all the time so I hope you have not looked elsewhere or are looking at any other man. I want you and intend to have you as my girl and future wife. I want you to know that. So no other men please till you try me. Hope Billy and you have worked everything out and are happy. Maybe your getting the big OOOOOOOOOO now? Or very close to it I hope. Love you and want you. I told my mum and dad that you did not want to go to New York, so they send you an invitation. The invitation is if you would like to spend Christmas with us? It'll be for six days. My sister will be with us as well. If we have not made it in to the bed together by then you can have your own room. Can't wait for our first date. Kiss x John Please say you will spend Christmas in Liverpool with the family and me?? J xxx

October

From: john smith <appledogstime@yahoo.co.uk>
Date: 2 October 12:29:37 BDT
To: Natasha <natasha_nw3@yahoo.co.uk>
Subject: My mum and dad were asking..

They were asking that if we hit it off do you want to spend Christmas with my family? As they plan they're Christmas early. I'm mad to meet you, so crazy for you. Write soon Kiss x John x

From: john smith <appledogstime@yahoo.co.uk>
Date: 3 October 11:34:25 BDT
To: Natasha <natasha_nw3@yahoo.co.uk>
Subject: I need to hear from you..

I don't want to upset my parents, I told them so much about you including that you wrote to my sister. I hope we are still meeting up? Kiss X John x

From: Natasha <natasha_nw3@yahoo.co.uk>
Date: 3 October 11:44:13 BDT
To: john smith <appledogstime@yahoo.co.uk>
Subject: The coming Christmas

Dear John,
It is very nice to be invited to spend Christmas with your family and I want you to thank your mum and dad for me, I do appreciate it. My work at the moment is
very hectic and I am unable to plan so far ahead so I will have to politely decline the offer. But I do want you to thank your parents for their kind offer. If I do get the time of work for a few days, which I doubt I should like to go home to see my mum but that is a decision which I will make nearer the time, depending on time off and on my financial situation
Speak soon, I'm off to Iceland with Billy in an hour. Don't know when I can write to you again. Not sure about availability of computers over there. love Natasha x
Ps: I try to make a point of going to the Midnight Mass every Christmas

October

REYKAVIK
Sunday 3rd October

The lothario and his lady were at the top of the world. We had arrived in Reykavik. My agent had informed me that there was a very good opportunity to photograph the amazingly charismatic, one-off Bjork as she was in between albums and at home with her pretty daughter.

So I took myself off with my cameras, hot and ready to go to the land of the midnight sun. The land of the blue lagoon. The land of the largest whale schools in the world. The land of the blowing geezers. Planning to have fun and make love at the highest point in the world and the nearest to the north pole I had ever been.

Our first vision of Iceland as we got on the coach to take us to the Floki in the centre of Reykavik was a land burnt black with volcanic eruptions. A landscape that was more like a moonscape than anything you could ever imagine. The journey took roughly an hour and a quarter to our hotel, and hardly a tree or a bush or even a bird was visible. Black earth rolled onto black earth. Piles of volcanic debri and black black mountains.

But the weather was warm, the sun was shining and we were to find out that the first visions were an illusion. In actual fact Reykavik and the rest of Iceland had the most amazing blue waterfalls, hot geezers that sprouted out at unexpected moments, the incredible Icelandic white ponies which were everywhere and the hot springs where the temperature was between 20 and 30, with hot volcanic lava floors for you to stand on, and water to drink that the Icelandic people believed was good for your health and kept you alive for up to a hundred years. The problem in Iceland was the country was one of the most expensive in the world. The majority of people worked a minimum of 12 hours a day. Both Natasha and I were incredibly shocked. A cup of tea was £4, egg, bacon and chips, £10, £20 for two people. But even though the country which is as large as England, or maybe even larger, has a population of less than a million people, the icelandics are very charming, kind and helpful and considerate. They have the most superb taste in fashion and beauty products.

Because of the weather that predominates the country for 7 months of every year, most of the fashion designers, dress makers and coat

makers worked in wool and leather, which in an Icelandic atmosphere, looks stunningly attractive.
Our hotel was friendly and we looked forward to our first meal which obviously again, had to be fish. The icelandics know more and serve more fish and shellfish than almost any other country I have been to in the world, except maybe Japan.

You need a mortgage, or you need to take one out to buy an evening for two with wine. Even the cheapest restaurant. The Icelandic girls are extremely beautiful with pale skin and blonde hair. Their skin is like alabaster, like marble statuettes. Many of the girls grow their hair very long, and put them in highly complex beautiful styles. The Eskimo influence is noticeable everywhere, with many of the woollen coats having bone fasteners. We walked down the main street of Reykavik, our equivalent of Regents Street, and were knocked out by the simple but veru effective window displays. Sometimes one beautiful woollen coat with a tiny spray of Icelandic flowers in a wooden vase at the foot.

The nights turned quite cold and the Icelandic people themselves say, the only thing you don't know about the weather in Iceland, is the weather. One minute it could be pouring heavily, torrentially with rain, and the next moment you could be basking in warm sunshine.

We decided to plan our time around the many excursions. I hired a car for 8 days, and the opportunity of course to photograph the legend herself Bjork.

On the first night there we did not make love as we had a silly row just before we went to sleep about the Icelandic sheets and bed linen, which I said, you had to sleep on top of with the duvet over you. Natasha for some reason got it into her head, that you slept on the mattress, and the sheet and duvet covered you in that fashion. I ended up sleeping on the sheet and she was on the mattress. Not a great start to our trip.

I could not believe when we reached the harbour, that bjork lived only 150 yards from it. She was a legend afterall, with millions of albums sold to her name, and I could see the influence of her country in her music.
London was now thousands of miles away from us, and we were lucky in the fact that we had arrived just in time for Icelandic fashion week, quite close to the parking and bus routes of

Hverfisgata, and the cultural house.

We were finding in our walk about the streets that the Icelandic people are avid readers. They had a passion for language and literature that had existed for centuries. Such a tiny city as Reykavik boasted more than 15 specialist bookshops.

On the second day, we decided to go out and see the whales. So we got a special cut price ticket and after one and a half hours, the boat drew to a close, turned off its engines as we stood quietly in the Icelandic sea. Then we saw it.

First his nose, then his sleek body, and then up out of the water, with spray falling in every direction, the sun glistening on him, and with a massive flip of his tail, back into the surface again. A giant minky whale. The captain had given us specific instructions, saying that we must treat the boat like a clock. The bow would be 12 o clock. The right hand side, 3 o clock, the left 9 o clock, and the stern 6 o clock, with all the hours in between. He was high up in the captain's observation post with high powered binoculars and a hailer system, which in not very good English, with a strong Icelandic accent, he would try to produce lyrical poetic expressions of the wonder of the Icelandic seascape. As there was an agreement by all his guests onboard, that if we did not see any whales we would not have to pay and could come back for a second day free, every so many minutes, he shouted out at the top of his voice, excitedly, and all 100 people onboard, heads swivelled almost off their neck and shoulders to look in the direction mentions. In 99% of the cases we would be too late.

'Minky whale at 2 o clock now! Minky whale at 5 o Clock now! Two Minkies at 2 o clock now!'

But yes, we did see them, and yes they did come up to greet us. Not as many as he indicated, but we did see them. He moved the boat a little forward, 3 r 4 miles, turned off the engine again and then we realised his strategy. Wherever the birds fed on the water, the whales also fed.

There was a large flock of seagulls ahead of us diving and rediving and skimming the sea, and within half and hour, very very close to the boat, at least 20 fairly large minky whales surfaced, swam around the boat, ducked and dived and returned to the sea. It was certainly an incredible experience.

We all got back to Reykavik excited with our cameras full of whales and seascapes.

That night, after a really nice meal of prawn and clams, we went to bed and I felt quite amorous and sexy. Although we did make love, and she did give into me, it was with some reluctance. I suddenly realised that she was missing writing to John Smith for all the time we would be in Iceland, there would be no e-mails from her to him or him to her. I had asked her repeatedly, when he comes back, are you planning to run off into the sunset with him. She had always stated,

'No I don't think I could stand him too long sexually, and his dominate, strong and manipulative personality would overpower me.'

But as usual with Natasha, she gave very little away, and it was quite obvious that she was very much in love with him, missing being able to communicate with him. I was sure that if he had suddenly appeared in Reykavik, she would have vanished off with him.

The next day she insisted that she wanted to be driven to see the geezers and the Gull-foss waterfall.

We took the long journey. I was exhausted driving over 300 km across the countryside to get there. Through Landmannalaugar and right across visiting many of the giant waterfalls and hot geezers. I was absolutely drenched and freezing cold one minute, and the next running around like a mad thing, camera in hand photographing the beautiful Icelandic ponies in their natural environment.

In the meantime we had found out where bjork lived and posted a letter through her door with all our details, contact numbers and addresses, both in England and in Reykavik.

On Sunday morning we visited Reykavik's flea market and on Sunday afternoon we went to the blue lagoon, which is probably one of the most incredible experience anyone can go through. Miles and miles of deep, heavy, blue, blue water, perfectly still with no waves, and you can wade up to your neck or even swim. The temperature reaching over 30 in some parts. The icelandics had been incredibly imaginative, building tiny little hot seats on the bed of the lagoon for people to sit down and enjoy the therapeutic effect of the waters.

Waiters stripped to the waist even served coffee, tea and

Icelandic drinks, wading out into the waters with tiny little bow ties around their necks, and not much else.

The icelandics, were very interesting people indeed. They also have considering the size of their population, a great deal of unmarried mothers, of which Bjork was one of them. I was quite surprised to learn she had a son of 19 years old, who she had with a previous band member.

Then I started to get goose pimples, so I told Natasha that I was going out to get something to eat quickly at the restaurant and she said, 'I'll see you in 15 minutes. We can catch the coach back after that.' We had been there for nearly 5 hours. Time had gone so quickly and we were about to have our first big row. I didn't know if this was because we were cooped up together 24 hours a day or the John Smith scenario or the fact that we were both tired at the intensiveness of the trip, with so much to see and driving to do, and so many places to go.

40 minutes later I was getting frantic. She had still not appeared and there was no way that they were going to let me back into the lagoon to look for her, as there was strict control over entry as vast numbers of coach people arrived and enjoyed the lagoon throughout the day continuously. It was fast becoming of the biggest attractions in the world.

It was now one hour and ten minutes, and there was no Natasha anywhere. I had walked to the coach station twice, been round all the restaurants and all the souvenir shops, asked two of the girls to go in and look for her, giving them detailed descriptions of how she looked, and still nothing. Finally she emerged looking hot and flustered, one hour and twenty five minutes after saying she would be out in fifteen.

I went berserk. Absolutely crazy and furious.

'Where the fuck have you been? I was looking for you everywhere!'

She did not have an excuse, nor a reason, and she was certainly not prepared to offer one. Needless to say, the coach trip back was one where we sat in separate seats in silence, and when we arrived back in the city, I went off on my own for the whole afternoon, leaving her to her own devices. That night we slept back to back without a word.

The next morning we both made an effort to rescue the

situation over a nice breakfast at a cute restaurant that we had found nearby.

We got quite excited to hear from the waitress that Bjork and her daughter had passed by just 5 minutes before, and was making her way down the main street. But I could see no sign of her. I was beginning to think I may not even recogise her even if I did see her, and contrary to what her agent had told my agent, I still had not receieved a phone call or a letter, or any form of communication as to when I would be allowed my precious 20 minutes with her.

The atmosphere started to improve and we got more and more lovey dovey, holding hands again, for the last five days of the holiday. We were seriously worried about the money as you had to be a millionaire to live in Reykavik. The price of a bacon sandwich was £11. It was unbelievable. But books, wool were cheap, and the clever icelandics had even set up a clever second hand business with second hand fashions and clothing and merchandise, even second hand bjork Cds which I bought 2 or 3 of. Considering that a beautiful woollen skirt, top and hat was around £300, a good quality second hand one which may only have been worn 1 or 2 times, cost £60. The Cds cost me the equivalent of £2 each. So we were learning to survive out in Iceland. We visited numerous museums, hot baths, hot swimming pools, in fact, all the water and heating and pools in Iceland are fed by the unique system that they have developed, harnessing the hot volcanic waters for use for their cities and towns. The only thing that put us off, and we did get used to it, is that when you take a bath or shower, you notice just the faintest smell of sulphur.

The last night was hot and passionate as we both made an effort to make the final evening good for both of us. So yes, we did have good sex and she enjoyed it, or appeared to as much as I. Maybe it was because she was happy knowing that she could get home at last after an enormous amount of time, in her book, of not having any contact with her beloved John. I could imagine her rushing into her flat and hitting her computer within minutes of me dropping her off.

Then we had another upset. Not between us two, but the coach failed to turn up to collect us at the airport. It was due at 4 o clock, and our plane back to Stanstead was at 7. At 5 o clock there as still no coach, so we had to hire a taxi and one other person joined us to make our way to Keflavik airport. We finally arrived there only 25 minutes before take off, and we were passed through customs quickly and efficiently and onto our little plane.

In the end, except for coming very close on four separate occasions, we never got to photograph Bjork, but we did have an unforgettable experience.We landed in Stanstead quite late, and were in London after 12:30 midnight. I hired a cab to take myself home and left her with her souvenirs, memories and whatever other dark secrets she may have had in her head, at her flat.

October

City of the North, Reykavik

We went on a visit to a city far north,
The sea rushed up to the big blue sky,
The boat it rocked, pitched and tossed, the wind it cried,
The stars twinkled and shone in the black autumn night.
I held you close, held you tight.
Our hearts were heavy so we managed to cry,
We thought of the dream we knew would die,
You told of the misery which in your heart dwelt,
My hand reached out to wipe your tear,
The boat passed the point of no return,
And you again, drew near,
When we return to England's shore,
Like in fairytale, you must go your way,
And I'll go mine, to find another day,
We will part forever til the end of time,
The city of Reykavik has had its way,
A woollen muffle on your ears,
You can no longer hear what I say,
And I look at you through a veil of tears.
City of light, snow and ice settles my fate,
To clear a path that we might see,
The pain will fade we'll lose our hearts,
But there'll be another day.
Tightly close your eyelids while I kiss your eyes,
Forget the love we used to know, remember now,
Rivers, waters, heights and cloudy spheres,
Seconds, minutes, weeks, months, centuries and years.

October

From: john smith <appledogstime@yahoo.co.uk>
Date: 12 October 11:03:28 BDT
To: Natasha <natasha_nw3@yahoo.co.uk>
Subject: Very, very disappointed

Dear Natasha I have been so upset (hence no reply), really sad that you turned my family and me down. Kiss x John

From: Natasha <natasha_nw3@yahoo.co.uk>
Date: 12 October 15:21:36 BDT
To: john smith <appledogstime@yahoo.co.uk>
Subject: Disappointed? Me too.

Dear John,

I am sorry that you are so very disappointed. I am disappointed too, but I can't make commitments which I may not be able to keep. I have just returned from Iceland, Reykavik with Billy, and I am up to my eyes in debt, I will have to work extra hard to pay it off now. The money I owe is more than I initially thought, which means that I can't even think about taking a holiday with you or your family because the tax people are on my back everyday. This is not a happy situation to be in. You will be with your family at Christmas, my mother will be alone so it makes sense, that if I do have any spare time (and funds which I doubt) I will go home and be with her. You would not expect me to leave her alone, would you?

Love Natasha

From: Natasha <natasha_nw3@yahoo.co.uk>
Date: 13 October 15:15:27 BDT
To: john smith <appledogstime@yahoo.co.uk>
Subject: How can you be so unreasonable?

Dear John,
Whatever - I also said that I would need sufficient time and sufficient funds to go home, or did you over look that. I strongly doubt that I will have either. I will probably be

spending the Jewish equivalent of Christmas in the kitchen and the rest of what is left probably on my own in my flat (as I have done on

many occasions before). Do spare a thought for me when you are with your family dear boy, having six days of holiday. This is the grim reality of my life. Paying off over seven thousand pounds which I don't have is not fun. Maybe you would like to sort this one out for me as well, as you seem to have a solution to everything else. It would be very nice if you showed a little bit of interest at least.

Love N

From: john smith <appledogstime@yahoo.co.uk>
Date: 13 October 22:59:45 BDT
To: Natasha <natasha_nw3@yahoo.co.uk>
Subject: A little bird told me...

A little bird told me that that there is a really beautiful Swedish chick after Billy and she is crazy for him? I also hear that he told you that he shagged her. Anyway good for him, he deserves some pleasure in life. After all he destroyed his marriage, left his wife and for what? For whom? Someone who gives him a really hard time all the time and everyone else she meets and talks to. I hope he wakes up soon and comes out of his trance the poor shit! Hope he goes where his heart should be..with someone who loves him, admires him and wants him. Not someone that gives the whole world a hard time as well as her self all the time. the You and your negativity. The other word positive has never been heard of! If you came to me to get your head sorted and I was a doctor, I would jump out of the window in desperation. God I wanted you so much but I never realised you were such a defeatist about life. You get a blow and you go down instead of fighting. Where are your guts? Where is your fight? Everything with you is always on the dark side all the time. My god..I hope he looks down on you as he is the only one left x
John

October

From: Natasha <Natasha_nw3@yahoo.co.uk>
Date: 13 October 23:37:23 BDT
To: john smith <appledogstime@yahoo.co.uk>
Subject: Very unreasonable!

John I need answers now not at Christmas. Your father cannot go through my books or would you like to tell your parents the truth about my past? Or have you already? The books are done and the figures are on paper, I simply just can't pay the final bill. This bit is simple. There is no other solution needed. Billy is not an accountant, when he needed one he employed one of the top accountants and they knew all the tricks in the book. But Billy doesn't need accountants anymore. But I remember in one of your very first letters to me you said if you ever need any help I am there for you... To your polite invitation I did ask you to thank your parents very much, that I value and appreciate their invitation, but have work commitments which I will have to keep. I am sure that if you tell that to your mum she will understand and not harbour hard feelings against me as it is normal that some people have to work over Christmas. You are just put out because I spoilt the second of your lovely plans. Contrary to what you might think I would love to have met them all and spent time with them but it is not to be. Instead I will be looking after the kitchen, the new born and two other children as well as the house and the other people I work for. And me and Billy? We are doing just fine, he is still the best lover I have ever had, he does it for me every time now, and according to him I am sex on legs as hot as the first day he shagged me (only hundred times better) his words not mine today, the bedroom department is at its best in years. He is a very sweet man and I am a very sweet woman. I still get short tempered and depressed at times (partly me partly medication) but that is me. People who do not like it can ... you know what. There is not quick fix in life for anything and if you don't like me the way
I am you don't like me full stop. How ever many promises and declarations of undying love for me you make. Eliza Dolittle said to Freddy: 'don't give me words SHOW ME'. Actions

speak louder then words. I have read lots of lovely words from you, just the action is or rather is not. Well it is non existent and that is a big shame my little boy ....
Kiss me
Ps: How is your health after the accident? Any lasting damage on your big spoilt head? Hope you are getting back to normal.

From: Natasha <natasha_nw3@yahoo.co.uk>
Date: 13 October 00:03:58 BDT
To: john smith <appledogstime@yahoo.co.uk>
Subject: The Little Bird.

Dear john,
Not breaking news to me, I know all about this lovely admiring lady. I knew her sister, who in case you are not up to speed about Billy bedded as well. Just wonder why Billy hasn't gone to her already? The opportunity is and has been there all this time. He has the opportunity to leave and move to Sweden when ever he feels ready to...Wonder why he hasn't yet?... But for now he has chosen to be with me. Really can't think why ... Maybe I am not as horrid, awful, shifty, self centred, living up my own bum, big headed, nasty so and so as the doctor diagnosed. Just normal me. I will sort out my problems myself as I have always done. A defeatist can't afford to be a defeatist at this moment as there are only words coming from you. As I said I am finding it hard to pay my bills. That is not a rocket science, no degrees required. I can't afford sweet words and marriage proposals as Billy says Words come easy ... Maybe you should call and tell me instead of writing it all down, you should scream it down the phone or do a naked fan dance and pray to the god of rain to stop the floods. Lets be stupid but not nasty again.
Sweetness and hugs me
P.S. You should not be so nasty to me or I may start believing that you really liked me once.

October

From: john smith <appledogstime@yahoo.co.uk>
Date: 14 October 14:39:55 BDT
To: Natasha <natasha_nw3@yahoo.co.uk>
Subject: Tomorrow I leave for Israel with Ruth

One month in the Promised Land with the little girl and then back for you. I return on my own on the twentieth of November. Shall be round to pick you up for your fist date on the 22nd of November and after all the trouble you gave me be ready for a sore bottom! Knickers pulled up between the cheeks and well spanked.. Before the nice stuff.. A long walk in the woods, kisses hugs etc. As I always promised, we shall meet at seven thirty on the 22nd of November. This is it at last after a long frustrating eight month wank thinking of you. Now you get me??? Every bit of me, completely. I'm flying out tomorrow morning at 3am. See you soon. Looking pretty and sexy and wearing my knickers you got with the dollars. Take care xx John

From: Natasha <natasha_nw3@yahoo.co.uk>
Date: 21 October 17:30:49 BDT
To: john smith <appledogstime@yahoo.co.uk>
Subject: Looking forward to the first day of the rest of my life with
you!
Dear John,
Looking forward to it, after all that hard time you have given ME, and that is not the hard time I enjoy. I am very jealous of you having a lovely sunny time in the promise land.
See you when you return from Israel. I can't wait. Finally.
Love end kisses
Natasha x

Ps: How good are you at keeping your word to me? Can't wait to talk to you, to see you, to be with you, meeting your parents and your sister, taking you home to where I was born and showing you all the secret places .... Is this finally true or am I just dreaming? Or is the first day of the rest of my life just about to really happen...

From: Natasha <natasha_nw3@yahoo.co.uk>
Date: 21 October 17:36:04 BDT
To: john smith <appledogstime@yahoo.co.uk>
Subject: Forgot to ask

Dear John,
Are you checking your mail at all? You might be having such a good time that you don't? Let me know how the holiday is going? Are you having a good time? Love Me x

From: john smith <appledogstime@yahoo.co.uk>
Date: 23 October 13:39:42 BDT
To: Natasha <natasha_nw3@yahoo.co.uk>
Subject: SHIT! SHIT! SHIT!

My holiday is shit, my life is shit and me?? Well me, I'm shit too!! I can't sleep, I still love you but Ruth... more shit!!! Especially her future. Don't ask... needless to say, I'm feeling shit, but SHIT what am I expected to do?!...

Natasha, I have a baby girl on the way!!!!

My life is the biggest load of fucking shit in the world!!! I am a fucking fool!! YES YES YES... you know that! Do I still love you and want to marry you?? YES! And where am I? I'm not with you, but here having a baby from a girl I don't love! A baby I wanted with you... She kept saying, let me come with you Johnny... let's come together Johnny... fuck me harder Johnny... come deep in me Johnny... Let's come together and cherish this moment forever Johnny... and here we are. I'm stuck with this for the next 18 months...

Will you wait for me another year or more Natasha? Fuck off John Smith! Go back to where you came from!! You are a big shit and a fool! I hear you say. Are you right? Yes you are. And how am I? No sleep... been thinking about you for the last three nights. And how is she??? What is she saying??? Love me John, love me! I'm going to be a little mummy, love me! But can I? No!! Do I want the little girl? Yes. But not by a

woman I no longer love. At least the baby will be Roman Catholic... I'm off to New York and she is coming with me. The company have offered me £500,000 a year to be the head of the New York office with a large flat in the centre thrown in too... Mum sold my flat in London, and she's having all the things shifted to the US. How do I feel? Shit. I want to be with you... We were so close... so very close... I'm thirty, mad, clever but crazy.
I will write to you again from New York in January if you want me to? Tell me to piss off if you don't. I know I'm a fucking fool. We all are sometimes... John xxx

From: Natasha <natasha_nw3@yahoo.co.uk>
Date: 23 October 15:13:02 BDT
To: john smith <appledogstime@yahoo.co.uk>
Subject:

How far gone is she and when is it due? As if it mattered anyway.

From: Natasha <natasha_nw3@yahoo.co.uk>
Date: 23 October 16:59:42 BDT
To: john smith <appledogstime@yahoo.co.uk>
Subject: Fwd: Seems like the rest of my life has already started

I am hurting after a night of two hours of sleep. Now I can't sleep, I cant eat, I am so unwell, I wish I wasn't anymore. Why I didn't want or couldn't go to New York with you and why I politely declined your invitation to Christmas in Liverpool. I couldn't think of a better and sweeter offer to Christmas then with people who wanted to know me and who went out of their way to invite me to their house. My Christmas has been crap for as long as I can remember. I will be alone as usual but the email will
explain. Anyway before I congratulate you on the good news and say thank you for hurting me to the depth of my being..I knew this was going to happen, had a feeling about it about a month ago, this was the only way she could keep you and she

succeeded. I waited my turn and I got nothing...Lucky you lucky her. Waiting for you for another 14 to 15 months? Tell me a good reason why, when you are going to shag her and set up home with her in your big house. I waited since your accident, you would not even talk to me on the phone when I begged you to. She's flying to New York to hold your hand. Enjoy! Enjoy! Enjoy! You have made a choice with your cock! What can I say, that is what you do best, and that is why you nearly killed yourself. Had I known that you were having unprotected sex with her all for those months I wouldn't have wanted to know you. But I tend to try to see the best in people. I waited for you to finish in peace with her and this is what I get for my patience, you didn't trust me, I trusted you implicitly with all my heart. Enjoy all the rows with her as much as you can! I would have given you my life but it would have been wasted on you! You deserve her and the fury of her family you do... You will have the little baby, lots of money, lovely flat, fat and grumpy woman in toe and you will shag every prostitute in town! After all you can afford it (I can't even pay my bills now and nobody will help me, there are days where I can't get up in the morning. I am so tired and unwell at the moment). You just go and enjoy your life. Your dad and mum will give you a lecture on how to be a responsible father with a woman you don't love. Go do it, you will drive yourself mad for few months till you can't stand it anymore. I have seen it before, sticking together for the sake of the kid? Good idea the kid really needs two people who are fighting day and night because they are unhappy, but at least you will have the little baby girl. Who cares! You will all be unhappy. You saw the little heart beat on the monitor and felt so proud. I wanted to be the one on the bed with the little blob inside

her. Your baby my baby our baby. Who knows babies sometimes sort the problems between two people out too but in your case I doubt it. I wanted a baby for the past ten years so much it would have made me the happiest woman on this earth, to have your child our child, but you wasted it! For what? A little daddy's spoilt Jewish girl? For five seconds of an orgasm with her? Did you enjoy it? I drive people mad with

the baby talk, I want a baby so much. The woman I work for is having a third one this week the due date is on Wednesday, she is preparing the nursery. Buying so many unnecessary things for the baby and I am so jealous of her, so very jealous. I don't know how to cope when the child is born as she
is Jewish as well. But normally I don't get what I want. I played by the rules here and it didn't pay off. I did as I was told by you for a year and you went and did this to me? Why did I trust you all these months? Why? I was looking for a wedding dress and baby clothes, planning my future with you, the walks in the woods, the holidays, the house and the nursery, growing old together, fighting, making up, me pregnant by the end of next year and our baby the following. The little girl I wanted since I was one, for what I wish you were dead and me too. You have made a bed for yourself but you didn't look as it was the wrong bed, the wrong woman, the wrong womb and now you sleep on it! Do me one last favour as I have never ever asked you for anything. Do not even think of forwarding this email to Billy. After all he wouldn't let me read yours, I think you have hurt him as well as a whole lot of other people. Me included enough.

Natasha xxx

Ps: Now I can tell you. When I told you about my financial problems I expected you to offer help. After all I was the woman you promised to share everything with all your life and all your worldly possessions (your words not mine) but you didn't. I would have paid you back it was just £5000. I paid the rest already but I don't like asking especially for money. Never have as I'd rather well go with out as I have been doing for so many years. I have always paid my own way, my daddy never gave me anything and never will. I even looked after Billy financially when he was not doing well still have the IOUs in the draw. I know Holidays with ex-girlfriends and babies are very expensive, now I know it. You could have at least offered but you were more worried about the holiday with Ruth. The reason I didn't want to go to New York with you (amongst others reasons you will read) was because I didn't feel right doing so. You jumping in to bed with me when your cock was still dripping come form Ruth. I have more respect for myself than that. I wanted to get to know you as a person before becoming your lover and then whatever, what does it matter? Forget the babies, the money, everything. What I didn't get and what I will miss most is the friend I had in you, our e-mails and endless letters. You were so near but now so far, maybe I was madly in love with the idea of the perfect man and for the past months it took your body but would you have ever measured up to it? No I don't think so. So you deserve everything that is coming your way for all the hurt you have caused and will cause in the future to people who were more than good to you. You were once my perfect man, I am very distraught for now but I will get over it and over you but you will be stuck with the woman you don't love and her kid from a broken home which you will create forever.

From: Natasha <natasha_nw3@yahoo.co.uk>
Date: 22 October 10:27:09 BDT
To: Billy Clayton <billy_clayton962@hotmail.com>
Subject: Seems like the rest of my life has already started

Dear Billy,

I want the whole truth from him. Why would he do this after all the promises of undying love and devotion and all else. All the promises, he said soon you will have your own big house to look after and the little girl which is as beautiful as her mother, loving straight talking husband, family, holidays in lovely places, loyalty, love, the engagement ring from Tiffanys, wedding in Liverpool Cathedral with a white dress like my mum and dads wedding, both our families there. I was going to do everything in my power to make him happy, to make it work. I would have been the most devoted wife. Why would he send you my letter with those words? Why? Why? Why? Only you know.... For the whole year I didn't look at another man, didn't even speak to another man. Did everything I was told, tried my damn hardest (paid for my own implant though I don't have much money) to please all the people around me again and where did that got me, I'll tell you where, fucking nowhere! As in this world it doesn't matter if you lie or tell the truth, the outcome is the same whatever route you chose. I want to believe that this statement is not true but it seems to be, at least applied to the last year. I told you everything was straight with you and with him, and look where I am, not even worth one letter of explanation. That is how precious I was to him, so he can't find the time and words to tell me. He must know that the news would have reached me by now, not a damn thing from him! So much for his trouble solving skills! Dealing with problems when they arise (as mummy and daddy taught him), courtesy and respect for people. I am still the last to hear. I won't believe it until he tells me, I can't stand this gossip from everywhere, I trusted him. Seems he sorted MORE than her head and her tears. I feel so betrayed, forgotten, used, sad, angry, outraged. I slept three hours last night and I can't sleep anymore. I am so tired of everything I have heard so many promises from everybody all through my life. From the people closest to me (you as well), and invariably it ends like this. Who will make a big effort to sort my head for me now, I feel that everything I touch turns to dust. I felt so special, so flattered when he invited me to his parents for Christmas, that was the best offer ever for years and years. I didn't care for diamond rings (though they are nice to have) as this meant more to me then all the money he has. His family invited me to their house, they wanted to meet me and call me by my name, get to know me, I felt special so special. I worried so much about them not liking me but I couldn't go for six days but I would have been able to make two maybe three. But now as usual I will be alone you will be at your kids and me here. My mother will be working all Christmas and the airfare is so expensive. Anyway, not worth it anymore. The money is unjustifiable. All my friends are going home or have other plans already. I don't know why I worry I have done it so many times including Christmas and the New Year. When I was waiting for you to tear yourself from your family, me sitting here on my own just waiting (mostly just crying and waiting like a good girl) you would come and tell me with grand gestures that it is just another day nothing special. Yes you are right it is just another day or two but these days you spent with your children and family. I was here on my own or to ease your conscience you would send me home on a plane. And now I was invited to somebody's house for whom I wasn't just a burden and a Christmas problem, but somebody they wanted to know and now it is not going to happen. I feel so alone so very alone again!!!!!!!!!!!!!!!! People think that I am a hard bitch, not really, underneath I am as soft as jelly and I feel left again and that hurts so much, I trusted the man, with all his sweet talk and sweet promises. I wanted to be with him, but I wanted to do right by you as well, to give you the last few gorgeous months that I felt I owed to you. I tried so hard. I told you everything about the situation. I wasn't lying to you unless the truth is a lie in it self. Going to New York was a lovely idea but nobody knows but you that I don't have more then one pair of shoes to my name and they are three years old. I have no money. How could I have gone to New York with all the pretty people there. I would have felt so stupid. I worked so hard for the tiny amount of money I have saved so hard and now most of it will go to pay of the tax man and the council tax. I should have spent it on me while I could have, put it towards the university course I wanted to study for years to make something of my self finally or buy some dresses and shoes, make myself look and feel better, go to a hairdressers in the west end instead of Kilburn. Well that is not going to happen either now... If I ever have the misfortune of meeting the little shit I swear I will draw blood.. Well my heart will be bleeding floods of tears but he is used to the water works the little cow produced enough of them over the year. Daddy's little girl, the lovely little Jewish princess, may God bless them both, may they live happily ever after in the land of John and Ruth and enjoy the special moments together. After all, now he has what he always wanted, a concrete reason why not to get rid of the woman he calls his soul mates and loves so much. He made a big song and dance about sorting her head out together with a huge lot of nastiness about her, maybe I should forward a few of his letters to her like he did with my E-mails. The e-mails he

called
her every name under the sun! How he couldn't stand her anymore. Well now it is sorted forever!!! He wanted a little girl he has a little girl Jewish girl forever and I will just have to get over it one day soon.

One day I will get my own washing machine Billy. If not with you then with someone...
Natasha

From: Natasha <natasha_nw3@yahoo.co.uk>
Date: 23 October 22:52:31 BDT
To: john smith <appledogstime@yahoo.co.uk>
Subject: Re: MY LAST WORDS

John I have never done this before but would you be able to help me financially with the tax I have to pay? I believe that is the least you could do for a girl you wanted to spend the rest of your life with and promised the world and after ten months took everything away from her in just two short emails. Just when she dared to believe, leaving her in total despair over you. I would be grateful. I wouldn't ask if I wasn't desperate. I may have to go to hospital tomorrow again.
I feel so very ill over it all.

But I will understand if you can't.

Natasha xxxxxxx

From: Natasha <natasha_nw3@yahoo.co.uk>
Date: 24 October 01:07:00 BDT
To: john smith <appledogstime@yahoo.co.uk>
Subject: My last words to a dear man (for now)

Dearest Darling John,

I have stopped crying for a while and had a think long and hard. Can't sleep so I will write to you maybe you will, maybe you won't read this. Who knows?

October

What ever happened happened and we as much as we would like to, can not change it. There is not one, not two, but three losers in this sorry saga. We all lost as we don't get what we wanted, you fucked up, I fucked up and she fucked up big time. This happens everyday of the week and we are three very unhappy people now. The main thing is that you have chosen to be there for her. As you said it wasn't to be. She got the man by underhanded tactics and she is the biggest looser in this. I am sure you are fond of her and as much as I hate thinking about it I have to admit you have no other choice but to stick by her and try and make it work with her, how ever hard it will be, and it will be I realise that, the kid is half yours. This will not be a bed of roses but we all made our bed and now we have to lye on it. I was too indecisive and proud and now I know, but I did make a decision in the end, but it was too late by then. Dearest darling man try to do your best by her however hard it is be kind and loving, that is what I would have wanted if it happened to me, if I was in her shoes, you are there for her and she needs you now, (this is not easy writing to write, when my whole being is screaming come back to me and leave the little scheming bitch alone! Now she has what she wanted) it is for the best that you stick by her and I think you are doing the right thing, though it is not the one you would have chosen by far. I will go and try to sort out and rebuild my life now,
cry a few more bitter tears and then make a few important decisions and look forward to what the future will bring. I want to get a proper job, study, party, make new friends, try to make some more money as now my money man is out of the picture. Forget the last email I sent you, I am not that desperate, I will pull a rabbit out of a heat and sort the money situation out somehow. I am sure that there are other ways and who knows one day we might still meet, I will be here, not sure whether I will be waiting for you exactly, you might find it very difficult to leave your baby when you have her, but I will be here, do you remember the end of the last story I sent you?

Hugs kisses and all my love. Try to be happy, make the best

of a bad situation my dearest boy, I will think about you when I am holding the new Jewish baby in my arms. I am so sorry it didn't work out how we planned it, so very sorry I can't tell you...

Love Natasha xxx

From: john smith <appledogstime@yahoo.co.uk>
Date: 26 October 22:35:33 BDT
To: Natasha <natasha_nw3@yahoo.co.uk>
Subject: The future

Please don't reply. I will never marry her. Kiss x John

From: john smith <appledogstime@yahoo.co.uk>
Date: 30 October 00:43:36 GMT
To: Natasha <natasha_nw3@yahoo.co.uk>
Subject: I can't get you out of my head. I'm at the office, it's 2am.

I want you so much, will have to work something out. One thought of you, one look at your picture and WOW!!!! Now what? Don't answer, I will write soon. Want you more then this muck.

I am up to my eyes in SHIT.
She has found all our e-mails to each other and read all of them.

From: john smith <appledogstime@yahoo.co.uk>
Date: 5 November 13:50:25 BDT
To: Natasha <natasha_nw3@yahoo.co.uk>
Subject: hi baby, sorry for all the mess ?

Will write soon, and looking forward to meeting you in the new year. Home is a million dollar, lux penthouse... but hell on earth to be there if ever the devil punished you for his sins, because he is on my case, big time. Home is hell, so I try not to be there too much. Meanwhile the queen is strong but on

her own in the palace. I have started to hate her and wish you were here with me, having a wonderful life together. I can't believe two fucks brought my life down and everything I wished for with you…
Been having real busy 20 hour days, but good for me as I don't have to think. This is a safe email. She can't get into this one, even the Chief Rabbi won't get her into this. Just worry about my little girl and what sort of future she will have… if you and I have a child, would you look after my other child with me sometimes?
I understand if you say fuck off and way back to the grind… and I mean work, not sex. John x

From: john smith <appledogstime@yahoo.co.uk>
Date: 7 November 00:45:36 BDT
To: Natasha <natasha_nw3@yahoo.co.uk>
Subject: every day every night I think of you and I want only you and no other

Busy, busy, busy John x

From: Natasha <natasha_nw3@yahoo.co.uk>
Date: 14 November 00:40:21 BDT
To: john smith <appledogstime@yahoo.co.uk>
Subject: How much do you know about me- everything and nothing

Dearest darling John,

I wanted to write to you sooner but I wasn't sure what to write as I feel like three people in one. Maybe you are right and I am schizophrenic.

Nevertheless I haven't written mainly because I am not surprised that you have hell on earth in your house if poor Ruth, and I mean poor Ruth, found all your and my emails. She must hate the whole world. The letters are very intimate and she couldn't have known how deeply we were involved. Why didn't you protect them? They were my deepest and most secret thoughts in those letters which I wouldn't share with anybody, and now the whole world is reciting them back to me. I don't understand why you didn't look after them with more care. Everything I have written is public knowledge. And the poor cow is beside herself. What good that is doing to the unborn child, God knows.

I am only writing because a Jewish baby has been induced today at 10am as it is two weeks overdue. By tomorrow we should have a baby and my head is all over the place thinking about you.

In your case- I feel like the scarlet woman, I am splitting your family up and taking the man away from the pregnant ex-girlfriend and their unborn child, stoking a fire which should have been extinguished weeks ago the minute I knew there was a child involved. This makes the writing to you almost impossible to justify, though I live for the short messages you send me.

You have no idea what is coming to you my dear man. You are on a war path now only because it is all a big shock baby on the way. New job, new everything. But you will work it out slowly… your job, your situation, but where will I be after that? Will you write me one more 'sorry Natasha, I didn't mean to hurt you'-letter? …We haven't even spoken, I don't know your voice, your smell, your hands… but you are the perfect man in my mind. I so want to speak to you John, but you and Ruth have a history of many happy and some unhappy years together and remember how hell bent you were on keeping her as a friend and soul mate before we were supposed to meet. You wouldn't see me before you sorted her head out. She was your first and foremost priority. Should you not try to sort… something with her? And at least be civilised to each other. You know full well that you will marry her one lovely June day and I will be a distant memory then.

There is so much stuff I want to tell you, I have been in a trance ever since… I can't move on, I am reminded of the reality every day in the Jewish family I work for.

Thinking about you every day
Natasha xxx

P.s. I joined your Yahoo! Messenger how safe that is I don't know. Not much I guess as you haven't replied.

From: john smith <appledogstime@yahoo.co.uk>
Date:15 November 10:05:11 BDT
To: Natasha <natasha_nw3@yahoo.co.uk>
Subject: Have been to church, my mind is in turmoil. but we can be friends forever

Went to see an R.C. bishop here in the big big church babe, can't sleep, want to do the best by everyone. Anyway, I'm a man who has to make his mind up and go for something right or wrong. I may spend my life regretting it and maybe I will, but with god's help there is a slim chance that it might just work out, so I asked Ruth last night to renounce her faith and convert to Roman Catholic for me and the child's sake, so the little girl has no problems growing up, and will be happy with two people who love her and care for her and at least one set of grandparents who love and care for both of us. After a lot of crying and tears she said yes. I don't know after meeting you in the soul and spiritual sense if I will be happy with her but we will just have to make the best of it. I still think of you when I fuck and would love to be your friend and talk on the internet to you and share jokes, and I hope, meet. I don't know if I will be able to keep it in my pants, but she will have to keep a blind eye to that. Since you, something has left the relationship and is out for a run. The sex is not the same anymore, but mum, dad and little mummy will be happy… so I will have made three people happy???? And life will go on, whatever way it goes. So it will happen and it will be a life, I can't expect more. Money will not get you happiness. It gets you freedom and that's all it gets you. In the end you are what you are.
So Ruth starts lessons next week. The little girl will be

baptised as a R.C. My dad is flying over next week. The wedding will be in mid-February... And may god help us all. And I hope you will find happiness with Billy or someone who loves you as much as he has.. and I'm sure will continue to do. Believe me I will always be your friend, and I will continue to be if you want that, and it's not too painful. I do hope we meet one day and can talk on the computer. Not much I can say now at this stage except we both got to know each other well, and as the song says from Pretty Woman... it might have been love, but it's over now, it might have been love, but I fucked up somehow... god bless you and take care of you sweet lady. And god is always good so no, you will be okay... I really know that. Work hard, really work hard, that's best. Think positive and good, and good things will come to you... try to get some property or land in your country or some where as soon as you can make money.. be strong and independent and good things will come to you, they always do. Men love strong women. It comes from when we are babies and they look after us and control us. We never get over it... so be strong and go for it, work and money.. the rest will come, take care darling kiss x John

From: john smith <appledogstime@yahoo.co.uk>
Date:16 November 15:45:00 BDT
To: Natasha <natasha_nw3@yahoo.co.uk>
Subject: Re: Have been to church, my mind is in turmoil. but we can be friends forever

I don't think I can marry her... I don't think I want to ... I'm going through the actions like a man in a trance... I really can't face it... the pressure is out of this world... I have to find a reason at the last moment to run... took ten valiums today for the first time. What's the fucking time in England. It's five fifteen here, fuck, go out and drown my sorrows. Fucking save yourself for me you fucking wonderful... grab hold of kiss and bite arse... out of my brain valium and champagne and pain. That's why they call it that I know now you get the pleasure. Sometimes the sex after she has had a bottle of it inside her... then the pain pain love love kiss x John

November

From: Natasha <natasha_nw3@yahoo.co.uk>
Date: 19 November 20:35:06 BDT
To: john smith <appledogstime@yahoo.co.uk>
Subject: A letter
A letter I wrote on Thursday after receiving your 'wedding to Ruth' e-mail.

My Dear John,
This is your life and you have to live it the way you feel comfortable with. You have a responsibility to your daughter and only to your daughter after she is born. Think before you do anything you will regret for the rest of your life. Once you marry her there is no going back.

Your parents are the problem and I feel for you on this score, losing and displeasing them would be a big thing for you but again they can't live your life for you. How will they justify making you marrying a woman you don't love and don't want to be with? How will you justify harming her in a moment of madness as you have done in the not too distant past? You are trying to do the noble thing and do the right thing, but how can they expect you to do this after their life has been filled with happiness and love for each other?

A slim chance of a successful marriage is not good enough, and you know it. Miracles do not happen, and I can't see you making enough compromises to make this work. You would have made promises in church you don't mean, and how would mum and dad feel about that?

Your daughter will be better off with two parents who respect each other, are civil to each other, but don't live together, than two parents who are at each others' throats every day fighting and shouting every waking hour of the day, mum upset, dad upset equals little girl very unhappy, and I know… I lived it every day of my life and still do today. What might seem a good, suits-all solution may well turn out to be the worst in the long run.

And as regards to your conscience you have to sort that out for yourself- but rest assured that marrying her just for the sake of the child is not a good enough reason. Do marry her by all means but only if you can truthfully answer all you are going to promise her on the wedding day. 1) Do you love her? 2) Do you love her enough to spend your entire life with her? 3) Will your honour her and forsake all others till death do you part? And if the answer to at least one of these is no, then don't do it. You are storing big problems for yourself, and your child, and the two sets of parents you have involved now... big problems.

You are looking after her as best as you can. She is warm and secure and looked after very well by you, you have not kicked her out and that is the best you can do for her, you have stuck by her in the most valuable time in her life and that is important. But letting her convert to your faith and running after she had done so would be cruel beyond belief, unless that is the point of it. These are my opinions, so take him or leave him. I am in the same mess as you, and I feel it as painfully as you.

Dear John, I can only tell you what I think and you will have to make the decisions for yourself. This is an emotional rollercoaster you are riding and I am riding it with you. I don't have access to valium or champagne though today I could have done with both of them as I was unable to work. Few more days like that and I will lose my job, so back to reality and get on with it my boy.

Today 20th November you should have been home from holiday and I am still expecting the date you promised me. I am sure that you do remember. Just one more thing, John, your Ruth will play dirty as she said to me a few weeks ago, until she gets what she wants, she is prepared to take any action necessary to get it all. Her child is not even here yet and she threatens everybody. The minute you marry her she will take you to the cleaners if she hasn't done so already and then we will see how important your money is to you. My dear

friend who passed on a few years ago used to say- 'take my money by all means but don't waste my time. I can make more money, but nobody will return time which is wasted.' And time is something I don't have.
Ruth Cohen is buying a new hat to go with her Catholic daughter's wedding, so I believe that you will marry the woman whatever the consequences and I don't want to be there when you do so. Make it work or get out.
Ps. Take care of yourself my dear John. If you want to talk I will e-mail you my phone number… if not I am still here for you for now…. But don't expect me to be here after you have married her. I have been a mistress for 10 years, but not anymore. Not to you. However much it hurt, and it does, believe me. Nxx
From: john smith <appledogstime@yahoo.co.uk>
Date: 20 November 21:08:41 BDT
To: Natasha <natasha_nw3@yahoo.co.uk>
Subject: I am and I will

Words are ok and you have lots of them as always. Is it the money???? I made a play for you, a big one. But you came back on, but you know my bad ways, but you expected them…. Easy… is it the money for you as well as a bit mercenary..? I now don't believe Ruth planned it. She wanted that job in Israel. Very much. But we are both where we are now… and the long words you spoke about marriage, missed out the most important words in the R.C. code for better or for worse till death do us part. Maybe you should think of that as well… for better or for worse. We went to church together and we saw the bishop together. He says the most important thing for the church is the child. Natasha, I don't want my child to be born a bastard. And any way neither do I want her to grow up with that stigma to her name, and I don't want her looking at me when she is sixteen years old and saying and saying, 'dad, tell me why you left mum before I was born? Why?... every girl's got a dad, why not me? Why did you marry mum, after five years with her, you said you loved her and wanted her… so why… I can't let that happen never, never, never. The bishop said that man and woman are two halves, but the child is the most important. So that's where I am. So I will marry for better or for worse, I will be your friend, and I hope we learn a lot on the journey we took together, I did... I also learnt we have to stick by our mistakes and put them right and make them better... so you should think about what you did to someone and put that right as well. Anyway will write soon, and yes it's for 14 February at St. Mark's Church, New York, Central Square, Manhattan. You may come if you wish. I will send you an air ticket. Hope we can be good friends, take care for now, I wish you only the best x John

From: Natasha <natasha_nw3@yahoo.co.uk>
Date: 20 November 12:00:29 BDT
To: john smith <appledogstime@yahoo.co.uk>
Subject: John

The money was part of the attraction, I can't deny that. But you made me believe in something I never dared to believe. You had something more than money to offer me dear John. Money is nice but I wanted you as a man with all your faults and you do have plenty. I am not mercenary and you should not believe that. If I was married to Jonny Brad Haydon, that man has way more money than you ever will. I am sure that you know who that is. He has been after me for years (with Billy's blessing) I never had anything with him, and don't think I ever will. He has all the money in the world, it was the man who spoke straight, who had principles, who didn't like, who I could trust, who was R.C like me, who was prepared to give it all and who wanted similar things to me, that is what I wanted from you and with you.

If you want to marry Ruth, do, You have my blessing, but the e-mail you sent me before this one speaks volumes. You did actually ask me to hold out and save myself for you if you remember.

John, throwing vases at your beloved pregnant girlfriend, staying away from home for days or nights, drinking, taking drugs to ease your pain, shagging around... what sort of devotion is that dear John? Maybe this is the worse you were talking about, and the better will come soon. How long will you keep it up? In my last e-mail I wrote is also a paragraph about your daughter. Maybe you should go and reread it... not just the bits about money. How will you explain to your little girl that her mummy is in the hospital with injuries daddy inflicted upon her in a temper? Just as long as she is Catholic and not a bastard that is ok. John, do as you think. I am sure that you will marry her 100% and never doubted it. And I am not trying to stop you, just think about it. Many children are born to parents who are not married and who do not live together, she wouldn't be the only one, so there is not longer a stigma attached to it.

As I said, I am here for you until you get married dearest John. You have to live your life the way you want it... I am all for that. But is it what you want or are you really just going through the motions as you have written of your dad and the church and Ruth? Us Catholics do the guilt very well that is for sure.
Enjoy the rest of the day
Love you as always
Nxx

From: john smith <appledogstime@yahoo.co.uk>
Date: 21 November 14:00:03 BDT
To: Natasha <natasha_nw3@yahoo.co.uk>
Subject: are you not worried that I will beat you up one day, and if not why not?

Anyway, my mind's made up now. I see the bishops every week and am in therapy for sex and violence, which I don't mind as part of my training. Ruth and I are in marriage guidance, before it actually happens because we are working to grow together and be together... play together... this is a 200 year old Irish expression that my mother told me as a small boy. 'Work together, play together, say your prayers together and stay together'. That's what I'm trying to do right now sweet Natasha. Take care and good bye xxx John

November

From: Natasha <natasha_nw3@yahoo.co.uk>
Date: 21 November 14:46:33 BDT
To: john smith <appledogstime@yahoo.co.uk>
Subject: I'm not worried

Do whatever you have to do my John. No I am not worried that you will beat me up one day.

I sincerely hope and pray not for me and you anymore, but for you and Ruth. Hope you sort it all out and the vase misses every time you throw it. And yes I will hold you to your promise and come to your wedding if you wish, to wish you both all the happiness in the world, and a long life together. You are welcome to write to me but just as a friend… no more 'please hold out for me' or 'I can't marry her because I will run at the last minute'. I have feelings too and they seriously need protecting now. I am sure you understand that. I do miss the friend I had in you before though…

And just in case you are in real need of a good friend one day, you know where I live as you've sent me flowers and birthday presents, so please pop round to me. You can always send me an e-mail to let me know you are coming. Love and kisses, Natasha x

Ps. You can't beat me up because I am miles away from you. Always have been and always will be in your dreams… it is better this way :-)

And if you never write to me again, do me one big favour and write to me in three years time and tell me that you have made a success of it all. If not, there will be hell to pay! I will find you and then it will be you who needs serious protecting!

November

From: john smith <appledogstime@yahoo.co.uk>
Date: 21 November 17:41:01 BDT
To: Natasha <natasha_nw3@yahoo.co.uk>
Subject: She won't have you at the wedding

She says no… she said she wants nothing to spoil her big day… so sorry, no best friend wedding. Thanks for the numbers… I might use them one day, who knows? For one thing or another. Anyway, have a good Christmas and New Year… and go to church… it is a good thing for your mind and body sometimes. I have made so many friends over here, just from the Sunday morning services.

Anyway, I won't write again… got a lot to concentrate on, both love-wise and work-wise. The New York people go mad at Christmas. It's a really big thing. Happy New Year and take care.

You will never, never hear from me again… I really have got to concentrate now on my future child and now that Ruth has finally decided to become a Roman Catholic and dedicate herself to making me and our child happy and to be a good mother, it is obvious that while you are there in the background, I will always be tempted. Always wanting to visit you, always thinking about you, knowing that every time I come to London, you may be available for me. I wish you a good life in the future and I do hope that we have both learnt a great deal from the times that we have spent together, exchanging words, romanticising, having sex together via this crazy machine, getting to know each other and falling in love.

I'm sorry, I truly am, that I fucked up at the end… but that's life. We all fuck up one way or another, somewhere or another.

Take care, sweet lady,
Sad as it is, you will not hear from me again... it would be too hurtful for both of us.
Kisses forever, John xxx

December

From: Billy Clayton <billy_clayton962@hotmail.com>
Date: 22 December 17:41:01 BDT
To: Natasha <natasha_nw3@yahoo.co.uk>
Subject: Dearest Natasha

Dearest Natasha

I know that nothing I say will take the pain that you felt after losing John, and probably after Christmas you will get rid of me as well. I hope you enjoyed Porgy and Bess and the presents I gave you. I told you that John was a figment of my imagination and that I dreamed him up because I could not stand to see you in so much pain. I hope that the present fits and that the sounds last you all of next year, and that the pain of John whether you believe in him or not, will finally grow less and that you will only remember the good times that the year brought both of us, and the many happy memories we shared.

Happy Christmas, Billy, All my love

My music tells the way I feel
Sadness tears for real
I was born
No name
Raised
Tempered
With the wind and rain
A pebble by the sea
A soul man
Sometimes we all search for love too long
The melody
A drum
A pipe
A flute or two
The harp
A sound
You and me

December

THE ROT SETS IN

John Smith died in her dreams, and with him so did I. I knew the writing was on the wall. In the end it really was one more e-mail, one more year. I had given her an i-pod for Christmas and a smart new woollen dress. We made love for the last time on the dining room table, and then on the bed. But the soul, spirit and feeling had gone out of it. It just wasn't the same any more! There was something there, of course; that would never die. She and I were close as the sea is to the sand on the shore, but big John Smith; he'd become a dream for her. A dream, a fantasy of something that she wanted desperately. But now the dream had ended, she was shattered and disappointed. There was no one to occupy her mind each night, no one to fantasise about, no one to dream about having babies with. Just old Billy and her work. I went home and started to close down all the e-mail addresses. John's, Fay's all them. Bad yes, manipulative, yes, but we'd had a great last year together.

I did not see her for a week or more; we had a big hole beneath the waterline and the sea was pouring in. Proud, majestic, beautiful, but sinking.

Ten days later in beginning of January, she phoned me to say she received a new e-mail from John Smith. I fell off my chair and felt the feeling of colour draining from my face. This was impossible... It couldn't be... If what she was telling me was true, whoever was writing to her would have her phone number and address as well.

Another ten days had passed, and she called again to say that she had received four more e-mails from him. She had said that he had become quite nasty and was threatening to destroy her and her friends. I advised her to block the e-mails and have nothing more to do with them. I told her to contact the police. She was getting upset and angry, and I explained that it was because she rejected him- he must be back in England, and she said that the e-mails had confirmed this, so I told her, 'Have nothing more to do with them'. Everything was looking very strange and it was now two months from the split. I took to phoning her to see that everything was okay and to visit occasionally, but she obviously kept me at a distance, not wanting the relationship to resume in any way- she was relieved that I couldn't get close to her again. Her and

I were high-tension electric cables, but if we started, it would only bring heartache again- we'd only cry again- say goodbye again.

The little Cancerian-crab was pulling in her claws, retreating into her shell, scuttling behind her rock. The storms, the winds and the tides of destiny that have washed her up to me were now taking her out to sea again, to bring her onto a new shore. Her eyelids closed, rivers, waters, boulders, centuries and years. Dragon faced dragon. Now the limp, wounded male had to retreat to fight another day. Water drips from her head and sparkles like dew in her hair. The sand is wet on her lashes, but pain is engraved in her heart.

As for me- a chisel, a golden bullet, like a vampire, destroyed. The parting will eat me up. I see only misery and sadness everywhere. Like the emptiness of the sea, she is stronger because this is her domain. The tide took her away from me again. There were so many problems, so many obstacles to mention. She was like a cork as she floated when initially she resisted the hazards and reached the shore and me. Now she was gone, in many ways unwillingly.

We had been to the theatre, but even Porgy and Bess did not make her happy. We spent the night together after, and she made love only as a thank you for the theatre, and not because she wanted to, or needed to. I told her stupidly that John Smith was a figment of my imagination. That I had dreamt every single bit of him up, his family, his job, everything, in order to have one more last beautiful year with her.

I could not bear to have her suffering so much for the loss of the man that was me, but she would not believe, could not believe and would never accept that I could ever be in her wildest dreams, John Smith.

From: john smith <appledogstime@yahoo.co.uk>
Date: 10 January 12:02:29 BDT
To: Natasha <natasha_nw3@yahoo.co.uk>
Subject: WE BOTH HOPE HE LEAVES YOU. IT WOULD MAKE US BOTH SO HAPPY…

Want to send us both a nice wedding present… yes, yes, yes. Then write and tell us both that Billy left you and we will both be over the moon. I asked Ruth as a woman what makes you happy, and what makes your friends happy? And she said it was to make her man happy, to see him with a big smile on his face or singing in the shower after he has enjoyed ravishing her body. All her friends feel the same… men love to please women, to take her nice places, get her clothes, underwear, restaurants etc… and in return, a woman, at least, MOST women love to give themselves to their man… it's a thank you gift and something that the enjoy as well…. But you have taken off Billy for ten years and he has given up everything for you… but we both bet the amount of sex, hot crazy sex you gave him, you could count on your two hands. And yet from what we have heard he tries to please you all the time, so where is the 'partnership' in that? You take, he gives. And how much of the one thing that every man wants from his girl, do you actually give to him? Ruth is on me all the time, and it's the one thing I really love her for…. I hoped you would be with me as well, but now I realise you are an ice cold frigid bitch, who opens her legs to pee, for her tampons and the rest for as little as possible. When was the last time you deep throated him?? Bet you can't remember… and this was the man who gave so much to the world as an artist… with his art, his photography… who has had so many beautiful women in his life… poor sod ending up with a cross legged creature like you. I pray to god that he leaves you and finds a hot sexy caring woman. We both do. John, Ruth

January

THE LIGHT ACROSS THE STREET
10th January

Simon Williams had always been an oddball, a loner, but not a loser. He was a mainframe computer expert on the linux system and his classification job-wise for many large companies throughout the UK, was an AS400 systems administrator. He had plenty of free time to indulge in many of his fantasies of which Natasha was becoming his final obsession.

Many women regarded him as devastatingly good looking. He was 6'2 with a nice body, but girls avoided him like the plague. Their natural instinct told them he was dangerous. He had an air of hidden aggression and temper hidden beneath the well tailored suits and crisp shirts. It was even apparent in the way he used his hands for expression when he was talking. A couple of girls he had taken out were deeply shocked when he'd lost his temper and even went berserk in restaurants and coffee bars, when the service was not what he justified as satisfactory. One of them, after only two weeks of romance and infatuation, soon made a hasty exit from his life after he slapped her round the face and screamed at her at her front door when she wore a mini dress that he felt was too revealing.

He had suffered from manic depression since the age of 15 and had been on various medications. He had spent some time in prison for violent and aggressive behaviour at 18 against two young girls of 16 and 19, coincidentally, both tall and blonde. Since then he had learnt to become more crafty and calculating. There had been other incidents in his life, now he was nearing 36, but he had managed to avoid detection. Whenever he could not get his own way with a woman, or she became cheeky or verbally, physically defiant, the usual result was a violent outburst.

One woman with which he was briefly involved, had ended up in hospital, and he nearly had a charge of grievous bodily harm made against him.

He had moved in to the large Victorian block of flats opposite Natasha's some three years before. He had been stalking and watching her every free moment, and yet he was very careful that she never noticed him. Whenever he followed her, he dressed down to look more discreet.

He had watched her undress through a set of military high-powered night-vision binoculars on many occasions. During the winter months when her light was on, she would sometimes forget to draw her blinds down fully, accidentally exposing herself. In the summer months when she left her blinds up and the windows open, he even managed to watch her then as the late evening sun shone into her room and illuminated it.

He tried everything to get close to her without her knowledge. At night, very late, sometimes after midnight, or even later in case he was caught by people coming home after late-night drinking sessions, he would go through her dustbins. He always knew her particular bags, because to save money she recycled her Sainsbury's shopping bags for her rubbish, instead of the standard black bin liners every other resident used. By this method of visiting her dustbins, the night before the refuge collectors were due, he had managed to obtain her home address in the Czech Republic, her sister's address, her date of birth, credit card numbers, and National Insurance number.

Towards the closing days of January the year before, he had hit the jackpot. The greatest prize of all. The one that he had been dreaming and scheming about. At the bottom of one of her Sainsbury's bags, he found, mixed up with old wrapping paper and vegetable lasagne boxes, seven or eight pages of e-mail print-outs. He had her e-mail address, and someone else's who she appeared to be writing to, and was possibly madly in love with. A man called John Smith.

A rare find indeed. This gave him the key, and he had retrieved enough information to be able to obtain entry to her computer and access all her e-mails.

Now he knew her every move and thought, and all her personal feelings that she kept for herself. He even knew when she was going out, entertaining a man or making love to the regular older man that visited her.

Lighting up time, at around 4:30 in the afternoon in the early winter months became some of his most favourite and exciting times, when she had not pulled her blinds down and the lights were still fully on. Sometimes she would light little candles on the table, and the fact that he used night vision binoculars, and could not quite see every detail of what was happening made it even more exciting.

Sometimes she would write to her internet lover John

Smith, telling him that she was planning to have sex with Billy the next day. He would fantasise in his head about himself replacing Billy one day. Biting, hurting her and having horrific, violent sex with her. He would wait in anticipation for her visitor to come, knowing of what he was about to see. There were a few occasions where Natasha's lover had stripped down to his pants and then pulled the blinds for some privacy, which made Simon so angry, that on one of these nights when this happened, he threw his table lamp across the room in frustration. When he could see the action, however, he became so excited, that he would start up his computer and read her e-mails, holding his binoculars with his left hand, watching her every move, and wank off furiously with his right, shouting out at the top of his voice.

'I'll fucking have you bitch! Bloody little whore! I'll have you one day!'

From: john smith <appledogstime@yahoo.co.uk>
Date: 11 January 13:00:42 BDT
To: Natasha <natasha_nw3@yahoo.co.uk>
Subject: SO WHAT A SELFISH NASTY PERSON YOU TURNED OUT TO BE

You certainly fooled me... but the working girls are born to act. And you DID ACT. Acted your knickers off when you told me what a nice sensitive person you were??? I should have realised sooner... Oh well, it's 8 in the morning here in the Big Apple. I had told Ruth from November that I was off with you forever, so she knew everything... but not YOU... you lied and deceived Billy all those months, and made him think it was not going to work between us, even though you very well know that if it was not for the baby I would be with you now. Natasha, how could you do that to Billy? He loves you so deeply. How can you make friends or have anyone in your life when you handle people in this really bad way, with no thought for their feelings or how much pain you are causing them???
He took you to the theatre two weeks ago, and you did not want to go home with him afterwards and when you gave him sex, you just lay there with your legs open, as if to say, 'get on with it and get it over quick' How could you treat a man like that who gave you so much... to not put your best into the sex when you were with him.

GOD, I had a lucky escape.

When you have someone, you don't want them and treat them like dirt. And when you can't have someone and you think you are going to lose them, you throw everything at them and give them EVERYTHING... a true Oedipus complex. I did not know you had it so bad. I wanted to be your friend forever, but now... NO WAY. I do not want to hear from you ever again. You are BAD NEWS. May god forgive what you did to that man Natasha. He had the misfortune to end up with you in the latter part of his life, but I hope he finds someone nice.

GOOD BYE NATASHA.

I hope you will find someone as nasty as you.
Birds of a feather flock together.
Then one day you will know the hurt you caused other people.
John

From: Natasha <natasha_nw3@yahoo.co.uk>
Date: 12 January 15:58:21 BDT
To: john smith <appledogstime@yahoo.co.uk>
Subject: John?

Why are you being so horrible...?

Is this your guilt...?

You are hurting me... please, no more... no more... no more...

????????

???????????????????????????

January

A FEW DAYS LATER

He paced up and down his flat naked, his binoculars in one hand and a broad smile on his face. It was early morning and the strong sunlight was shining directly into Natasha's tiny room. He smiled with satisfaction. Her blinds were all up, her windows open and it was very warm for this time of year.

Simon was very excited. She had just taken her pyjama bottoms off followed by her knickers. He watched her wrap a towel around herself, and waited in anticipation for her to return to the room that she had just left, knowing that she would be coming back fresh and wet from the shower. He imagined her soaping herself all over.

He listened to the music coming from her open windows; the radio was playing Magic 105.4, and took to the idea of playing the same radio station. He danced around his room naked, wanking while he waited for her, so very pleased with himself, and so very happy knowing that in a few seconds she would be naked too. He knew she was getting his e-mails, and he also knew that she believed he was John Smith.

Then she appeared. She dropped her towel and stood in her room naked. He almost made himself cum. She bent over and tore her hair up with her hands. It was a wonderful sight for him. She collapsed all over the place, wringing her hands in despair, pulling chunks of her own hair out, falling on the bed, throwing her face deep into her cushions and hugging her teddy bear. There was nothing he loved more than to see a naked woman crying, upset, hurting, sad and destroying herself.

John Smith had finished with her a few days before, and now he himself put the boot in to make her suffer even more. All his sadistic tendencies came gushing out, doing all he could to hurt her with the e-mails he sent to her, while the John Smith was locked up in New York with his future wife and child. He knew there was still a risk that John would write to her again from New York, but he felt supremely confident that he would still get away with his façade, as she would just write a nasty reply back, thinking that all the e-mails had come from the real John.

Now he would have her, and he was sure of it. Now she was going to be his. He had been for a drink some months before with an Indian gentleman who lived five doors from him in the same block, happily married with two children. After quite a few pints, the man confessed without giving too much away, that he had been with Natasha on a number of occasions. Simon cross-questioned him to try and learn as much about his obsession as he could, but the Indian man was very cagey, and all he would let him know, was that she was the best thing in bed, the best in the sack that he had ever experienced.

Yesterday was a happy day for him. He'd seen Billy take her out for half an hour in the car, and through his binoculars, when they returned, he saw her slam the door so hard that it almost came off its hinges. They were obviously not getting along very well either. She lost one man on the internet, and now she was about to lose the other.

He made up his mind to try the 'softly, softly, hard and nasty, softly, softly' approach, hurting her badly one day, sending her the most terrible e-mails, throwing in the odd nice word to bring her back, then hurting her with words again. His moment was fast approaching, like a Scorpio with his sting at the ready at the end of his tail. He knew that his long wait and patience was about to pay off.

January

From: john smith <appledogstime@yahoo.co.uk>
Date: 13 January 22:32:28 BDT
To: Natasha <natasha_nw3@yahoo.co.uk>
Subject: happy new year
Well hers wishing you a happy xmas, hope you're doing okay and have all those that you love with you or sending you love… I think of you often… it must have been love but we lost it somehow…. I am tonight only 100 yards from your house … I wish you could come and visit me here till Thursday morning, but if you did, I know I would rape you. I could not help myself… you would be well and truly raped. The want and the feelings are too strong, and it's been so long. I would force you down on the bed and tear your knickers off you and eat you poor Natasha… no pussy left for the New Year. But there you go. I am mad, I am mad but so are you as you feel the wet in your knickers. Have a Happy New Year you bitch X John.

From: Natasha <natasha_nw3@yahoo.co.uk>
Date: 14 January 12:08:53 BDT
To: john smith <appledogstime@yahoo.co.uk>
Subject: Re: happy new year
Dear John,
So you are in London now and only 100 yards from my house. For the New Year call me on my home no. You know them all or call round asap so we can talk about the script for our meeting and your new found nastiness...
If you want to meet call me you have all the numbers or just pop round.
A bit late for New Year's celebrations isn't it?
Love Nxx

From: john smith <appledogstime@yahoo.co.uk>
Date: 15 January 09:18:07 BDT
To: Natasha <natasha_nw3@yahoo.co.uk>
Subject: Re: happy new year
And the same to you my dearest child. I'm glad I did not phone you or get in touch and that I was strong as I would have become weak and I would have ended up on a rape

charge as I slid into your tight little wet pussy, so thank god we did not meet. It would have been the end of me.
Anyway happy new year to you miss, and I hope you find what you're looking for. By the way I don't exist. That will help you to get over me. Also I suspect that is the by-product of Billy's overactive imagination. Nothing changes. Still playing with your life plots and counter plots with Russia etc... I expect it brightens up your life while a few other people get hurt in the process. Maybe I can fly one person over for my wedding and introduce him to some beautiful girls from the USA and take some of his pain away., still dishing it out to... oh well. You won't change. Glad you don't believe in me so bye for now from the man who is now here X John

From: john smith <appledogstime@yahoo.co.uk>
Date: 16 January 13:53:21 BDT
To: Natasha <natasha_nw3@yahoo.co.uk>
Subject: Happy New Year You Wonderful Bitch... and I know I'm late but at least you're getting it.

Hi hi creamy, pussy girl... keep that pussy for me, and one day I promise you I will be in it. This is my New Year's resolution... Everyone has a price. Even you. So I may have to pay you a lot of money, but you're worth it. I hope Billy fills you up with enough cock for the New Year. Have a nice one you little horny sexy slut and keep your mouth open when you swallow. HAPPY FUCKING NEW YEAR YOU DIRTY SLAG XXX JOHN

From: john smith <appledogstime@yahoo.co.uk>
Date: 18 January 12:20:48 BDT
To: Natasha <natasha_nw3@yahoo.co.uk>
Subject: It's one year today, still think of you since we started it

Glad you think I'm not real. It makes your life easier and not so painful... good luck this year........ from the man who is not real. Kiss John x

January

From: john smith <appledogstime@yahoo.co.uk>
Date: 18 January 14:48:28 BDT
To: Natasha <natasha_nw3@yahoo.co.uk>
Subject: Are you still alive? Hope so still... shit. I am back in England.
Lots of money, but no real love in my life. John x

From: john smith <appledogstime@yahoo.co.uk>
Date: 20 January 09:41:57 BDT
To: Natasha <natasha_nw3@yahoo.co.uk>
Subject: Will make a sentiment leaving her. She has become an RC but I can't stand to be with her...

She will stay in New York with the child and the flat paid for by me. I'm coming back to England to live. Have a place near you in Swiss Cottage x John
P.S. Will come and see you very soon

From: john smith <appledogstime@yahoo.co.uk>
Date: 23 January 08:23:10 BDT
To: Natasha <natasha_nw3@yahoo.co.uk>
Subject: Back in England.

I will come and get you, my little slut. X John

From: john smith <appledogstime@yahoo.co.uk>
Date: 24 January 10:28:21 BDT
To: Natasha <natasha_nw3@yahoo.co.uk>
Subject: Exchange in two weeks time.

Three bedroom flat next street to you... See you soon you wonderful bitch. Get ready get ready. Get your knickers on for the spring and me x John

February

From: john smith <appledogstime@yahoo.co.uk>
Date: 6 February 09:41:39 BDT
To: Natasha <natasha_nw3@yahoo.co.uk>
Subject: I will be looking...

You will hear from me but in my office capacity very soon. X John (you are a fucking shit slut, and you know it) If I ever fucked you I would fuck you sore and then leave you on the bed covered in my cum you sick whore. I might just knock on your door tonight...

February

AT LAST

He had spent days planning it all. He had specially abstained and refused to wank for at least a week. He was going to give the bitch every thing he had. He was going to make her suffer. Pain and pleasure, both at the same time. He had spent hours and hours planning it. Earlier on, he had been to the showroom in Bond Street, and had spent over £15, 000 with insurance and everything else to hire it for one week. A bright red, top of the range Ferrari, with the number plate flashing 'JS1'. It was 6 o clock, and he could hardly tamper his impatience for his time to go. He had hidden the car around the corner in the garage that belonged to the flat, and he knew that he had to wait for his moment.

One e-mail wrong… one letter, one phone call and he would blow it. He had been to drama lessons for weeks now at the Central School of Speech and Drama at Swiss Cottage. He had perfected his Irish accent down to the last degree, and was now passable and had tried out numerous dummy runs by paying frequent visits to Kilburn, and many hours of bullshitting in the local Irish pubs to old Irishmen, telling them 'I'm from County Cork to be sure, to be sure!' and he had passed the test. No doubt about it. The Swiss Cottage school of Speech and Drama is probably one of the best in the world, and his tutors had been very good.

He put on an extra pair of tight white pants, as the hardness in his trousers was becoming uncomfortable, and his excitement was reaching fever pitch. He knew that every night she came home and would appear on the street where she lived, coming home from work just round the corner, where she cleaned for a lady with three children.

He planned to visit her, but when? When? When? Everything comes to those who wait.

February

CONCLUSION

The door bell buzzed loudly and Natasha jumped, with shock. Her bell hardly ever rang, And then if it did, only because a pizza man or mini cab driver rung her bell in mistake for the bell above.

It was Friday night at eight o'clock and she was expected her friend Lily May Of course this is not her real name, this is just a nick name. Her real name was Kamilery, also she came from Moravia. She usually came to stay once a month, for a maximum of five or six days.

She was nick named Lily May but she was far from being as graceful as a Lily at twenty stone in weight, or as we are in the European community now around about 110 kilos. She loved her junk food but she had only phoned twenty minutes before to say she will not be there until 11:30 as there had been a delay on the trains from Manchester. Anyway, she had her own key. Natasha never answered the door, unless she knew exactly who was down there, as she had to come down three flights of stars if it wasn't night, she would look out her window to try to see who was at her door. Usually all her friends always phone, to her first to say they are coming.

In ten years she had never answered the door to any demon or imaginary assassin that might be waiting for her.

What made her go down this time? She will never know. If it was fate, it had finally caught her. But down she went anyway. She had just come out of the bath, wearing a big thick white towelling dressing gown. The only garment covering her naked body.

She opened the first door, and then the second and looked up in shock and disbelief.

He stood six foot five tall, and this time he was dressed immaculately in a fine dark, light weight wool suit. Nothing like the cheap casual wear which she had seen in the pictures that he had sent her.

His large blue eyes stared into hers intently with a twinkle in them, together with a lopsided puppy dog grin on his face. Somewhat cheeky with no care in the world.

Her legs turned to jelly, and she felt her face go red... The rush of blood turned her cheeks to bright crimson, she felt hot all over as if she was going to faint, also embarrassingly she felt a spurt a wetness around the top of her thighs. And the beginning of a slow trickle running down, her leg towards her knee.

She could not utter a single word. Her voice left her completely, the back of her throat felt dry and her whole body began to shake with fear and anticipation.

His blue eyes sunk into her as if he knew her thoughts and desires, her wetness, everything.

The close, very close proximity of the burning flame of unbridled desire. He breathed and gasped at seeing her for real .after all this time. The sensual inhalation of a long lingering glance as he beheld her from the top of her blond hair to the tip of her six and a half inch size slippers. She could see the bright gleam in his blue, blue eyes and imagined in just those few seconds his thick white sperm, flow into her body and impregnating her as he has promised.

She thought, 'God, I wanted him so much. I could die.' he reached out his hand and in spite of everything that had happened she felt her hand meet his. She had no control over her body. All her reason had gone. It was as if like a serpent he had hypnotised her. It became all too simple for words, as desire engulfed and took over her whole body.

He spoke his first words, 'I have come for you, Natasha. I told you I would.'

He looked her up and down. She recognised the look in his eyes, she had dreamt about it. People fall in love and lust for many crazy reasons, the hair colour, the tone of voice, the mannerisms, the smell. He repeated himself,

'I have come for you, Natasha.'

This was crazy! She wanted him to fuck her so much. She was so afraid, so afraid. The thought crossed her mind, 'I am the object of his desire. My pussy hurts its burning for him. I am soaking wet.'

Her eyes filled with tears. She felt desperate. Her legs could hardly support her anymore.

Finally the words came out.

'But you are not real. You don't exist. You are just a figment of my twisted ex-boyfriend's imagination. He just though you up so that I could sleep with him again. You cannot be real. You cannot be here. He just used a model from a model book. You know you are not him. Ruth's pregnancy was just dreamed up to kill you off so that I could not have you anymore and made me give you up in my mind. You were just something of his bizarre twisted imagination. Just something he did so that he could keep me for a little while longer. He told me so just before Christmas.' She could not get the words out quick enough.

She was aware that the dressing gowned had fallen open exposing the whole of her body up to her navel. His eyes were devouring her. He spoke again in his thick Irish brogue.

'Is that what he said? Was it, to be sure? So he still wants to keep you despite realising that he lost you to me. He must have been bloody desperate. He is a clever bastard, that Billy.'

'Well, I am here right enough, what's more, you and I know, you are about to find out how real I am.'

'What a glorious feeling that this could be after a bloody year. Behave yourself girly.'

She backed away from the door as he moved forward.

In a complete trance. She let him in. His eyes never left her.

How could you get me out of your head. More to the point, girl, how can I get you out my head until we know?

He bent to kiss her and his lips devoured her mouth, first at her bottom lip and then her top lip and then his tongue run the whole length of her lips from one side to the other, flicking and teasing. His hand slid beneath the dressing gowned, to her buttocks to stop her from shaking and to kiss her and hold her into sweet surrender. Desire overwhelming her. Emotional and sexual gratification sung in her brain. His hand pressing her buttocks. She knew he felt her wetness even there, and he held them and her tightly.

'Oh God.'

Her pussy went into over drive. She smelt her own sex and his after shave and self maintenance, so clean.

How many times had she orgasmed to the thought of him and now it is real.

They made there way to the third floor of her safe haven and heaven. She couldn't remember even getting to her room. It was as if she had floated there.

Outside, Billy's car pulled up some twenty minutes later. A long sleek, light blue Jaguar Mark II with spoke wheels. Since the final break up, he popped in not all that often just to see her from time to time. Just to make sure she was alright. He had not even sent her a Valentine's card this year. What was the point? The gesture would have meant nothing to her, in the mood she was now in.

He got out and walks toward the flat, removing his mobile to phone her, knowing she would not answer the door unless he called first.

And then he saw it!

The most beautiful car he has ever seen. It must have been worth a hundred and fifty thousand pounds, a sexual transporter of power and energy, bright red, the finest Ferrari he had ever seen, right outside her flat with the number plate, JS1.

He glanced up at the flat, at her open window on the top floor. The white roller blinds were down. But the unmistakable sound of hard, violent, passionate sex could be heard clearly even though the flat was thirty feet above.

The voice of a woman, who is crying and screaming at the top of her voice like a fox bitch on heat. Loud, orgasmic cries of pleasure and pain going on and on.

Billy imagined the spectacle happening above, the seizing of skin in teeth, the wild beast, hungry for her white flesh. The little flicks of his tongue reaching every one of her pleasure zones, drinking her like rich wine, drinking her like a vampire drinks blood.

In John's madness and his desire for her actually drawing blood on her white skin as he bites her breasts and belly. Billy imagines him whispering after a year of gain of loss of regain, of loss again and finally he whispers, 'You are mine.'

She was screaming louder and more intensely than before, as if she was in real pain. Billy, momentarily, his eyes blinded in tears. A hard pain cut into him like a blade. He got into his car, turned up his Neal Diamond CD and started the engine. The wind screen wipers started to work even though it was not raining. He wanted to sleep, he wanted to vomit. He wanted to scream. Time to drive back to his ex-wife if she would take him.

When your heart stops beating, it doesn't hurt anymore. The car started to pull away for the last time to drown the screams still coming from above Billy turned up Neil Diamond full blast.

Melinda was mine
Till the time
That I found her
Holding Jim
Loving him...
Don't know that I will
But until I can find me
The girl that will stay
And won't play games behind me
I'll be what I am
A solitary man,
Solitary man

"Solitary Man" by Neil Diamond
from "The Best of Neil Diamond", MCA Records Inc, 1996

The End

Angel

Where it began we chased the flowers,
We can't think to wonder,
No one in this world,
Knows who you really are,
And I will remain a fantasy for many as well.
But the important thing for history, life and the readers,
Is that we lived, existed and shared our love,
And only we knew the truth.

The End

Billy's Poems To Natasha

The Pretty Girl
Walks down a sunlit street
A pretty dress
The flowers at her feet
Happiness
Reaches up for the skies
The birds will listen
And stop to sigh
The stars fall
Open up her eyes
And she can see
It's me

The pretty girl
Shops in Baker Street
I long to meet
Trafalgar pigeons
At her feet
Ken Livingston
Sent them away
Big Ben is striking ten
As she walks by
The birds
Take to the sky
She can finally see
It's me

Please Understand

Please understand,
When I stare into space,
The cat's on the rug,
And you're in my place,
I'm thinking, do I love you?
But I dare not tell,
For if I told you the truth,
We would both hurt like hell.,
And you would say,
Billy, no sex tonight,
My knickers stay in place,
I've a headache, please don't fight.

I'm Billy The Capricorn Goat

I'm no ordinary Billy,
Munching my grass,
I might look silly,
But I'm no arse,
I'm sure-footed, you know,
My ambition is high,
There's no hill too steep,
Nor no mountain too high,
Success, wit and charm,
I have in my hands,
But I am a dreamer,
Who can do no harm,
The fool I play,
So that you may relax,
But be careful the rivals,
Who I slay with my axe.

Words Words Words

Why I want to know,
What are words for?
Confused am I so much,
And why we cannot touch,
The reasons that you give,
The things that you say,
If they're not important,
Make the words go away.
Is there a dictionary
Around today?
A thesaurus
Would make the problems
Go away
Who can put them right?
Please answer me each day,
Why the pain, why the strife?
And the reasons we have seasons,
And the seasons for the reasons,
And the people that we know
And the people that we don't
Why are we here?
What's it all for?
You tell me you love me,
I love you too.
Can't you be with me,
Every day, every night,
Every single moment.
Where is our life?

Time

As time goes by, the winter comes,
The night grows cold and long.
My love for you is still as strong.

Let's be friends, we have so much we can't forget,
Let's be friends, the falling leaves turn b rown and gold,
Let's be friends, I see your face, the smile of old,
Let's be friends, the past is done, and we are bold,
The memories we have are for life,
They will give us pleasure,
You're not with me,
But always in my heart,
And one thing I will say for sure,
I wish you happiness and joy,
I wish you love,
What can I say?
My soul is part of you,
Until my dying day.

Seagulls Over Reykavik

What happens when a seagull cries,
And dives at the sea?
When the sea is the sound,
Of a woman having an orgasm?
You'd better come,
And have some fun,
There's only one night of the year,
When there's a party,
There's lots of birds to spare,
And gulls are going free.

Fruity

An orange, an apple,
A pear, a plum.
These are sweet fruits
Not as sweet as your bum.
It seems so soft
Like a nice tangerine.

Your tits are like cherries,
The nicest I've seen,
Give me your bottom,
For a lick and a bite,
That's surely the best fruit
Of all in the night.

The Wind In Her Hair

The wind in the reeds
All I want to hear
Look at me
Look at you

Blossoms from the trees
Fall on lips you turn to me
Look at me
Look at you

Look see the sky
With your pretty pretty eyes
Eyes of blue
Yours are too
We hear the stream
Falling through the night
Kiss me more
Hold me tight

Your love brings me
Pleasure of the spring
You must fly
Fly away
Before you go
We will kiss on words
And wings of sin

Kiss and cry
Kiss and sigh

There is just one day now
And I must say goodbye
Fields of corn and wheat
The sand, the sea, the air
Are at our feet

I let down your hair

Satin dress like silk
I touch your face

So soft
Like milk

You hold me close
I go far away
And as at last I go
Please have no regrets

This is life
It is so

Tears from my eyes
Hide the pain
Of our goodbyes
As when true love dies
Flocks of white doves
Fill the sky
And we fly on the wind

One day in a high and cloudy sphere
I'll look for you
And there'll be angels here
And we will miss the wind

When You Whisper

Whisper what I like to hear my love
You're waiting there when things go right or wrong
I pray that you are always near
And when you are you sing my song

So when I feel now, feel a little lonely
You're the lover who becomes my one and only
Every day, come what may
You move a little closer to my heart
You move a little closer to my heart
And here it beats I love you so

Whisper what I like to hear my love
Your voice floating in my ear
Your dreams at night
Scatter your dress and when you do to wild delight

Whisper what I like to hear
As Autumn comes
And we're a little bit lonely
Leaves start to fall
Are you still my one and only?
The roses are all stripped and bare
The petals falling through the air

Rainbows

Show me a rainbow
You love me still
Grey is the sky
When I'm not with you
Blue is the colour
That makes me feel
Black is what's left
When you're far away
The colours of the rainbow
Show them to me now
Every single colour
That we could hope to see
Dreams in your eyes
Hopes in your smile
All the colours tell me
That you love me
Sing me a rainbow
Yellow and warm
Red is the colour
Your lips keep me warm
Pink are your cheeks
Green are your eyes
I love you my darling
Won't tell you no lies
Sing me a rainbow
You lay next to me
And as we make love
All the colours we see
Your my pot of gold
To have and to hold
We'll stay together
Till we both grow old

Epilogue

Imagine was the song
That made the whole think
We all thought about what it said
But not the kitchen sink
John Lennon was the greatest
A king of broken hearts
So I'm glad that it's the epilogue
And not a maid with tarts
Like Imagine, the song
There's something for each new day
There was only one of you for me to share
But now it's gone away
I'm a lonely one
You may be too
What's it like?
To be an only one
Since I've been with you

EPILOGUE

Billy Clayton

Two years after our story ends, our hero went abroad knowing that the only way to sever the ties completely was to put physical distance and time between them both. Like many great artists, one day having attained a great age, in a fit of depression, thinking about all the lost loves, labours and masterpieces that had slipped by in his life as well as his many accomplishments, by this time, his photographs, paintings and poetry hanging in many museums and art galleries around the world, never having being brave at the thought of pain and fearing the end might be near, at his own request he wanted no friends or family near him, believing that you should not make the rest of the world unhappy by your suffering and that you should pass away alone, as all cats love to do. he finally took an overdose of sleeping pills and died happily, surrounded by pussy (his three cats).

Natasha Monika Nemcova

Natasha Monika Nemcova survived a terrible sexual experience and sadistic treatment that Simon Williams administered to her, keeping her a virtual prisoner for nearly 48 hours, repeatedly beating, raping and sexually abusing her. As she had invited him in willingly he got off scot-free on this occasion, but with a severe caution. She was in hospital for nearly 6 months with damage to her cervix and her body badly marked with his vicious bites and various other atrocities that he inflicted on her in his extreme sexual deviation. After coming out of hospital, she met and fell in love, not even believing it herself, with a six foot three, black baseball player who did not believe in marriage. She had a mixed race child by him and he left her. After a year of pleading by her, he came back and again made her pregnant. To this day, she has never learnt to drive and has never been to see the professor of Gastroenterology as Billy had always pleaded with her, to clear up her health problems caused by a lack of self-confidence and acute nervousness. Her father had always made her feel inadequate and a failure, and try as she may to deny it, she continues to be insecure.

Simon Williams

Three years after the attack on Natasha, Simon Williams was arrested on charges of multiple rape and grievous bodily harm.

At the time of writing this epilogue, he is currently languishing in one of HRH's institutions for the criminally insane.

John Smith

John Smith settled happily in New York with his daughter and Ruth and grew more and more erratic. His dealings with the stock market became more and more risky. He consulted for long periods of time, various top analysts for the severe mental problems he started to suffer from, included one of self-destruction. One day towards the close of 2008, due to over-indulgence of the American mortgage companies and banks, on a black Monday morning, the market crashed. Many millions of Americans had borrowed more money than they could ever hope to pay back. John, in a fit of madness, smashed himself to pieces on the freeway in his Ferrari. Ruth and the child went back to living in Golders Green, and the last news heard from them was that the little girl helped her mother in a nail salon. (That is if you believe that John Smith ever existed to begin with)

Printed in the United Kingdom
by Lightning Source UK Ltd.
124164UK00001B/1-30/A